Community-based Maternity Care

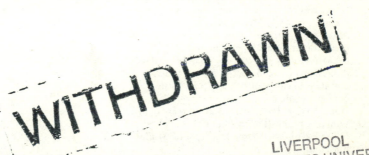

OXFORD GENERAL PRACTICE SERIES
Editorial Board

Andrew Chivers, Godfrey Fowler, Jacky Hayden, Iona Heath, and Clare Wilkinson

Community-based Maternity Care

Oxford General Practice Series

Edited by

Geoffrey Marsh
General Practitioner (retired), Co. Durham

and

Mary Renfrew
Professor of Midwifery Studies,
University of Leeds

Oxford : New York : Tokyo

OXFORD UNIVERSITY PRESS

1999

Oxford University Press, Great Clarendon Street, Oxford OX2 6DP

Oxford New York

Athens Auckland Bangkok Bogota Buenos Aires Calcutta
Cape Town Chennai Dar es Salaam Delhi Florence Hong Kong Istanbul
Karachi Kuala Lumpur Madrid Melbourne Mexico City Mumbai
Nairobi Paris São Paolo Singapore Taipei Tokyo Toronto Warsaw
and associated companies in
Berlin Ibadan

Oxford is a trade mark of Oxford University Press

Published in the United States
by Oxford University Press Inc., New York

British Library Cataloguing in Publication Data
Data available

Library of Congress Cataloging in Publication Data

Community-based maternity care/edited by Geoffrey Marsh and Mary Renfrew.
(Oxford general practice series: 43) (Oxford medical publications)
Includes bibliographical references and index.
1. Maternal health services. 2. Community health services for
children. I. Marsh, G. N. (Geoffrey Norman) II. Renfrew, Mary.
1955– . III. Series. IV. Series: Oxford medical publications.
[DNLM: 1. Maternal Health Services. 2. Community Health Services.
W1OX55 v.43 1999]
RG940.C65 1999 362.1'982—dc21 98-21742

ISBN 0 19 262768 6

Typeset by Joshua Associates Ltd., Oxford
Printed in Great Britain by Biddles Ltd, Guildford & King's Lynn

FOREWORD

Mary Newburn

Head of Policy Research,
National Childbirth Trust

This important book brings together much of the evidence and under-standing that is fundamental to good, community-based maternity care. At their best, family doctors and midwives based in the community have the opportunity of ensuring that women and their partners have an experience of pregnancy, birth, and early parenthood that enriches their lives.

I grew up as the second of four children who were all born at home. My mother taught me that giving birth and breastfeeding a baby was a wonderful, worthwhile thing to do; a pleasurable and normal thing. She said so now and again, but mostly she showed it. We lived in a remote Cumbrian valley and the women looked to each other for help with new babies. The health visitor didn't get up our way all that often and the doctor was an hour's drive down roads often blocked by snow in winter and tourist traffic in summer. So people made do without professional advice a lot of the time. My mum admired the screwed-up faces and urgent little limbs of the new babies brought to visit her and reassured new, younger mothers that they were doing really well. My fondest memory is of her bathing my brother and then soothing his plaintive cries with a warm breast, the air fragrant with baby powder. I just longed to be that kind of mother one day.

So, my first knowledge of the world of pregnancy and new babies was home and neighbours, not a maternity ward. My mum learnt what she knew from her mother, from her sister who trained as a midwife at the London Hospital, and from the National Childbirth Trust. She taught that you should trust your instincts and do what feels right; that during labour, unless there is a good reason to complicate matters, you are better off getting on with things simply and quietly with a minimum of intervention; and that after the birth you need someone to help keep the house warm and clean and to cook nourishing meals while you rest up with the new baby.

In the decades since my brother was born maternity care has become more medicalized and more hospital based. It didn't really occur to me to ask for a home birth when I was expecting my first baby. In any case, such an idea was virtually out of the question where I lived in the 1970s. However, I felt fortunate to be booked into the local GP unit. In the event, I gave birth in the specialist unit and had such an excruciating and miserable time that I have been a campaigner ever since. Twenty years on, I still vividly recall having been reduced to tears by an exhausted and disillusioned house officer, how my partner was sent home and I was left alone, in pain, strapped to a monitor with anonymous midwives flitting in and out, chatting to each other, and ignoring me.

It is so important for women that midwives and doctors are respectful and kind to them. Women continue to tell us that they have difficulty finding out what they need to know during pregnancy and that some doctors and midwives are authoritarian and insensitive. Thankfully, many also tell us that they have trusting and supportive relationships. Too much 'care' has had unintended and unwelcome consequences, creating problems rather than preventing or solving them. Community-based maternity care is intended to be close to women's homes and part of their local culture; provided by familiar, trusted people; and we can hope that it will reduce the use of iatrogenic advice and treatment. Providers of community-based care should strive to be seen as one of 'us' rather than one of 'them', and to combine the valued aspects of traditional care with the use of research-based knowledge, appropriate skills, and technology which helps rather than hinders.

Is the current focus on community-based care a misguided attempt to recreate a fictional golden age? I believe firmly that it is not. We should never expect things to stay the same. 'Traditional' ways of doing things are not necessarily best, but neither do 'modern' ways automatically represent progress. Fortunately, we now have a growing expectation within maternity care that services will be audited so that their effectiveness can be assessed and debated. It is also expected that new treatments and procedures should be evaluated systematically *before* they are launched wholesale on an unsuspecting public. (It is now possible for subscribers to the Cochrane Library to look up the available clinical evidence on a specific topic by simply turning to the computer screen.) By making use of research and audit we can recreate a maternity service which builds on known strengths and allows individuals to make conscious, informed decisions. We should use this opportunity to keep reviewing how maternity outcomes and opportunities shape up against our policy objectives.

For several years, those of us providing information to pregnant women and local networks of parents have found the pamphlet from the Association for Community-based Maternity Care, *The case for community-based maternity care*, a useful guide to the available research and changing policies. I hope that through this book evidence on community-based care will now reach a very wide audience.

One of the book's great strengths is that it has been written and edited by a multidisciplinary team. A number of opinion-leaders in maternity care see multidisciplinary education as a crucial step on the path towards less conflict between specialties and greater cooperation. As attitudes are formed during training, when ways of thinking and responding to clinical situations are established, there is much to be said for future obstetricians, paediatricians, general practitioners, and midwives learning together. Let us hope that if they have the opportunity to develop shared values and approaches to clinical practice through joint learning, that they will be better equipped to attempt to provide maternity care in a mutually supportive way which meets the needs of women and their families.

Mary Newburn

CONTENTS

Contents

CONTRIBUTORS

The editors

Before his retirement, **Geoffrey Marsh** was a general practitioner in Stockton-on-Tees for 35 years, working in a comprehensive primary health care team. His study of the team's work resulted in an MD from Newcastle University in 1974. Throughout his practising life, he audited the team's care of approximately 1500 pregnant women, most of whom had their babies in the nearby general practitioner unit or at home. In 1974 and 1978, he was a visiting Professor in Iowa, USA, and Montreal, Canada.

Mary Renfrew qualified as a midwife in Edinburgh in 1978. She completed her PhD with the MRC Reproductive Biology Unit in Edinburgh in 1982. She has worked in Scotland, England, and Canada in midwifery practice, research, and education. She established the Midwifery Research Programme at the National Perinatal Epidemiology Unit in Oxford. She was Co-editor of the Cochrane Pregnancy and Childbirth Group from 1990–1996. She is now Professor of Midwifery Studies and Director of the Mother and Infant Research Unit at the University of Leeds.

The chapter contributors

Jo Alexander qualified as a midwife in 1977. She has worked in midwifery practice and education. She wrote her PhD on antenatal preparation for breastfeeding. She is currently Head of the Centre for Midwifery Studies at the University of Portsmouth.

Sarah Clement completed her PhD in psychology at London University in 1990, and has carried out research in maternity care since then. She is currently a Lecturer in Health Services Research at Guy's and St Thomas's United Medical and Dental School and works for the South Thames Primary Care Research Network.

Tony Dowell was, until recently, Senior Lecturer in General Practice at the University of Leeds and a general practitioner in that city. His academic interests include the primary health care team and he has had clinical obstetric and maternity care experience in the United Kingdom, New Zealand, and Africa. He is now Professor of General Practice in Wellington, New Zealand.

Jean Duerden qualified as a midwife in 1973 and practised in the North West until 1996, predominately in the community. She was Midwifery Manager for the Community Midwifery Service in Salford and subsequently their Midwifery Development Project Leader. She undertook an audit of the supervision of midwives throughout the North West Regional Health Authority and is just completing an ENB/UKCC-funded project with a research team at Sheffield University. She is now LSA Midwifery Officer for the Yorkshire sector of the Northern and Yorkshire Region.

Maggie Eisner is a General Practitioner in Shipley, Yorkshire. She is a GP trainer and undergraduate tutor and has a special interest in women's health in general and maternity care in particular.

Sandra Elliott was a practising clinical psychologist for 15 years, and has also carried out research into postnatal depression. She is now a Senior Lecturer in Psychology at the University of Greenwich and the Perinatal Mental Health Education Unit, University of Keele, with a clinical practice at the Maudsley Hospital.

Chloe Fisher was until her retirement a Clinical Specialist in Infant Feeding and a Vice-President of the Royal College of Midwives (UK). She is an Advisor to La Leche League (Great Britain), the Association of Breastfeeding Mothers, and the International Lactation Consultants Association. She is a UNICEF Consultant for Croatia and Bosnia.

Jo Garcia works as a Social Scientist at the National Perinatal Epidemiology Unit, Oxford. The main theme of her research has been women's views and experiences of maternity care. Currently, she is working on aspects of postnatal health, randomized controlled trials, and maternity care organization.

Frances Griffiths, Paddy O'Neill, and **David White** (GP partners), and **Ann Jackson** (community midwife), work together in a primary health care team in Stockton-on-Tees. They provide general medical and antenatal care for all their pregnant women. They use the integrated GP/consultant delivery suite for low-risk deliveries. None of the GPs have a special interest in obstetrics, their contributions being rooted in their routine practice. They do have special interests in factors influencing the uptake of hormone replacement treatment, psoriasis, and accreditation of Senior House Officer posts in psychiatry. They exemplify the broad horizons of 'ordinary' general practice.

Erica Haimes is Professor of Sociology at the University of Newcastle. Her main interest is the relationship between the state, medicine, and the family, with a focus on the new technologies of assisted conception.

Marion Hall is a Consultant Obstetrician and Gynaecologist in Aberdeen. She wrote her MD on folic acid deficiency in pregnancy and has studied and written extensively on antenatal care. She has chaired the Royal College of Obstetricians and Gynaecologists' Audit Committee and has served on the Central Research and Development Committee for the NHS.

Cath Henson has a background in health visiting and neonatal nursing. She is now a Family Care Coordinator in the Nottingham Neonatal Service. She qualified as a Lactation Consultant in 1993.

Mary Hepburn first trained as a General Practitioner and then as an Obstetrician and Gynaecologist. She established and is Consultant in Charge of the Women's Reproductive Health Service for women with social problems. She is a Senior Lecturer in Women's Reproductive Health and Honorary Consultant Obstetrician and Gynaecologist in Glasgow.

Janet Hirst trained and practised as a nurse and midwife at Bradford and completed her MSc degree in1991. She works as a lecturer at the University of Leeds, and is planning to submit her PhD, which examines maternity care given to women from minority ethnic communities, in 1998.

Sally Inch is a midwife working in the Oxford Breastfeeding Clinic. She has written widely on the subject of breastfeeding. She is also a Baby Friendly hospital assessor.

David Jewell has been a Senior Lecturer in Primary Care at the University of Bristol for almost 10 years. He is a reviewer for the Cochrane Pregnancy and Childbirth Group, and founder member of the Association for Community-based Maternity Care.

Sheila MacPhail is a Senior Lecturer in Obstetrics and Gynaecology and Subspecialist in Fetal and Maternal Medicine in Newcastle upon Tyne. Her PhD was awarded in 1994 for a study of changes in red-call membrane function during human pregnancy.

Rosemary Mander is Senior Lecturer at the University of Edinburgh. Her doctoral thesis was on midwives' employment decisions. She has carried out research and published in loss in child-bearing and is currently focusing on pain in the child-bearing cycle.

Sally Marchant trained as a midwife in Perth, Scotland. She is currently working as a Research Midwife at the National Perinatal Epidemiology Unit, Oxford, studying aspects of postnatal care.

Michael Maresh qualified in medicine in London in 1975. His subsequent interest in perinatal audit resulted in him developing a computerized perinatal information system. He is now a Consultant Obstetrician in

Manchester with a special interest in materno–fetal medicine. Since 1991, he has been Honorary Director of the Royal College of Obstetricians and Gynaecologists' Clinical Audit Unit.

Bernardette Modell is Professor of Community Genetics and Wellcome Principal Research Fellow, Department of Primary Care and Population Sciences, University College, London. In collaboration with the World Health Organization, she developed the concept of 'community genetics', and her present remit is to help primary care workers deliver genetics services.

Michael Modell, following 30 years in north London general practices, is now Professor of Primary Health Care at University College Medical School. His interests include child health, community aspects of genetics, innovative undergraduate education, and asthma.

James Neilson worked in Glasgow, Zimbabwe, and Edinburgh before taking up the Chair of Obstetrics and Gynaecology in Liverpool in 1993. His major interests are in fetal assessment, clinical epidemiology, and tropical reproductive health. He is Coordinating Editor of the Cochrane Pregnancy and Childbirth Group.

Louise Parker graduated in physiology from Newcastle University and was awarded a PhD in 1988. She is now a Senior Lecturer in Epidemiology at the Department of Child Health in Newcastle, and is a principal investigator on the new study of the Newcastle 'Thousand Families'.

Helene Price is qualified nurse and midwife. She works freelance in primary care both within and outside of the NHS, providing training and consultancy advice. She is a National Trainer for the Health Education Authority.

Peter Selman is Head of Department of Social Policy at Newcastle University. His current research is in the areas of family planning services, teenage pregnancy, and adoption. He was Chair of Newcastle Community Health Council from 1988–1992 and is currently Chair of the British Advisory Board on Intercountry Adoption.

Nigel Simpson qualified in medicine in London in 1986. He has a particular interest in the process of placentation and the physiological control of labour. His MD thesis is on the developing uteroplacental and fetal circulation in the macaque monkey. He is a Lecturer in Obstetrics and Gynaecology in Leeds.

Lindsay Smith is a rural General Practitioner providing support to women giving birth both at home and in hospital. He is Chair of the Association of Community-based Maternity Care. His doctorate is from Bristol and his Masters degree is from the University of Western Ontario. He is a part-time Senior Lecturer in London and Chair of the Clinical and Quality Network of the Royal College of General Practitioners. He has published widely and has particular research interests in women's health issues and in education.

Janet Tucker has worked in maternity health services research since 1981 and is now a Lecturer in Perinatal Epidemiology and Child Health in Dundee. Her recent research into who delivers antenatal care resulted in her PhD in 1997.

Sara Twaddle graduated with an MSc from York in 1987, and since then has worked as a Health Economist. For the last three years she has been Contracts Manager for women's acute services in Glasgow. She obtained a PhD from the University of Strathclyde in 1996 on the economic implications of alternative forms of care in obstetrics.

James Walker qualified in Glasgow in 1976. His MD thesis was on the aetiology, presentation, and management of pre-eclampsia. He has pioneered the development of Day Assessment Units for high-risk pregnancies. He is Professor of Obstetrics and Gynaecology in Leeds.

Steve Walkinshaw is a Consultant in Maternal and Fetal Medicine in Liverpool. He coordinates the services provided for high-risk pregnancies within central Liverpool and has responsibility for the care of women requiring preterm delivery transferred from other hospitals in the Mersey region. His research is focused on pragmatic, randomized clinical trials and he is a reviewer for the Cochrane Pregnancy and Childbirth Group.

Stuart Walton is a Consultant Obstetrician and Gynaecologist in Stockton-on-Tees and has worked in Kenya and New Zealand. His primary interests are hysteroscopic surgery, family planning, and postgraduate training. He is currently Northern Region RCOG Advisor and Chair to the Higher Specialist Training Committee of the Faculty of Family Planning.

Sara Watkin is a Consultant Paediatrician in Nottingham. Her work is principally in neonatology. Her particular interests are new methods of ventilation and the role of the nurse practitioner in neonatal intensive care units.

Denise Young graduated in economics from the University of Strathclyde in 1993. She obtained an MSc in Health Economics from York in 1996 and now works at the Greater Glasgow Health Board.

Gavin Young is a country doctor in Cumbria. He was co-founder of the Association for Community-based Maternity Care and was the General Practitioner in the Expert Maternity Group which produced *Changing Childbirth*. He is a reviewer for the Cochrane Pregnancy and Childbirth Group.

ACKNOWLEDGEMENTS

Books would never get written without secretaries and we thank Limota Vaughan and Charlotte Tomkies for their excellent perseverance; staff at Oxford University Press who have been extraordinarily patient; all the chapter authors who worked hard and cheerfully to keep the book as close to the timetable as they could; and Mary's colleagues who did not have as much of her time as they would have, had she not been working on this! Special thanks also to her children, Jamie and Calum, who shared her time with this book and who reminded her to keep life balanced between work and home; and Geoffrey's wife, Jean, for her constant loving support and being, as ever, his literary 'second opinion'.

CHAPTER ONE

Introduction

Geoffrey N. Marsh and Mary J. Renfrew

In brief

This book makes the case quite unashamedly for placing the majority of maternity care in the setting of the community. It reviews the components of that care, it discusses today's major issues and challenges, and it indicates the way forward.

It is written by a group of care providers whose multidisciplinary background allows them to reflect on the future of shared midwifery and medical and nursing education, research, and service. Each chapter is an extensive digest substantiated by comprehensive referencing.

After reading this book, midwives, general practitioners (GPs), and obstetricians should find the theory that underpins their work more sharply and accurately defined and evidence based, and the work itself more effective.

Changing times

Change, turbulence, turmoil, revolution, and counter-revolution have been the continuing norms for health care during the last decade. The National Health Service (NHS) has been shaken up almost beyond recognition. Maternity care has not been excepted – indeed it has probably been at the forefront. Only 30 years ago nearly 30% of babies were born in their own homes. Ten years ago the figure was under 1%. Recent deliberations and policy changes are now resulting in an increase in birth in the home again.

Not only has the setting of childbirth changed, but so too have the carers. Thirty years ago pregnant women rarely saw a specialist obstetrician; they received care from their GP and the community midwife who usually worked separately. Ten years ago about 90% of women, including a high proportion of women with normal pregnancies and births, saw a specialist obstetrician – frequently even a consultant – and care by midwives and GPs in the community was dwindling. Today the midwife in the community is a pivotal carer in over 80% of pregnancies and GPs are struggling to redefine their role. Increasingly, specialists are involved only by referral.

The care itself has experienced great change. Thirty years ago pregnant women were told what to do and what they should expect. Ten years ago the earlier rumblings of discontent at this ordained care had become an uproar. Nowadays care is aiming to be woman centred and provided according to women's choice – alternatives should be available.

So everyone has been caught up in and participated in this huge change. As a result, community-based, woman-centred care is becoming accepted as the norm for the majority of women. So it seemed important to us – a GP and a midwife – to edit a well-referenced work that describes and discusses the current situation, airs the important issues that need to be addressed now, and indicates how maternity care will evolve in the early years of the new millennium.

Just as we were in the final stages of this book, and we thought that calmer waters were ahead for the organization of maternity care, a number of new policy changes emerged. These include the White Paper: 'The New NHS: Modern-Dependable' (1997), the Green Paper 'Our Healthier Nation' (1998), and the NHS Executive report on R&D in Primary Care (the Mant Report, 1997). Each of these documents will have a major impact on primary care in general. What their effect will be on maternity care is impossible to assess at this point; but it is clear that coping with organizational change will continue to be an essential feature of the work of primary caregivers in the coming years.

The book itself

The Preface is all encouragement and appropriately written by a mother of four children. That she is also a senior member of staff of the National Childbirth Trust, representing tens of thousands of women, gives our book a very special credence.

The first section considers the three main participants in community-based maternity care: the woman, the midwife, and the GP. It begins with a chapter written by the founder and first chairman of the Association for Community-Based Maternity Care. Central to that Association are midwives, and Chapter 3 is a major declaration of their potential. This is followed by a somewhat sobering account of the present, rather enfeebled role of the GP from an analysis of recent literature. An account of multidisciplinary team care follows with its varieties of strengths and weaknesses. Women's experiences of maternity care and the difficulties experienced in offering choices about care ends the first section.

The second section discusses four major contemporary issues. Maternity care has to be viewed against a radically changing social background and this is described first. Finances are not infinite for maternity care – value for money is essential – so the next chapter tackles the economics of care and the difficulties of evaluating these. Audit, a relatively new concept in many areas of health, has long been used in maternity care; it is discussed next. Education of the carers, with the emphasis on a multidisciplinary approach, concludes this section.

In Section 3 we decided to tackle what we considered to be the major clinical challenges in maternity care. Firstly, what can be done to reduce the differences in morbidity and mortality which seem to be perpetually associated with differences in age, social class, and ethnicity. Next, and closely linked with that, a chapter on the care of women who have special needs, including the very young, the homeless, the very poor, and those engaging in risky behaviour including drug use and prostitution. Although inner-city practices have a disproportionate number of women with special needs, virtually all practices have some. The major clinical cause of neonatal morbidity and mortality – being born too soon and/or too small – receives attention in the next chapter and indicates ways that midwives and GPs may try to prevent this. The high prevalence of technology – one in four babies in the United Kingdom still appear to require some form of 'extraction' from their mother – receives sanguine appraisal by a specialist who, like GPs and midwives, feels that something is awry. The section concludes tangentially but nevertheless importantly with the new and exciting concept of the fetal origins of adult disease.

In the final section we turn to the clinical care carried out by GPs and midwives themselves. A chapter on the psychology and psychopathology of childbearing is followed by one from practising GPs on the treatment of clinical illness in pregnancy. There follow chapters on the care of the mother during and after birth, and her newborn baby, including an all-important piece on how to resuscitate the baby that fails to breath – the nightmare scenario of every midwife, GP, and specialist obstetrician. We make no apologies for a whole chapter on breastfeeding. The great majority of babies do not feed from their mothers beyond six weeks. Midwives and GPs implementing Chapter 24 could change that.

In the conclusion we analyse what these GP and midwife editors have learned from scrutinizing what is written in this book. We anticipate the resolution of the current tensions between midwife, GP, and obstetrician. We describe their roles more clearly and we highlight their cooperation and collaboration which will arise from the mutual respect accruing from joint service, education, audit, and research. For the mother and baby – the fourth and fifth partners in the process – we see a responsive, effective, sensitive service in the next millennium.

References

NHS Executive (1997). *Research and development in primary care*, National Working Group Report (The Mant Report). The Stationery Office, London.

(1998) *Our Healthier Nation. A Contract for Health*. Green Paper. The Stationery Office, London.

(1997) *The New NHS: Modern-Dependable*. White Paper. The Stationery Office, London.

SECTION ONE

THE MOTHER, THE MIDWIFE, AND THE GP

CHAPTER TWO

The case for community-based maternity care

Gavin Young

Why do I propose that maternity care be based in the community? I believe that is where it belongs and that it is in the interests of most women and their families that maternity care is based within their community.

It is necessary to argue the case because throughout this century, in technologically advanced countries, care in pregnancy and, in particular, childbirth has become increasingly something hospitals provide. It appears then that I am arguing in favour of reversing an almost universal trend of many decades. I am. This trend has been one of the major social changes of the twentieth century – the hospitalization of one of the most private and crucial aspects of our existence – giving birth, as well as care before and after childbirth.

Where we have come from

I shall concentrate on place of birth because the hospitalization of childbirth is the leading example of how maternity care was taken over by specialists working in hospitals.

In 1927, when reliable data were first collected in England and Wales, only 15% of babies were born in an 'institution'. By 1937 one third were, and by the 1950s two thirds. By 1992 only 1% of births took place at home (Campbell and Macfarlane 1994).

Some have stated that the move to hospital birth was driven by obstetricians building their empires. This may in part be true but such a view lacks respect for obstetricians, many of whom genuinely believed that hospital was, and still must be, the safest place to give birth. It also underestimates the importance of other forces, not least the views of women themselves, some of whom chose hospital because of the availability of anaesthesia and better analgesia, for the provision of rest, food, and warmth, and because hospital was perceived as safer.

However, until the Second World War most doctors probably considered home was at least as safe as hospital. Certainly the British Medical Association thought so: '. . . all the available evidence demonstrates that normal confinements . . . can be more safely conducted at home than in hospital' (British Medical Association 1936). Even the obstetricians agreed that 'adequate hospital provision for all cases could only be made at great expense; the results of domiciliary midwifery do not warrant such expenditure' (British College of Obstetricians and Gynaecologists 1936).

Up to this time maternal mortality had stayed fairly constant through the twentieth century – four mothers died for every 1000 births. Over the next decade, including the war years, there was a dramatic decline (Figure 2.1). We do not know what caused this sudden decline, but it seems unlikely that it was improved social conditions. A possible explanation may be the simultaneous arrival of safer anaesthesia, blood transfusions, caesarian sections, and the use of antibiotics.

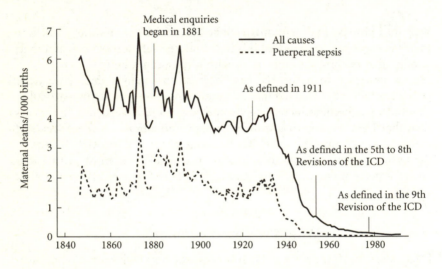

Figure 2.1 *Maternal mortality, England and Wales, 1847–1992. (Source: OPCS mortality statistics.)*

Whatever the reason for the sudden fall in maternal deaths, many became convinced of the benefits of hospital. By 1959 the Cranbrook Committee recommended:

'sufficient hospital maternity beds to provide for . . . 70% of all confinements . . . to meet the needs of all women in whose case the balance of advantage appears to favour confinement in hospital' (Ministry of Health 1959).

It was largely hospital specialists who, at that time and for the next 30 years, held influence over government committees which recommended hospital birth. However, many women themselves wished to avail themselves of their new rights within the National Health Service. The Association for Improvements in the Maternity Services (AIMS) was founded in 1960 primarily to fight for more hospital beds. This is a far cry from AIMS' stance today, but is consistent in that they have struggled to obtain for women that which they could not obtain for themselves.

Ten years later the prevailing view was further polarized in the Peel report:

'We think that sufficient facilities should be provided to allow for 100% hospital delivery. The greater safety of hospital confinement for mother and child justifies this objective' (Peel 1970).

By the next decade those holding the reins had convinced themselves they had driven in the right direction:

'The practice of delivering nearly all babies in hospital has contributed to the dramatic reduction in stillbirths and neonatal deaths, and to the avoidance of many child handicaps' (Maternity Services Advisory Committee 1984).

It is true that perinatal mortality had fallen dramatically (Figure 2.2) at the same time as the percentage of home births had fallen (Figure 2.3). However, it is more likely that this association was casual rather than causal (see Section 2). Moreover, even more startling in its blind confidence is the 1984 report's statement about the avoidance of many child handicaps. I have yet to see evidence that there had been *any* reduction in birth-related child handicap, let alone that the incidence of any handicap had been influenced by hospital birth. In particular, the incidence of cerebral palsy has remained unaltered throughout this century at approximately two per 1000 births (Pharaoh 1990).

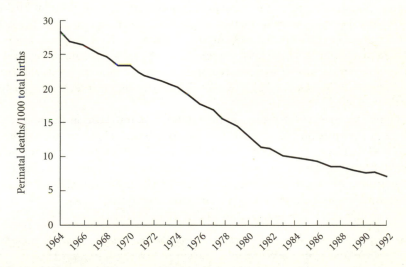

Figure 2.2 *Perinatal mortality, England and Wales, 1964–1992. (Source: OPCS mortality statistics, series DH3.)*

By 1990 less than 1% of babies were born at home. What was the evidence put forward to support this move to hospital?

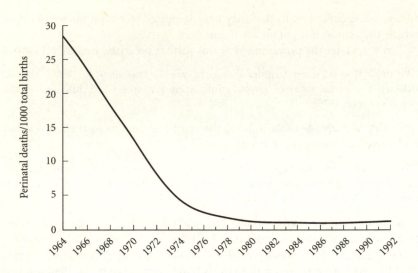

Figure 2.3 *Percentage of deliveries at home, England and Wales, 1964–1992. (Source: OPCS birth statistics, series FM1.)*

The case for the shift to hospital

The major evidence laid before government committees was the fall in maternal and, later, perinatal mortality rates coincident with hospital births increasing. Few people seemed either bright or brave enough to argue against the change. One exception was Archie Cochrane: 'It is surprising how successive committees have been content to accept trends as something God-given which must be followed, instead of demanding a more rigorous analysis of causality' (Cochrane 1972). He, like Schubert, was not much listened to until after his death.

Other evidence was that perinatal mortality rose for births at home in the 1970s at the same time as it was falling for total births. However, there was a probable explanation for this (Campbell *et al.* 1984). As more women delivered in hospital the proportion of those giving birth at home fell, but the proportion of those choosing birth at home unintentionally (usually prematurely), or without any previous care (unbooked), rose. These two latter groups have high perinatal mortality rates (PNMR) – see Table 2.1.

Table 2.1 *Differences in perinatal mortality between planned and unplanned home births*

Planned place of birth	% of total births at home	PNMR
Booked for home	67	4.1
Booked for hospital	21	67.5
Unbooked deliveries	3	196.6

Source: Campbell *et al.* (1984).

As the percentage of booked home births fell, so the overall PNMR rose (Table 2.1). In all the hullabaloo about women choosing home birth, it is surprising how little attention has been paid to the tragic outcome for the women with unbooked deliveries.

The third and perhaps most potent category of evidence was personal anecdote. Many hospital specialists could remember instances of 'chloroform and Keillands in the kitchen' or similar horrors which stuck hard and fast in the memory. These were reinforced by serious events happening to women within hospital who were then rescued by prompt intervention. The presumption then made was that such an event would also have happened to them had they delivered at home, but the rescuing intervention could not have occurred.

The increasing use of sophisticated technology, in particular continuous electronic fetal monitoring in labour, led to the almost universal view that hospital must be safer.

Is hospital safer?

The only certain way of answering this question would be a randomized controlled trial (RCT). This could have been done in the 1950s but, as far as I know, such a trial of home versus hospital was not suggested. Such a suggestion has now been made (Dowswell *et al.* 1996) but it would require 500 000 women in a trial to answer the safety question (Lilford 1987). This is patently impossible so we make do with data which may suffer from the bias that women choosing home birth may be different from women choosing hospital, however well one may try to match them. Nevertheless, one can look at the outcomes in relation to place of birth. One of the first to do so was Marjorie Tew, a statistician working at Nottingham Medical School. In her large-scale and detailed study, she analysed data from the 1970 British Births Survey and compared perinatal death rates in different places of birth (Tew 1985). She recognized that one would expect more 'high-risk' deliveries in hospitals than at home. Tew attempted to control for this by using both antenatal and labour prediction scores to categorize expected risk. These scores had been measured as part of the 1970 survey, but had not been presented in the published reports. Tew found that babies were more likely to survive if born in a GP unit or at home, rather than in hospital, at all levels of risk scores. Only at the very highest level of risk were the better results at home and in GP units *not* statistically significant. Tew had great difficulty finding a medical journal which would publish these results, as they went against medical 'wisdom'. It is possible that Tew's results may show that prediction scores do not foretell problems. They were not, however, her scores but were provided by obstetricians. Tew's results have not been refuted and the 1970 survey data do not support the then prevailing view that hospital was safer. Tew has displayed great courage over the years, initially being one voice crying in the wilderness; she can now take pride in her part in getting people to question that prevailing view.

Studies from other countries support Tew's results. In New Zealand, small rural units staffed by GPs and midwives had lower birthweight-specific perinatal mortality rates in all but the very lowest birthweight group (Rosenblatt *et al.* 1985). There was no evidence that a satisfactory outcome depended on a minimum number of deliveries. The study was done at a time when the New Zealand government was considering (and did, despite the study results!) closing the smaller rural units, believing them to be unsafe if delivering less than 100 women per year. A small rural unit is not the same as home, but as regards the matter of safety and facilities, the differences may be very small. Rural units will have midwives available, should have a neonatal resuscitation trolley, and may have better ambulance access than some homes. Very few have facilities for Caesarean section.

The Netherlands, alone of all European countries, has maintained that home is the place for uncomplicated births. Approximately one third of Dutch women give birth at home. A prospective study of midwifery care in Wormerveer from 1969–1983 (Van Alten *et al.* 1989) showed that midwives were good at selecting women at high risk during pregnancy and referring them to obstetricians. The women who continued under midwifery care, either at home or in small midwifery units, had a perinatal mortality rate of 2.3, including those transferred in labour. UK data give similar results. My own study of the small unit at Penrith, for example, showed a PNMR of 4.7 (Young 1987).

The prevailing view of small units was that, like home, they were unsafe. In the Bath district, 'low-risk' births in small rural units were matched against similar births in the big central unit from 1985–87 (Sangala *et al.* 1990), and the results appeared to support this view in that the PNMR for the women booked to deliver in the small units was 4.8 compared with 2.8 in Bath. However, the majority of the perinatal deaths occurred before the onset of labour. The difference ascribable to place of birth was less than one per 1000, not statistically significant, and a smaller difference than that found between different UK regions. Later PNMRs in 1988–90 were 3.0 for the small units and 2.6 for the central consultant unit and, again, most of this difference resulted from intrauterine deaths before labour.

In summary, if there is any difference in perinatal mortality because of place of birth, it is likely to be less than one per 1000, and we cannot say in which direction the difference lies. Interpretations of the data vary widely. Some believe that hospital is safer than home (Settatree 1996), others believe that it is not (Northern Region Perinatal Mortality Survey Group 1996). Campbell and Macfarlane conclude succinctly:

'There is no evidence to support the claim that the safest policy is for all women to give birth in hospital'

and

'The policy of closing small obstetric units on the grounds of safety or cost is not supported by the available evidence' (Campbell and Macfarlane 1994).

I have dealt at length with the subject of place of birth and this may seem unjustified to some readers. However, the issue of place of birth epitomizes many issues in maternity care, such as: Who should best provide the care? How should the care be provided, and where? These questions seem to arouse emotion rather than fact. 'Midwifery is an unusually emotive subject so, a priori, a very high standard of statistical analysis or experimental approach would not be expected' (Cochrane 1972).

Much of the emotion probably has to do with inter-professional power struggles which are not likely to improve care. However, the questions raised above are frequently answered by stating that safety is paramount, hence hospital care from specialists must be best.

Is safety paramount?

It may seem heretical in the context of childbirth, where we are concerned with the lives and health of young women and of babies, even to ask this question, but unabashed I will proceed to ask it. I suggest that though most of us often say safety is paramount, we do not really mean it. *If* safety was paramount, women would choose to remain childless, as they are more likely to die from pregnancy and childbirth than from contraceptive use. Many of us are prepared to accept risk-associated actions because we consider they are balanced by 'benefits', for example: BSE v. the taste of beef sirloin, drowning v. the excitement of dinghy sailing or ocean racing, multiple fractures v. the exhilaration of climbing a difficult rock face. If we really believe safety is paramount we should – I am told – all buy Saabs. We do not.

At this point, some doctors – paediatricians in particular – will say 'Ah, that's all very well, but there is a second person to consider – the baby'. There is here an unfortunate implication that either the baby's mother doesn't care as much about her baby as the paediatrician does, or just lacks knowledge of what is best for her baby. But even considering the baby, which in my experience pregnant women do all the time, I cannot see that we should persuade most women against home birth as (a) we do not have the data to support such dissuasion and (b) even if there was a very small difference in safety in favour of hospital birth, it is for the woman, with her partner, to decide what form of care she wishes for herself and her baby. I am surprised by the vehemence with which some doctors, sadly often the woman's own GP, will try and talk (or shout!) the woman out of home birth on the grounds that it is putting the baby at risk, when months earlier the woman has the freedom to end the life of her fetus altogether. Years later she has the freedom to endanger her child's life by taking him or her canoeing, mountaineering, or on holiday to Florida.

Yes, safety matters, but most of the time most of us do not act as if it is paramount and we should not, therefore, insist that pregnant women must adhere to such an imposed view of safety. Our role is to provide information and support, not to impose. This was well expressed in the *Changing Childbirth* report:

'Whether a mother with an uncomplicated pregnancy is putting herself and her child at any greater risk by choosing to have her baby away from a general hospital maternity unit is a topic that has been argued with vehemence and emotion for decades. The inability to reach agreement after this length of time suggests that there is no clear answer. Furthermore, professionals cannot quantify the enriching experience which some women feel when they have their baby in a place of their choice. The job of midwives and doctors, therefore, must be to provide the woman with as much accurate and objective information as possible, while avoiding personal bias or preference' (Department of Health 1993).

For many years the imposed views of professionals were, on the whole, accepted by women. As described above, hospitals were perceived as safer; specialists knew more than family doctors; technology led to the development of sophisticated techniques designed to assess the well-being of the unborn baby. These tended to be available only in hospital. But it was not just the birth that moved from home to hospital – almost all aspects of maternity care did so. From the 1950s to the 1980s large, impersonal, 'cattle-market' antenatal and postnatal clinics developed. Many women found these degrading.

The reversal of this trend was largely a result of women themselves reacting against such impersonal and often inappropriate care. This unease became so great that in April 1991 the House of Commons Health Committee chose to look at maternity services. Unlike all the previous government reports (see earlier), the Winterton report made extensive use of the views of users of the service. Indeed it concluded:

'Above all, it requires an affirmation that the needs of mothers and babies are placed in the centre, from which it follows that the maternity services must be fashioned around them and not the other way round' (House of Commons Health Committee 1992).

What do women want?

Maternity care can only achieve its aims if it adapts to what women ask of it. This may seem obvious, but the phrase 'woman-centred care' has been greeted with derision by some professionals or, maybe worse, with the response that 'we've been providing that for years', despite women's views never having been sought. My own belief is that some of the ferocity of the reaction from professionals to the Winterton (House of Commons Health Committee 1992) and Cumberlege (Department of Health 1993) reports result from the fact that they were 'women centred'. As a member of the group which produced the *Changing Childbirth* report (Department of Health 1993), I am proud of our evidence-based efforts. What was different about the Winterton and Cumberlege reports from previous reports on the maternity services was that part of the evidence base was the views of women. In Cumberlege these emanated from a speciallycommissioned MORI survey. Such views are sometimes uncomfortable, and some professionals have tried to discredit the evidence from users' organizations such as the National

Childbirth Trust (NCT), the Maternity Alliance, and the Association for Improvements in the Maternity Services (AIMS). They suggest that they do not present a balanced view of what women want. It seems to me that they are more likely to get closer to what women want than the Royal Colleges.

Common themes kept recurring in the evidence given by women and their user organizations. The Winterton report stressed three strong elements:

(1) the need for continuity of care

(2) the desire for choice of care and place of delivery

(3) the right to control over their bodies at all stages of pregnancy and birth (House of Commons Health Committee 1992).

Continuity

The importance of continuity was well expressed by the NCT in the evidence to Winterton:

'During the antenatal period women feel devalued and demoralized if they see a succession of different personnel who know nothing about their history and, because of lack of continuity, are inclined to give different prognoses and contradictory advice' (NCT evidence to the House of Commons Health Committee 1992).

The Maternity Alliance recommended similarly:

'There should be a clear recognition of the social importance of a community setting for antenatal care, which will sow the seeds of the postnatal support which is vital to the needs of mother and baby. Antenatal care should be regarded as one phase within a continuous web of care which is provided, as far as possible, by the same small group of professionals and within the woman's own community' (Maternity Alliance evidence to the House of Commons Health Committee 1992).

Women in pregnancy have clearly expressed a wish for continuity of care (Mori 1993). They often ask for continuity of *carer* (i.e. a person), not just the continuity of a system of care. It is not impossible for hospital staff to provide such continuity of carer, and some large units have made real advances in providing individualized midwifery care based in the hospital (Hundley *et al.* 1996; Turnbull *et al.* 1996). Those of us working in the community must be wary of assuming we provide what women want. McVicar, when talking about the Leicester 'Home from Home' scheme (MacVicar *et al.* 1993), quotes a woman who preferred the hospital clinic to her community one, as she had to wait less to be seen. Similarly, a woman with cerebral palsy at a *Changing Childbirth* meeting spoke eloquently about her preference for hospital because she felt known and understood there. Nonetheless, it is likely that continuity of carer can more readily be provided in the community.

What do I mean by 'the community'? Community means many different things, but what unites the meanings is a core to do with belonging and sharing. One of the characteristic features of hospital is that most people feel them as 'other' and often a rather frightening other, where they neither feel they belong, nor do they wish to. Many people do not feel they belong in doctors' surgeries or midwifery clinics either, but they are likely to see the local facility as *less* alien – it is more likely that they will visit it for advice, minor illness or injury, immunizations, and contraception. 'Patient groups' are becoming commoner around general practices, engendering a feeling of belonging. Hospitals are seen as largely for those who are ill. Few pregnant women are ill, though again we must not go overboard in our desire for community care. Some women, particularly those with high-risk pregnancies, may well feel and be much more secure with hospital care.

I do not intend to enter the rather fruitless argument as to whether the GP or the midwife should provide antenatal care. That decision should be one the woman makes. At present, few systems offer the flexibility for the woman to have any choice and it takes maturity and a certain magnanimity to accept that another professional may be preferred to oneself. How often do any of us offer women the chance to plan who they see?

There is an argument for midwives providing a greater part of the care if the midwife is going to be able to attend the birth. However, I am uncertain how important this is to women. There are some midwifery projects which allow women to get to know one or two midwives who will provide care before, during, and after birth (for example, Page *et al.* 1994). Given all the other aspects of a general practitioner's job, it is unlikely that a GP can ever provide care right through labour, as a midwife does. Nonetheless, women do value their GP's occasional presence in labour and also birth. Only a very small proportion of women in this country are attended at birth by a midwife they have met before, let alone know. Some midwifery schemes attempt to introduce the woman to all members of the team antenatally so that she will 'know' the midwife who is present at the birth. I consider that this is disrupting antenatal care for false gain. Having coffee with a midwife *once* during pregnancy is not 'knowing' her, and it is not what was meant by the fifth indicator of success in *Changing Childbirth*:

'At least 75% of women should know the person who cares for them during delivery' (Department of Health 1993).

If it is possible for midwifery to move into the community to be 'mit Weib', 'with woman', then midwives may be able to provide real continuity. However, a MORI poll found GPs appeared to offer better continuity in antenatal care than community midwives. Eighty-five per cent of respondents saw the same GP, compared with 68% seeing the same midwife (MORI 1993). Midwives need not be surprised. Women usually know their doctors before pregnancy and may, indeed, have known them all their lives. I once met a Norfolk GP who had that day attended the birth of the third generation of one family. Imagine being able to say to a young girl, 'I saw you, your mother, and your granny born'; inter-generational continuity. We do not know how best to provide continuity of care or carer, and different systems will suit different women and different places. We do know we should be aiming to improve continuity. In the MORI poll described above, the question was asked of over 1000 women, 'If you went through pregnancy and birth again, what would matter most to you in terms of the care you were given?' The commonest single response was 'continuity of care', followed by 'more support', and equally 'more explanation' (MORI 1993).

I have deliberately spent some time on the subject of continuity because it is such an important part of the argument for placing more maternity care in the community. However, not all women want the same thing. I shall now look at the second major area which Winterton highlighted.

Choice

Until recently, health care has been provided 'as the doctor ordered'. Choice was available as it was for the Model-T Ford – 'Any colour, so long as it's black'. Several factors have changed this position. One of the advantages of the move towards evidence-based care is that defining islands of what we know has revealed oceans of what we do not know. This may be uncomfortable, but has the merit of honesty. The publication of *Effective care in pregnancy and childbirth* (Chalmers *et al.* 1989) will, I believe, be seen as one of the most important steps in medical publishing ever. The parallel publication of a condensed paperback version may be more important, as it enables pregnant women to discover which forms of care work and which do not. This major shift towards making knowledge and ignorance public was followed by a crucial electronic publication, the Cochrane Collaboration Pregnancy and Childbirth Database (CCPC), and, more recently, the Cochrane Library. This is available on computer disks and carries systematic reviews of all the known randomized controlled trials in the subject (Cochrane Library 1997). The availability of meticulously examined evidence enabled the Midwives' Information and Research Service (MIDIRS) in Bristol and the NHS Centre for Reviews and Dissemination in York to produce a set of 'Informed Choice' leaflets for professionals and for women, covering such subjects as support in labour, ultrasound scans, and fetal monitoring in labour. Giving women information allows them to make choices for themselves.

Midwives and GPs can offer an alternative to care in hospital, particularly antenatally. This shift may not only make care more accessible to women, particularly those who have difficulties reaching hospital and those with preschool children, it may also be better care. The Sighthill project in Edinburgh, where antenatal care was shifted from hospital into the community, was associated with an impressive fall in perinatal mortality (Sighthill Maternity Team 1982). Obstetricians' insistence that they must see every woman at least once during pregnancy is beginning to fade, as it should; it is considered to be a 'form(s) of care unlikely to be beneficial' (Enkin *et al.* 1995). Similarly rated is routinely involving doctors – GPs take note!.

Women should be offered the choice of seeing an obstetrician or not. Some will wish to do so, however much the GP or the midwife feels it unnecessary. If obstetricians' skills become focused on women with complicated pregnancies, then these women can have the proper attention and continuity of carer they require. The obstetrician's time is best not diluted amongst those who do not benefit from it.

For women to make well-informed choices, they need both clear information and, perhaps more difficult for carers to provide, the sense of freedom and trust which allows the woman to ask questions. The MORI poll found that 51% of women agreed that the hospital doctor gave clear information, compared with 71% for the hospital midwife, 70% for the GP, and 86% for the community midwife. When it came to feeling they could ask all the questions they wanted to, 63% agreed they could ask the hospital doctor, 82% the hospital midwife, 79% the GP, and 89% the community midwife (MORI 1993). Doctors in the community appear to perform better in the area of inviting questions and information-giving than hospital doctors. Similarly, midwives in the community do better than hospital midwives and, overall, midwives do better in this area than doctors. The MORI poll was unable to examine whether the clear information was correct information, but I have no evidence that midwives purvey misinformation any more or less than doctors.

Information-giving was shown to be poor in an Aberdeen study in 1980–83 (Hall *et al.* 1985). In 62% of hospital antenatal consultations, women asked no questions at all. Perhaps allowing time for questions has been considered of lesser importance than the routine check-ups of antenatal care. Much of the latter is ineffective. A London professor of obstetrics wrote: 'Almost all of these routine antenatal procedures are of dubious value' (Steer 1993). One of the major aims of antenatal care is to detect babies who are not growing well in the womb. In the Aberdeen study mentioned above, only 44% of the babies with birthweights below the 10th percentile had been assessed as small before birth (Hall *et al.* 1985). Perhaps more humbling for those of us trying to assess fetal growth by measuring the fundal height is that for each *true* small baby, 2.5 were said to be small but weighed above the 10th percentile. In other words, this method of detecting small babies has poor predictive value and causes much needless anxiety. This is a great pity as there is now an effective way of assessing whether high-risk babies *are* actually running into difficulties – Doppler ultrasound (Neilson and Alfrevic 1996). At present, though, we have no practical way of detecting which babies might benefit from Doppler studies. This problem conjures up visions of all women being subjected to an investigation whether they might benefit or not, a similar position to that reached with continuous electronic fetal monitoring in labour; but more of that later.

In addition, women are being offered many more investigations in pregnancy – ultrasound and serum screening to name two of the commonest. They cannot make choices without information. In some areas it is apparent that they do *not* make choices; how can one area of the country have a 95% take-up rate for serum screening for Down's syndrome and another 50%? An example of good practice is Kevan Thorley's practice in Staffordshire (Department of Health 1993). Here the first half of the antenatal clinic is group discussion and the second is talking privately with the doctor and/or midwife. The focus is on what the woman wants to ask and when (Thorley and Rowse 1993).

Perhaps the greatest prerequisite for good communications is the ability to listen. It is not easy to provide written examples of this!

There have been attempts to reduce the frequency of antenatal appointments, but a recent study of traditional antenatal care in south London versus a reduced schedule showed the traditional group were less worried about the baby before and after birth, and had a more positive attitude to the baby (Sikorski *et al.* 1996). As Steer implies (see above), there is scant evidence that our present antenatal care has much impact on perinatal or maternal mortality but we must not make the nihilistic leap to say that care does not matter.

The availability of community maternity care makes information more accessible to women. Obviously it makes the *choice* of local care possible, not only antenatally but also for birth itself. After birth it allows choice regarding time of discharge from hospital. Winterton noted how choice of place of birth had been effectively removed for most women:

'Women in this country have been deprived of effective choice about where they give birth. Small maternity units have been closed because health authorities have decided, without pausing to consider the evidence too closely, that these are unsafe, expensive, or both. They have then set about ensuring that they become more expensive by introducing policies designed to reduce their use further' (House of Commons Health Committee 1992).

It is a sadness for me that there are large rural areas of the UK, particularly Scotland, with *no* maternity units. This in turn leads to deskilling of community midwives and GPs so that there are large chunks of the UK where there are no carers competent to deliver a baby.

Sadly and finally, MORI found that the majority of women questioned as to how much choice the GP had offered about place of birth answered 'no choice at all' (MORI 1993). We know from a recent survey that 8% of women would like to have a home birth yet only about 1% do so (National Council of Women of Great Britain 1990). It is apparent, especially to user groups from whom women seek help and advice, that women requesting home birth can be met with open hostility.

'The Expert Group heard accounts of some GPs who asked women and their families to transfer to another GP's list . . . This is clearly a distressing experience for the women . . . It is an unacceptable practice which must cease (Department of Health 1993).

Such an attitude on the part of a normally caring family doctor is unjustified. It betrays an ignorance of the epidemiological evidence and the role of the midwife, as well as a failure to place the wishes of the woman ahead of the irrational fears of the doctor. This attitude was not helped by an unfortunate document from the General Medical Services Committee

(General Medical Services Committee 1995) which, whilst not denying women choice, helped to perpetuate the very negative attitude to home birth commonly held by GPs (Young 1996). More recent advice from the Committee, however, has offered a more positive attitude.

Control

I no more like the idea of women controlling their carers than the other way round. What the House of Commons Committee meant was that women should feel in control over what is happening to them. This is closely bound up with choice and this in turn has much to do with how much the woman can trust her carer, which in turn is related to continuity of carer. It is not possible to feel in control if one is not offered any choice as to what is done to one. There is a long, sad litany of things done routinely to women without their being offered any choice – some now, happily, abandoned, some alas not: enema in labour, shaving, routine episiotomy at birth, withholding food and drink in labour, directed pushing, encouraging breath-holding. All these are forms of care 'unlikely to be beneficial' (Enkin *et al.* 1995).

Even forms of care we, as professionals, may think helpful may reduce a woman's sense of control. Routine electronic fetal monitoring, early amniotomy, and early use of oxytocin are all widely practised, yet the benefits are either non-existent or so small that they are counterbalanced by drawbacks. Thornton and Lilford conclude:

'. . . it is the presence of a companion in labour, rather than amniotomy or early use of oxytocin, which is the effective ingredient of an active management package' (Thornton and Lilford 1994).

It is becoming increasingly clear that continuous support in labour has many beneficial effects (Hodnett 1996). All the following are reduced: duration of labour, likelihood of medication for pain relief, rates of operative vaginal delivery, the rate of Caesarean section, negative ratings of the childbirth experience, post-partum depression, and an increase in personal control in labour.

Much of what we do is *not* clearly beneficial and women should be allowed to decide what kind of care they receive. As the Association for Community-Based Maternity Care said in evidence to Winterton:

'Discussions concerning maternity care have been distorted in the past by attention paid to opinion and not to scientific evidence. Unfortunately, evidence on many issues is lacking. Where this is so, we believe extra attention should be paid to women's wishes . . . As professionals we do not believe we should dictate the pattern where science cannot support such a pattern' (House of Commons 1992).

The option of carrying their own notes is one way to increase women's feelings of being in control (Hodnett 1995). Women prefer to carry them and they lose them less than the hospitals did in one of the two randomized trials listed by Hodnett.

What has community-based care to offer to women to help their sense of control? Women carrying their own notes is a good example here. The benefits are not confined to community-based care but it enables such care to be more effective when doctors and midwives outside hospital can write in the real notes. Given the evidence from the MORI poll that such staff spend more time *explaining* than hospital staff do, interpreting what is written in the notes by hospital staff may also matter.

One of the findings in an early matched-pairs study, comparing delivery in the GP/midwife unit in Oxford with consultant care, showed less induction, assisted delivery, and augmentation, whilst showing more intact perineums, mobility in labour, and breastfeeding, with no apparent ill-effects (Klein *et al.* 1983). The preliminary findings of a one-to-one midwifery scheme in London showed similar results (Page *et al.* 1994).

Some interventions during childbirth may be life-saving, but it is apparent that many which are used very frequently, if not routinely, are of doubtful benefit, or even harmful. Electronic fetal monitoring falls into both these categories, of possible benefit in high-risk labours but likely to lead to more harm than good in low-risk labours. Community midwives and GPs tend to use such monitoring rarely, if at all. The Northern Regional Home Birth Study showed the commonest reason given for wanting a home birth was because the woman wished to feel in control (Davies *et al.* 1996). The more things done to one, even by considerate staff, the less one is likely to feel in control. I have given up listening to the fetal heart in antenatal checks once the mother begins to feel movements from 20 weeks unless she wishes me to listen as I believe it sends an implicit message that a woman needs a check-up to tell if her baby is alive. This is almost always untrue if movement is reported, and listening to the heartbeat in pregnancy implies to the woman that we can tell something she cannot. Professor Marc Keirse, former co-editor of the Cochrane Pregnancy and Childbirth Group, often tells his audiences that the prime carer for the pregnant woman and her unborn baby is the woman herself. One of our roles is to increase her ability to do this and increase her self-esteem, in part to enable her better to be the baby's main carer *after* birth.

The future

Maternity care in the UK has come a long way this century – maternal and perinatal mortality have fallen dramatically in the past 50 years. Before the Second World War, data from many countries indicated that delivery was safest at home with a midwife and that hospitals and doctors were likely to *cause* problems (Loudon 1988). This may still be true for a percentage of women with low-risk pregnancies. However, many women have reason to be grateful for highly technical specialist care. The continuing problem is to know which women will benefit from such special input (Chapter 13). Yet all women will benefit from considerate care from midwives and doctors if such staff can help the woman's knowledge, understanding, and self-esteem. There will be a continuing shift to more community-based care, especially in pregnancy, but also to a certain extent in childbirth too, though this may be limited for fiscal reasons unless the organization of midwifery can adjust to the increasing demand for home birth.

Midwifery needs to continue to find new and better ways to provide this care without lowering standards of care and, if possible, at the same time enhancing job satisfaction. The role of GPs is less certain though it seems likely that they will continue to play an important role in antenatal and postnatal care. Few GPs are involved in care at birth, though a GMSC survey in 1992 indicated that 27% said they would like to be. Altering training might encourage GPs rather than discourage them as at present (Smith 1991; see Chapter 4). A training based on understanding the normal, and therefore being able to recognize the abnormal, would help. Midwives could play an important part here. Continued experience, education, and support are needed to maintain competence and confidence. In these areas the outlook is brighter – the Association for Community-Based Maternity Care, founded in 1989, is a unique forum for GPs, midwives, and obstetricians to plan and encourage community-based care. From 1997 an emergencies updating course with a high practical content has become available in the UK (Gibson 1997). This course, Advanced Life Support Obstetrics, will provide experience in simulated emergencies such as shoulder dystocia and post-partum haemorrhage.

However much midwives become able to provide real continuity, I believe it would not be to the benefit of women in the UK if family doctors reached the point of having no knowledge and experience of childbirth. A further, very recent, role for the GP may be in *purchasing* maternity care. 1996 saw the start of pilot projects in total fundholding, and extended fundholding specifically to purchase maternity care. These schemes are being evaluated in a study based in the Edinburgh University Primary Care Research Unit. Fundholding has in some instances been a real force for change, leading to innovation and improved services. This may also happen if GPs begin to purchase maternity services. However, most fundholders have *not* been innovative, nor has the system overall proved cost-effective (Audit Commission 1996). Many doctors consider that fundholding has made the NHS less equitable and welcome the change to commissioning groups under the new Labour government. It remains to be seen who will be involved in the commissioning of maternity care.

Perinatal mortality, like most other measures of health, shows an inverse relationship to income. Government could do much to help here, if it had the will, by changing our education system (which fails many UK children, some of whom will become young mothers) and by altering the benefits system so that low-income mothers could afford healthy, fresh food and could afford to take time off work long enough to breastfeed their babies. These seem unlikely to occur with the Government's 'Welfare to Work' scheme. Banning cigarette advertising could perhaps do more for maternal and child health than any other single action and it is disheartening to note that the Government appears less committed to doing this than it appeared to be when in opposition.

All this may seem to have little to do with community-based care. Quite the contrary. We, as carers, have a duty to try and improve the health of those to whom we provide care. One way of doing this is to bring to the attention of the Government how it can help improve health, especially by reducing social inequality (Watt 1996; see Chapter 11).

Meanwhile, community-based maternity care can provide accessible continuing care to women in ways which enhance the woman's ability to care for herself and her future child. It is flexible enough to adjust to local needs and close enough to women to fit individual needs. Therein is its strength.

References

Audit Commission (1996). *What the doctor ordered – A study of GP fundholders in England and Wales.* National Audit Office, HMSO, London.

Australian and New Zealand Perinatal Societies (1995). The origins of cerebral palsy. *The Medical Journal of Australia*, **162**, 85–9.

British College of Obstetricians and Gynaecologists (later Royal College of Obstetricians and Gynaecologists) (1936). *Outline of a scheme for a national maternity service.* BCOG, London.

British Medical Association (1936). The British Medical Association and maternity services. *British Medical Journal*, **1**, 656.

Campbell, R., Macdonald Davies, I., Macfarlane, A., and Beral, V. (1984). Home births in England and Wales, 1979: perinatal mortality according to intended place of delivery. *British Medical Journal*, **289**, 722.

Campbell, R. and Macfarlane, A. (1994). *Where to be born? The debate and the evidence* (2nd edn). National Perinatal Epidemiology Unit, Oxford.

Chalmers, I., Enkin, M., and Keirse, M. J. N. C. (1989). *Effective care in pregnancy and childbirth.* Oxford University Press, Oxford.

Cochrane, A. L. (1972). *Effectiveness and efficiency: random reflections on the health service.* Nuffield Provincial Hospitals Trust, London. (Reprinted 1989, jointly by British Medical Journal and NPHT.)

Cochrane Library. In: Neilson, J. P., Crowther, C. A., Hodnett, E. D., and Hofmeyr, G. J. (ed.) Pregnancy and Childbirth Module. of the Cochrane Database of Systematic Reviews. The Cochrane Collaboration, Issue 4, Oxford. Update Software, 1997. Updated quarterly.

Davies, J., Hey, E., Reid, W., and Young, G. (1996). Prospective regional study of planned home births. *British Medical Journal.* 313,1302–5.

Department of Health (1993). *Changing childbirth, Part I. Report of the Expert Maternity Group (Cumberlege report).* HMSO, London.

Department of Health (1993). *Changing childbirth, Part II. Survey of good communication practice in maternity services,* pp. 17–18. HMSO, London.

Dowswell, T., Thornton, J. G., Hewison, J., and Lilford, R. J. L. (1996). Measuring outcomes other than safety is feasible. *British Medical Journal*, 312, 753.

Enkin, M., Keirse, M. J. N. C., Renfrew, M. J., and Neilson, J. (1995). *A guide to effective care in pregnancy and childbirth* (2nd edn), p. 406. Oxford University Press, Oxford.

General Medical Services Committee (1995). *Maternity medical services: legal advice for GPs*. British Medical Association, London.

General Medical Services Committee (1997). *General practitioners and intrapartum care: interim guidance*. British Medical Association, London.

Gibson, J. (1997). ALSO (Advanced Life Support Obstetrics). UK office: Primary Care Development Office, Newcastle General Hospital, Westgate Road, Newcastle upon Tyne NE4 6BE. Tel: 0191 256 3281.

Grant, A., O'Brien, N., Joy, M-T., Hennessy, E., and MacDonald, D. (1989). Cerebral palsy among children born during the Dublin randomized trial of intrapartum monitoring. *Lancet*, 2, 1233–5.

Hall, M., MacIntyre, S., and Porter, M. (1985). *Antenatal care assessed*, p.57. Aberdeen University Press, Aberdeen.

Hodnett, E. D. (1993). *Women carrying their own casenotes during pregnancy* (revised May 1995) In: Enkin, M. W., Keirse, M. J. N. C., Renfrew, M. J., Neilson, J. P., and Crowther, C. A. (ed.) Pregnancy and Childbirth Module. of the Cochrane Pregnancy and Childbirth Database. The Cochrane Collaboration, Issue 2, Oxford. Update Software, 1995.

Hodnett, E. D. (1996). *Support from caregivers during childbirth* (updated 5 December 1996). In: Neilson, J. P., and Crowther, C. A., Hodnett, E. D., Hofmeyr, G. S. (ed.) Pregnancy and Childbirth Module of the Cochrane Database. of Systematic Reviews. The Cochrane Collaboration, Issue 4, Oxford. Update Software, 1997. Updated quarterly.

House of Commons Health Committee (1992). Second Report: *Maternity services*. Vol. 1. HMSO, London.

Hundley, V. A. *et al.* (1994). Midwife-managed delivery unit: a randomized controlled comparison with consultant-led care. *British Medical Journal*, 309, 1400–4.

Klein, M., Lloyd, I., Redman, C., Bull, M., and Turnbull, A. C. (1983). A comparison of low-risk women booked for delivery in two different systems of care. *British Journal of Obstetrics and Gynaecology*, 90, 118–28.

Lilford, R. (1987). Clinical experimentation in obstetrics. *British Medical Journal*, 295, 1298–300.

Loudon, I. (1988). Maternal mortality: 1880–1950. Some regional and international comparisons. *The Social History of Medicine*,1(2),183–228.

MacDonald, D., Grant, A., Sheridan-Pereira, M., Boylan, P., and Chalmers, I. (1985). The Dublin randomized trial of intrapartum fetal monitoring. *American Journal of Obstetrics and Gynecology*, 152, 524–39.

MacVicar, J., Dobbie, G., Owen-Johnstone, L., Jagger, C., Hopkins, M., and Kennedy, J. (1993). Simulated home delivery in hospital: a randomized controlled trial. *British Journal of Obstetrics and Gynaecology*, 100, 316–23.

Maternity Services Advisory Committee (1984). *Maternity care in action,Part II. Care during childbirth: a guide to good practice and a plan for action.* HMSO, London.

Ministry of Health (1959). *Report of the Maternity Services Committee (Chairman, Lord Cranbrook).* HMSO, London.

MORI (Market and Opinion Research International) (1993). *Maternity services research study conducted for Department of Health, April-May 1993.* MORI, London SE1 0HX.

National Council of Women of Great Britain (1990). *Are we fit for the 90s?* London.

Neilson, J. P. and Alfrievic, Z. *Doppler ultrasound in high-risk pregnancies* (updated 5 December 1996). In: Neilson, J. P., Crowther, C. A., Hodnett, E. D., Hofmeyer G. J., and Keirse, M. J. N. C. (ed.) Pregnancy and Childbirth Module. of the Cochrane Database of Systematic Reviews. The Cochrane Collaboration, Issue 4, Oxford. Update Software, 1997. Updated quarterly.

Northern Region Perinatal Mortality Survey Group (1996). Perinatal loss of planned and unplanned home births. *British Medical Journal.* In press.

Page, L. A., Jones, B., Cooke, P., Harding, M., Stevens, T., and Wilkins, R. (1994). One-to-one midwifery practice. *British Journal of Midwifery*, 2(9), 444–7.

Peel, J. (1970). See Standing Maternity and Midwifery Advisory Committee (later).

Pharaoh, P. O. D., *et al.* (1990). Birthweight-specific trends in cerebral palsy. *Archives of Diseases in Childhood*, 65, 602–6.

Rosenblatt, R. A., Reinken, J., and Shoemack, P. (1985). Is obstetrics safe in small hospitals? Evidence from New Zealand's regionalized perinatal system. *Lancet*, 1, 429–33.

Sangala, V., Dunster, G., Bohin, S., and Osborne, J. P. (1990). Perinatal mortality rates in isolated general practitioner maternity units. *British Medical Journal*, 310, 418–20.

Settatree, R. S. (1996). Mortality is still important and hospital is safer. *British Medical Journal*, 312, 756–7

Sighthill Maternity Team (1982). Community antenatal care – the way forward. *Scottish Medicine*, 2, 5–7.

Sikorski, J., Wilson, J., Clement, C., Das, S., and Smeeton, N. (1996). A randomized controlled trial comparing two schedules of antenatal visits: the antenatal care project. *British Medical Journal*, 312, 546–53.

Smith, L. F. P. (1991). GP trainees' views on hospital obstetric vocational training. *British Medical Journal*, 303, 1447–52.

Standing Maternity and Midwifery Advisory Committee (Chairman J. Peel) (1970). *Domiciliary midwifery and maternity bed needs.* HMSO, London.

Steer, P. (1993). Rituals in antenatal care – do we need them? *British Medical Journal*, 307, 697–8.

Tew, M. (1985). Place of birth and perinatal mortality. *Journal of the Royal College of General Practitioners*, 35, 390–4.

Thorley, K. and Rowse, T. (1993). Seeing mothers as partners in antenatal care. *British Journal of Midwifery*, 1, 216–19.

Thornton, J. G. and Lilford, R. (1994). Active management of labour: current knowledge and research issues. *British Medical Journal*, **309**, 366–9.

Turnbull, D., *et al.* (1996). Randomized controlled trial of efficacy of midwife-managed care. *Lancet*, **348**, 213–18.

Van Alten, D., Eskes, M., and Treffers, P. E. (1989). Midwifery in the Netherlands. The Wormerveer study: selection, mode of delivery, perinatal mortality, and infant morbidity. *British Journal of Obstetrics and Gynaecology*, **96**, 656–62.

Watt, G. C. M. (1996). All together now: why social deprivation matters to everyone. *British Medical Journal*, **312**, 1026–9.

(Data available from) Wiltshire Health Committee Area NHS Trust, St John's Hospital, Trowbridge BA14 0QU.

Young, G. (1987). Are isolated maternity units run by general practitioners dangerous? *British Medical Journal*, **294**, 744–6.

Young, G. (1996). General practitioners and home birth. *Journal of the Diplomats of the Royal College of Obstetricians and Gynaecologists*, **June 1996**, 144–9.

CHAPTER THREE

The midwife's potential – from ritual to radical

Jean Duerden

This chapter will look at developments in midwifery, especially within the community setting, and suggest where the community midwifery service should be going in light of primary care development. It is important to remember that maternity services across the country vary tremendously and there can be no set pattern of care as the differing populations and geographic settings determine contrasting systems.

The midwife is qualified to monitor the health and well-being of mothers and babies and the progress of women through pregnancy, birth, and the post-delivery period, with the ability to recognize deviations from normal which require referral to a medical practitioner. She is the only health professional trained specifically for both the advisory and the clinical aspects of pregnancy, labour, and the puerperium (Chalmers, *et al.* 1989) so, at the same time as offering physical care, she educates women according to their needs. She is the focus of a woman's midwifery care and has been so since time immemorial. A fascinating account of the practice of midwives over many centuries and in many parts of the globe can be found in Marland's *The art of midwifery* (1993). Leap and Hunter (1993) have collated an oral history from handywoman to professional midwife in *The midwife's tale*. This gives an account of midwifery in the early years of this century, before the National Health Service (NHS), when doctors were rarely involved at births of working-class women as the families could not afford to pay, and midwifery care was given only in labour and the immediate postnatal period.

The 1936 Midwives Act entitled every woman to the free services of a qualified midwife, and the postnatal care extended to 10–14 days after delivery. After the introduction of the NHS in 1948, midwifery care continued to be offered predominantly in the community until obstetrics moved more and more into the hospital setting and home birth was declared to be unsafe, according to the Peel report (DHSS 1970) which advocated 100% hospital delivery. Local authorities provided the domiciliary midwifery services in this country with the Medical Officer of Health at the helm, and in 1936 the Midwives Act required local supervising authorities (LSAs) to provide the domiciliary midwives. The National Health Service Act 1946 made the local health authority the LSA, employing certificated midwives.

Allison's excellent account of the domiciliary midwifery service in Nottingham from 1948 to 1972 (Allison 1996) gives a rich description of the district midwife's role at a time when up to 50% of women gave birth at home. The government recommended an annual case-load of 55 women per midwife, but many are reported in this study to have attended up to 200 home births in a year, and some midwives recount delivering up to seven babies in periods of 48 hours. Off-duty hours were literally that; 18 hours off would mean one night a week not on call, and 38 hours off duty would mean no on-call from 8 a.m. Saturday until Sunday evening. The care given to women at that time epitomized the principles of *Changing Childbirth*, but no community midwife today could contain such a workload within her working week.

Ritual

The postnatal care given to women followed a ritualized pattern which was prescribed by the *Midwives' rules* (Central Midwives Board 1962). This rigid regime continued until the rules changed in 1986 (United Kingdom Central Council for Nursing, Midwifery, and Health Visiting 1986). The ritual involved twice-daily postnatal visits for three days and daily visits until at least the tenth postnatal day, with the flexibility to continue visiting until 28 days after delivery. At each visit the mother's temperature and pulse were taken and recorded, the fundal height measured for involution, and the lochia and perineum checked. The baby also had a top to toe examination at each visit and cord care given. Baby baths were part of the ritual. Despite the fact that the rules changed over 10 years ago, and the current rules merely refer to the postnatal period as 'a period of not less than 10 and not more than 28 days after the end of labour, during which the continued attendance of a midwife on the mother and baby is requisite' (United Kingdom Central Council for Nursing, Midwifery, and Health Visiting 1993), there are many midwives still giving prescriptive care.

Continuity of care

Continuity has become the buzz-word of the nineties in midwifery, yet district midwives offered this for many years, originally with predominantly a home birth service when the NHS was introduced in 1948, and more recently with domino (DOMiciliary IN Out) or GP unit schemes introduced in the late sixties. Each midwife had a case-load of women, either according to her geographical patch or a GP attachment. These women were booked for either shared care with hospital delivery, or total GP/midwife care with a domino booking where the woman gave birth in a hospital delivery bed but was attended by her district midwife and discharged soon after, or she gave birth in a dedicated GP unit, again with her own district midwife attending the birth and a subsequent early discharge. The GPs were available but rarely attended for delivery. The district midwife would work opposite a colleague midwife from a neighbouring practice, being on call four nights one week and three the next. The colleague midwife would cover her case-load when the named midwife was off duty and vice versa. This relief midwife would have met the woman on antenatal clinic days and a list of the midwives' home telephone numbers would be left with the woman from about 36 weeks of pregnancy.

When the woman went into labour she would ring the midwife at home and a home visit would be made by the midwife to assess labour before transferring the woman to the GP/midwife maternity unit. Many false alarms were tucked back into bed, without ever having to wait it out in a hospital bed. When established labour was ascertained by vaginal examination, the midwife took the woman in her car to the GP/midwife or maternity unit for delivery.

Many GP/midwife units were staffed at night just by a nursing auxiliary and, after the birth, mother and baby would be left in her care as the midwife returned to bed. In the maternity units, the hospital staff would care for the woman until approximately six hours after delivery when the midwife would return to see the woman home. She was taken home by ambulance, on a stretcher, and carried up the stairs to bed, where she would stay for the next three days at least. All postnatal care was carried out over the next 10–14 days by the same district midwife, but on her days off the colleague midwife would attend. The only time a third midwife would enter the framework would be when the midwife, or her relief, was on annual leave. The continuity demonstrated here could be seen as an ideal of *Changing Childbirth*, although treating the newly delivered women as an invalid is less than ideal.

This style of domiciliary midwifery continued for many years, but the on-call was replaced by a duty rota soon after NHS reorganization (DHSS 1972). Shared care became normal practice, district midwives became community midwives, and the community midwifery service became part of the maternity hospital management system. These changes caused much dissatisfaction and personal worry for many midwives as they had to form new teams and off-duty rotas. On-call cover reduced over the years to as few as one midwife on night duty for the whole community midwifery service, depending on its geographical size.

Today, a duty community midwife might work in a GP or maternity unit on a shift system, so that any woman going into labour has a slim chance of being delivered by her own community midwife, and a slightly better chance of being delivered by a midwife she has met previously. After giving birth she will be taken home in her partner's or friend's car, or even a taxi. She will be visited by one of the 'team midwives' daily in the first instance, but thereafter selective visiting will be the norm. This should be at the mother's request but, more often than not, is according to the needs of the service. Realistically, it could mean a total of four home visits in the postnatal period, by four different midwives.

Changing Childbirth and its influence on community midwifery

The community midwife was, and can be, the focus of community care. Much evidence was collected for the Winterton report (House of Commons 1992) and the *Changing Childbirth* report (Department of Health 1993) demonstrating that women want continuity of care and carer. The community midwife is best placed to offer such continuity, but Sandall's study to examine the impact of *Changing Childbirth* on midwives' work and personal life (Sandall 1997) showed that models of care such as personal case-loads may be more sustainable in terms of personal accomplishment, and cause less burn-out, than team case-loads. The personal case-load means that the woman has one midwife to relate to, and all community midwifery care is focused on her. The community midwife is seen at the first antenatal visit at the GP surgery and at most subsequent antenatal visits, and the same midwife does the home postnatal care. In ideal situations, the same midwife may have some involvement in intrapartum care.

There are many examples across the country of how the community midwifery service has been reorganized to achieve the principles of *Changing Childbirth*: choice, continuity, and control. Green *et al.* (1998) have examined the evaluations of these schemes and it would appear that few could be used as development tools in other areas, taking into consideration the differing needs of each geographical area, its client load, and its midwifery staff. The One to One midwifery project in West London, set up jointly by Hammersmith Hospital NHS Trust and Thames Valley University (McCourt and Page 1996), has been hailed as a success (Cresswell 1997), but before replicating the service in other centres, more rigorous evaluation, examining sustainablility of the service, is needed.

Many pilot schemes in other parts of the country have been abandoned because they could not be rolled out across the entire maternity service as far more midwives were needed to make the scheme work. It is evident from the current shortage that the required number of midwives would not be available for work and trusts could not fund them if they were. Of those midwives who were available, few would be able to commit themselves to the required on-call. As midwifery managers desperately try to recruit staff from a rapidly diminishing pool, trusts need to make working conditions attractive to those midwives with young families returning to work. Job share, crèche facilities, and hours that fit in with nursery hours will attract these midwives, while four nights a week on-call will not.

Warwick offers excellent small-group practices, based at King's Healthcare Trust, London, which have been very successful, but she also acknowledges that it is not possible to provide continuity of care for all (Warwick 1997) and she admits the schemes need more midwives. However, she challenges trusts to consider continuity of care schemes which are affordable and to ruthlessly target those women who experience worst pregnancy outcomes. She believes there is mileage in looking at schemes which offer excellent continuity in the antenatal and postnatal period.

Bradshaw and Bradshaw's study of heads of midwifery in Yorkshire (Bradshaw and Bradshaw 1997) found that *Changing Childbirth* policies were not being introduced because of a lack of earmarked resources, and the required reorganization of services could not be implemented within existing cash limits. The extra expense quoted by the heads of midwifery in this study included travel costs, extra duty payments, and the cost of additional equipment, and in the current climate of financial constraint within the NHS there was no funding for these.

The *Changing Childbirth* report (Department of Health 1993) appeared to herald new opportunities for community midwives. It recognized the confidence which women have in midwives, the specialist skills of midwives, and their ability to practise independently. The indicators of success were achievable in most aspects, apart from the fifth one which required that 'at least 75% of women should know the person who cares for them during delivery'. The only way this could be addressed was to introduce teams so that the woman could get to know the team members, who would then be available on a rota basis to give intrapartum care to a large number of women. How well the woman would know the midwife who attended her was debatable, and the resultant burn-out from trying to be all things to all people is well documented (Wraight *et al.* 1993; Chadda 1996; Bradshaw and Bradshaw 1997; Sandall 1997). Wraight *et al.*, in Mapping Team Midwifery, showed little evidence that units providing team midwifery achieved improved levels of care. The cost implications of introducing such schemes have been prohibitive (Henderson 1997) and where funding was available for pilot schemes, it was not recurrent and the schemes were suspended when the funding ceased (Duerden 1997, Warwick 1997).

The principles of *Changing Childbirth* can be interpreted into a community framework. If community midwives who worked in the community prior to the NHS reorganization (DHSS 1972) reflect on the care they gave at that time, the question 'Isn't it what we always had?' is inevitable. Smith argues that the enhancement of the role of the traditional community midwife could provide a care system of the highest quality (Smith 1997) and highlights the need to change the indicator of success which advocates a known midwife for delivery. A woman in labour is more concerned that she is cared for by a midwife with whom she feels safe and secure than the fact that she has met the midwife before (Stewart 1995). Smith's concern is that 'the indicator of success will result in a regime to satisfy the indicator itself, and not the needs of the woman' and that the continuity of care offered to women in the community for many years will be compromised by disseminating a case-load of women to a team of midwives.

The district midwife of the past worked in partnerships rather than teams (Allison 1997). However, the long spans of duty necessary to achieve this care are not suited to the personal circumstances of every midwife. The hours of duty undertaken by district midwives of old would not suit a family life where one's own children require on-call availability such as 'Mum's taxi service' for their individual needs. A recent study undertaken by Sandall (1997) showed exactly this. It looked at midwives' burn-out as the impact of *Changing Childbirth* on midwives' work and personal lives was examined. Sandall looked at three different models of community-based care: a group practice, traditional community midwifery, and a community team. The women's experience of continuity from traditional community midwifery was greater than that of the community team, but less than that of the group practice. The GP-attached community midwives had large case-loads, but were able to develop meaningful relationships with women and experienced greater job satisfaction. Their sacrifice was not being able to attend the birth of the majority of their case-load. The team midwives found the most stressful part of their work was being on call and not 'knowing' the women.

Another recent study from the midwives' perspective (Fleissig and Kroll 1997) examined the views of community midwives on the continuity of care and carer they provided after a new system of group practice midwifery had been introduced to the community, with pairs of named midwives belonging to a team of eight. All of them felt the quality of care given to local women was worse than that given to women in the previous domino service. The authors believe that these views reflected not only their previous midwifery experience but also their domestic commitments. They emphasized that the 'one-to-one' midwives had applied for, and been especially selected for, this service, again endorsing the fact that this type of midwifery is not appropriate for all community midwives as it requires radical changes in the way they have to work. They need to be flexible and committed, and the authors believe there is a risk of midwives 'expecting too much of themselves'. They conclude that the first priority for midwives should be to give a service offering supportive, personal, and consistent care.

When *Changing Childbirth* was introduced, midwives were full of optimism and hope, yet the Audit Commission report (Audit Commission 1997) shows that eight out of 12 health authorities have no strategy for maternity services and some have refused to fund *Changing Childbirth* pilots. The gratifying aspect of the report is that 90% of the women surveyed said they were happy with their midwifery care. Considering the staff shortages which were highlighted, which meant that many women did not have one-to-one midwifery support in labour, this says a lot for the abilities of the midwives involved. The postnatal care given in the home was quoted as being 'highly popular', another example of the satisfaction with the community midwifery service.

Selective visiting

After the movement into hospital for the majority of births, the community midwife's role changed. Most women stayed in hospital for several days after giving birth, so midwives provided postnatal care for a large number of women over a short period of time. As a result, the numbers of midwives practising in the community reduced. In 1942 there were 12 250 district midwives working in the community; in 1985 this had reduced to 3906 community-based midwives (DHSS 1987). Over the last 20 years, hospital stay after birth has reduced dramatically, until even women who have had Caesarean sections will sometimes be returned home on the third post-operative day. The numbers of women requiring home postnatal visits has escalated so much that static, existing community midwifery staff cannot sustain the workload. Government statistics for 1995–96 (Department of Health Statistics Division 1996) demonstrate that since 1988–89 the total number of antenatal contacts at midwife-only clinics has increased by 74%, reflecting the growing trend for midwife-led care. There was also a 1% increase in antenatal domiciliary visits over that period, but the postnatal contacts fell by 13%. The antenatal contacts per maternity rose from 4.7 in 1988–89 to 7.1 in 1995–96, while the postnatal contacts per maternity fell from 9.2 to 8.4 in those respective periods. Seventeen per cent of these contacts in the postnatal period are made by health visitors, as are 12% of the antenatal contacts.

Reduced funding and staffing levels mean that postnatal care has been radically changed. The community midwifery service in the UK offers a more extensive home visiting service than most countries; in fact many countries do not provide home postnatal visits, and criticism of selective visiting may be unfounded. There is much potential to use this wisely and effectively. The value of a daily visit of routine examination in the absence of problems can be questioned, and one study revealed that women complained about the number and timing of visits (Murphy-Black 1994), as did the women surveyed by the Audit Commission (Audit Commission 1997). In the later survey, one in five complained that the frequency of visits was not right for them, and the Commission therefore recommends developing guidelines for matching home visiting to the needs of mothers and their families. Daily visits may be welcomed by a first-time mother but, for those with other children, such visits have been seen as a tiresome intrusion into a busy family schedule.

The most important aspect of selective visiting is to ensure that women know how to request an unplanned visit and from whom they should seek emergency advice or a home visit. The 24-hour helpline provided by most community midwifery services is a lifeline to many distraught women in the middle of the night. The anxiety may seem trivial to the experienced mother, but to someone having their first experience of an inconsolable crying baby, or a bleeding cord, and no one at home with whom to share that anxiety, the reassurance of a professional opinion and the offer of a home visit will do much to alleviate the acute problem. Selective visiting can not, therefore, have a prescriptive pattern, and it must be in accord with the individual needs of each woman. Extended families are no longer in close proximity and more women are being visited who have no previous experience with babies.

Education and training

Midwifery education and training is discussed in detail in Chapter 10. When training was divided into two parts, part one involved instruction in normal and abnormal midwifery in a school of midwifery attached to the maternity unit. The role of the hospital midwife was emphasized and midwifery tutors worked in the clinical environment with the pupils, having their own antenatal clinics, and their expertise was never questioned. For part two, many of the students (previously known as pupils) lived and worked in the community and instruction emphasized public health and domiciliary midwifery. Some will recollect the lectures on sanitation, housing, and social services with visits to local establishments, such as a work centre for the handicapped, disinfestation centres, and the sewage works to complete the district picture. Social and domestic responsibilities were emphasized and a common talk to the part two pupils by the local supervisor of midwives would be instruction in improvisation and social etiquette, such as being told never to refuse hospitality, as it would offend, and that tea was made with boiling water so should be relatively sterile.

This changed slowly over time and the picture today is very different as midwifery education is a continuous course, delivered often a great distance from the maternity unit in which the student midwife will practice. The clinical instruction is given by senior midwives in the work area, and the public health emphasis is not so rigorous. Allison (1996) regrets the demise of medical students being trained by district midwives and obstetricians teaching student midwives, believing that the opportunity for first-hand witness of the interplay between district carers and the public health function is lost as ties with close colleagues are severed.

All midwifery education establishments have moved into universities which has meant amalgamation of local, hospital-attached midwifery schools. The midwifery programmes are set at diploma or, increasingly, at degree level. The focus has changed to one of self-directed learning with a combination of hospital and community assessors at the practice base. There is no specific training for community midwifery which means that midwives are influenced purely by their community experience which may not have been with a long-established community midwife.

Skills of the midwife in the community

One must never overlook the need for specific skills as a community midwife. It is not possible to 'put an old head on young shoulders' and a hospital midwife cannot be expected to work in the community on the assumption that she has the knowledge and experience to accommodate the change in practice. A midwife first going out into the community has many anxieties. Experienced community midwives who are used to carrying case-loads with many women booked for home birth are now approaching retirement and the younger, less experienced workforce may well have implications for the home birth service as midwives may feel humiliated in asking for help from their GP or hospital colleagues.

Good communication skills are probably the most fundamental requirement of a community midwife who has to liaise with many different health professionals in determining the best care for the women on her case-load. She also has to relate to women of varied backgrounds and ethnicity, and to act as their advocate. Hunt tells us:

'When communication is good, women are more likely to feel in control of the childbirth experience and more able to understand the implications of the choices that are available to them' (Hunt 1996).

The community midwife needs to be a good decision-maker (Page 1995) as she is challenged to make sound clinical judgement and to diagnose the abnormal, at the same time involving the woman in that decision-making and ensuring she has her consent (Kirkham 1989). The community midwife, as all midwives, should respect confidentiality and consider the environment in which she shares information with other professionals. The difficulty is maintaining confidentiality whilst ensuring that such information as necessary is available to the clinicians responsible for their care (Department of Health 1996).

A community midwife also needs to be a good navigator! Just learning the way around the geographic area involved causes serious worry, and this area gets larger and larger as the service is no longer local, but an economically centralized service.

Relationships

If multi-professional teams are to come together to provide high-quality services that make the best use of the specialist skills and experience of the staff involved, creating the seamless service demanded in the Government White Paper, A Service with Ambitions (Department of Health 1996), then establishing good working relationships with all professionals involved in maternity care is vital (see Chapter 5). Primary care meetings are essential to the smooth running of the service and much can be gained from these multidisciplinary meetings, not least knowing who are the other practitioners involved in the care of women on the case-load. Liaison with all these individuals is so much easier when they are personal acquaintances and not just a voice on the other end of a telephone.

Centralization of the maternity services has meant that few community midwives see themselves as part of the primary care team, but this should not be an issue. Being employed by an acute trust should not deprive community midwives of membership of the primary care team, neither should such membership marginalize the midwife from colleagues at the base hospital. In the author's experience, it is possible to carry out both roles effectively, without compromising either service. In this way the midwife acts as a conduit between the hospital maternity service and the community maternity service, removing the seams.

The involvement of the health visitor in the community maternity service is particularly crucial as she plays an important role in the welfare of the family and her involvement antenatally is to be encouraged. The line of communication here should be from community midwife to health visitor and many opportunities exist for collaborative working which will enhance the care which mothers and babies receive. Patterns of postnatal care vary in each area and the handover of care to the health visitor occurs at different stages of the postnatal period, according to local protocols. As postnatal care becomes more fragmented, it is important that a smooth transition of care from midwife to health visitor takes place. This transition is enhanced if the midwife has involved the health visitor antenatally. If midwives are visiting beyond the tenth postnatal day, according to *Changing Childbirth*, the mother should be able to choose which of the two health professionals should be the prime care provider (Department of Health 1993). This is not a cue for inter-professional rivalry, but for closer collaboration and a consistency of advice which has been notoriously conflicting in the past. This consistency cannot be achieved without regular contact and discussion amongst these primary carers who are usually employed by different trusts, which may lead to reduced opportunities for regular contact.

Excellent communication with the GP is essential if most of the antenatal and postnatal care is to be given by the community midwife. Many GPs fear the loss of contact with women during their pregnancy, but these fears can be allayed if there is a shared approach to care in the antenatal period and if the midwife maintains a professional relationship with the doctor. This must be a two-way relationship as the GP knows the medical background of the women on the midwife's case-load. One approach would be for the GP to carry out one scheduled antenatal examination per trimester (see Chapters 19 and 25).

The doctor/midwife/obstetrician relationship is crucial to establishing optimum community maternity services (see Chapter 2). There is overlap in the roles and responsibilities of each (Kroll 1994) and the boundaries need clearer definition. Inter-professional cooperation should underpin the service and the midwife can act as an effective liaison between hospital and community. She can refer women directly to obstetricians. Maternity payments have contributed to the duplication of care offered. The new guidelines, *General practitioners and intrapartum care: interim guidance* (General Medical Services Committee 1997), will hopefully resolve this issue. It is accepted that general practitioner obstetricians are a dying breed (Bull 1994) and their involvement in intrapartum work has diminished for many reasons (see Chapter 4), but through effective partnership with the community midwife, excellent results can be achieved.

Communication with obstetricians is of similar significance. Direct referral from a community midwife should now be commonplace as obstetricians recognize her autonomy and clinical skills, but there are tremendous variations as to how referrals are made. A referral can be made by telephone, and with the introduction of antenatal day-care assessment centres, women should be seen straight away rather than awaiting a clinic appointment, if the midwife feels the referral should be immediate. The midwife in charge of the fetal assessment unit may well take a midwife-to-midwife referral, and accept the woman for assessment and then notify the obstetrician after she has been assessed on the unit. (Management of the post-mature woman would be an excellent example.) This type of liaison is to be encouraged and bodes well for the future community midwifery service. Similarly, if antenatal visits at the hospital are to be effectively reduced, a respect for the community midwife's clinical judgement by obstetricians is crucial.

Satisfactory relationships within primary care underpin the community service. There is little room for conflict, yet in a survey of the three pilot group practices in South East Thames (Allen *et al.* 1997) some of the midwives described conflicts both within the groups and with other colleagues. Some women in the study were concerned about the negative attitude towards GP care by some of the midwives. As has been highlighted in other studies, some of the midwives were reluctant to hand over care to colleagues and suffered guilt for not being available all of the time. The GPs were particularly concerned about the lack of consultation with them as the pilots were set up, they felt communication was poor and that their contact with the women had been reduced by the group practices. If good community schemes are to be implemented, GP consultation and cooperation is vital.

The midwife/mother relationship cannot be taken for granted. The social circumstances of the mother may inhibit the midwife in forming a constructive and helpful relationship and she may make false assumptions about the necessity of passing on relevant information and fail to communicate effectively (Kirkham 1993). Even without the social conflict, equality is difficult to achieve in the clinical environment, such as in busy antenatal clinics. In contrast, a very strong and loving relationship can build up between mother and midwife and severance of those ties at the end of the postnatal period can make the mother feel utterly bereft. The skilled community midwife can find the appropriate level of communication for each individual, and much can be learned from listening to others and observing (Kirkham 1993; Hunt and Symonds 1995).

The teaching role of the midwife in the community

As normal midwifery features throughout the early modules of the current midwifery education programmes, it is often considered appropriate for the student midwife to have her first placement with the midwife in the community. This provides a wonderful opportunity for the student to experience first hand a complete package of care for women. She will be accompanied at all times by the community midwife and consequently have ample opportunity to observe all aspects of antenatal and postnatal care in a normal pregnancy. Identifying the abnormal will also be demonstrated. Depending on the area, there may also be opportunities to witness intrapartum care and normal births. Foundations for a holistic approach to midwifery care can be made during this formative experience.

Many midwives in the community have expressed concern about mentoring undergraduate midwives, feeling inadequate to teach at that level. They should not need reassuring that their own practical experience gives them the authority to teach with confidence. It is very rare to hear a student midwife complain about her community placement or a lack of learning opportunities. The importance of the relationship between the midwife and the student cannot be overemphasized when this long clinical placement is considered, and the rewards are great as the community midwife is able to watch the student develop under her supervision.

Supervision of midwives in the community

When the supervision of midwives related purely to district midwives, pre 1977, the supervisors were clinically linked and district based (Allison 1997). From the introduction of the 1902 Midwives Act, supervision was carried out rigorously in the community, in the first instance by inspectors appointed by the medical officer and after 1936 by non-medical supervisors who had practised as midwives for at least three years, and at least one of those years as a district midwife. It was not until 1977 that supervision of all midwives, including midwives working in hospital, was introduced. As a result, the emphasis of the supervision of midwives has been on community midwives, and the history of a three-monthly visit to check bags and records, and a visit to the midwife's home to check the secure storage of drugs within a locked box within a locked cupboard, was a reality until a relatively short time ago. The supervision offered now to community midwives is from a named supervisor, not necessarily a community midwife or manager, with emphasis on an annual supervisory review during which the midwives' professional development needs will be discussed. A confidential environment is provided for the midwife to discuss any anxieties about her own practice or midwifery practice generally.

An on-call service is provided 24 hours a day by the supervisors in each trust on a rota basis, and advice can be sought at any time by community staff (Duerden 1995). This advice is often sought by midwives who are concerned that the choices that some women make are potentially life-threatening, although, happily, this is a rare event. When it does occur, the supervisor will provide support for the midwife, perhaps carry out a shared home visit with her to discuss options with the woman concerned, and also enlist the help of an obstetrician if the woman remains determined in her decision.

Independent midwives

Independent midwives have for many years offered a community-based midwifery service which provides the choice, continuity, and control advocated by the *Changing Childbirth* report (Department of Health 1993).

Sadly, this service has been seen as a threat by some community midwives, rather than a service to those women who want a guaranteed named midwife to care for them throughout their pregnancy, birth, and postnatal period, and to receive a tailor-made service which allows all their choices to be taken into consideration and granted wherever possible. The independent midwives have a good track record of providing such a service with excellent outcomes (Weig 1993). Unfortunately, the present nationwide increase in obstetric litigation has made many trusts wary of accepting vicarious liability for independent midwives practising within their trust premises. As a result, if a woman being cared for by an independent midwife needs to be transferred to hospital, she may not be able to continue to care for her once she enters the hospital doors, and can only stay as a supporter. This interruption of continuity can cause unnecessary distress to the woman concerned, and smacks of a lack of trust in the independent midwife. Thankfully, several trusts are happy to continue providing honorary or bank contracts to these midwives, but unfortunately with the result that women have to travel further afield when being transferred into hospital in an emergency situation. This is far from ideal and needs to be addressed urgently by trust managers and supervisors of midwives.

Community issues

Murphy-Black's study of care in the community during the postnatal period (Murphy-Black 1994) found one of the common themes to be conflicting advice. The women complained that all the midwives had different ways of doing things and they gave opposing advice on feeding and how to handle a crying baby. This is not surprising, as it is a regular complaint of the midwives themselves that their colleagues follow them in at the next visit and contradict all the good advice given by them at the previous visit. If there has been this awareness for so long, why does the situation continue? It is possible to give continuity of advice, as midwives in Bournemouth have achieved (Walker 1996). Here, women interviewed to evaluate the service at the Royal Bournemouth Hospital said 'They all say the same thing'.

Midwives have easy access to evidence from studies into all aspects of midwifery practice. Why are they not using the Cochrane Library or reading *A guide to effective care in pregnancy and childbirth* (Enkin *et al.* 1995) or even putting into practice what is read in the midwifery journals? The conflicting advice was read as criticism by several women in Murphy-Black's study and she emphasizes the impact that a single midwife can make on a woman during a very sensitive period in her life. The starting point for new advice should surely be with that which was given at the previous visit and by evaluating its efficacy. Similarly, the advice which the community midwife gives in the home should be consistent with that given in hospital. If the same quality of care is given by all carers then continuity of care is assured (Nunnerley 1990).

Fragmented and routinized care was another theme which emerged from

Murphy-Black's study. Women recognized that the midwives were pressed for time. The researcher believes that the midwife should concentrate on assessing the needs of the woman, offering a more efficient and appropriate service during the home visit rather than concentrating on routine tasks. If the midwife decides whether or not the blood pressure needs to be measured, she can also make the same decision about maternal temperature and pulse.

The recent audit report, First Class Delivery (Audit Commission 1997), showed that some aspects of care, in particular postnatal care, were less satisfactory than care in the antenatal period and in labour. This was most marked in hospital where the availability of staff was of particular concern, in contrast to women's views of postnatal care in the home which was 'highly popular'. Within the community, around 80% of the women interviewed said they were encouraged to ask questions, felt they were listened to, felt someone got to know them, and felt the staff gave them confidence, whereas in the hospital the percentages were between 35 and 65. Clearly, the midwifery service in the community is highly valued by women. Continuity of care was shown to be important to all women, but continuity of carer was only important to some. The Audit Commission recommend that in pregnancy 'trusts should aim to base the care of these women in the community with care provided by midwives and GPs. Not only does community care cost significantly less than traditional, obstetrician-led, shared care, but it is more appropriate and probably more satisfactory for many of these women' (p.17). The Audit Commission's recommendations for postnatal care are that 'trusts should review the efficiency and quality of postnatal hospital care and target postnatal community services where they are most needed' (p.50).

Problem families

Almost one third of Britain's babies are born into relative poverty (Allison 1997). The Nottingham study showed that before 1972 the district midwifery service was biased towards poor families. The situation is the converse today. It is predominantly articulate, middle-class women who seek the services of a community midwife for a home birth. However, community-based midwives are in the best position, because of their access to community-based carers, to assist women whose problems may be very diverse and may include drug or alcohol abuse, malnutrition, non-attendance for antenatal care, lack of family or social service support, mental or physical illness, homelessness, itineracy, child abuse, and many others (see Chapter 12).

Child protection is a growing issue and community midwives must be aware of the Children Act of 1989 and its implications. Home conditions may indicate potential problems, especially health issues. The community midwife is uniquely placed to observe family dynamics and is often the first to report concerns about possible child abuse or non-accidental injury.

Community-based maternity care and its future

When considering community schemes, the organizational priorities must first be determined and options have to be considered both for women and midwives when establishing working patterns and deciding priorities. Managers need to look at what can be practically achieved within the available resources. The thorn in the flesh will always be trying to provide continuity of carer for the birth. Definitions are needed of ways to achieve continuity of care and carer as one looks at the advantages of case-load holding over teams (Green *et al.*, 1997).

It is extremely difficult to break down centralized care to give continuity of care in the community. No one expected in 1976 that we would lose that continuity offered by the community midwifery service when the service became centralized. We have come full circle and now have to consider where the service is going. With the current emphasis on primary care, the opportunities to develop community-based maternity care should be boundless. *Primary care: delivering the future* (Department of Health 1996) offers support for community-based schemes which are experimental alternatives to the single national contract for general practitioners (Coulter and Mays 1997). In theory, community midwives could set up a practice and employ salaried doctors with a chance to develop new models of care, but the risks are considerable and the health authorities who are charged by the legislation to regulate the pilot schemes may not look favourably on a scheme which only covers a limited group from a general practitioner's case-load. Some schemes have been proposed which involve midwives as well as nurses, therapists, counsellors, care managers, social workers, and GPs (Coulter and Mays 1997). Only one midwifery-led bid has been submitted as these are difficult to prepare when the Government insists that any pilots must incorporate all the services which patients are entitled to (Royal College of Midwives 1997). Midwives must therefore seek to be involved in the first wave of pilots. If the aim of primary-led care is the provision of 'one-stop health shops', midwives must consider how they can contribute to this facility and how they can ensure that women-centred care is not impeded by any new structural changes (Silverton 1997).

Whatever service is developed it must be woman-centred and maintain the principles of *Changing Childbirth*. Determining the woman's needs accurately will not be easy if they are still not understood by service users (Bradshaw and Bradshaw 1997), and midwifery leaders are not all convinced that their clients either wish for or understand what the report proposed. This author has strong recollections of a community midwife lamenting, after a string of booking visits in the home, that each of her clients when offered a wide choice for delivery (home, GP/midwife unit, midwife-led unit, shared care, or consultant care) responded by saying 'I want my baby in hospital'.

Involving lay people in planning professional services is very commendable, but many maternity service liaison committees are struggling to find lay representation, and how can one be sure that those who do attend represent all service users? Articulating the needs of those affected by poverty, one third of all users, is very difficult and determining consumers' views of maternity care is equally a struggle (Garcia 1989). What is without doubt is that the community midwife is well placed to help those women who often fail to get the best from the system (Walton and Hamilton 1995), such as the very young, the ethnic minorities, the disabled, those with poor social circumstances, and travellers. As the model of midwifery care is now based on health rather than illness, community midwives have the opportunity to undo some of the harm caused by the medicalization of birth (Hunt and Symonds 1996).

Conclusion

Community midwives are said to be born not trained (Aspinall *et al.* 1997), and it must be understood that some midwives feel more suited to working in hospital while others determine early on in their training that the community is where they wish to develop their midwifery career. A simple analogy would be the doctor who chooses to be a GP rather than a hospital specialist. For midwives to be successful in the community they need to be assertive in agreeing clear expectations of work and practice with colleagues, women, and at home (Sandall 1997). Those with support at work and at home and with clearly defined time off work will, according to Sandall's study, be able to establish meaningful relationships with women.

The target of an equitable, nationwide, seamless service between hospital and home still seems out of reach, but if trusts evaluate the evidence from the many studies into community-based maternity care and create realistic, manageable, and regularly monitored case-loads, a promising service can be achieved which does not cause unnecessary stress. One way of achieving this is to provide an adequate back-up and relief service, rather than utilizing existing team members to stand in for sickness, study leave, holidays, and maternity leave, further stretching an overburdened workload.

There is no longer an untapped pool of midwives waiting to be recruited to the service. Gone are the days of student midwives unable to gain employment upon qualification. Fewer students are applying for midwifery education as registered nurses are unwilling to reduce their income and move on to an educational contract. In order to compensate for the reduction of available midwives, it is likely that the role of the health care assistant (HCA) will be reviewed. Midwives' former reservations about using them now needs reconsideration.

Management ideals for the community maternity service must be realistic. Implementation of all the 10 indicators of success listed in the *Changing Childbirth* report must now be acknowledged to be unrealistic and impossible within every trust. This author tried to implement team midwifery as a community midwifery manager – with an unwilling workforce, this is virtually impossible. Having separate systems of care within one centralized service marginalizes midwives as well as women. What can easily be achieved, however, is an expert community maternity team, very locally based, offering continuity of care and a home birth service. This has been achieved for years, but more recently, in an endeavour to implement the *Changing Childbirth* recommendations, there have been experiments to improve the service. These experimental schemes have been evaluated (Green, *et al.* 1997) and it is now time to acknowledge and respond to that evaluation by learning lessons from the past, using the knowledge we now have from experience and evaluation, to produce a community maternity service which is good for women and midwives alike. The onus is, therefore, on the leaders of the profession to provide the necessary support for an effective community midwifery service which works closely with all others in the primary health care team, ensuring that organizational boundaries do not get in the way of care for women.

References

Allen, I., Bourke Dowling, S., and Williams, S. (1997). A leading role for midwives: evaluation of midwifery group practice development projects. Policy Studies Institute, London.

Allison, J. (1996). *Delivered at home*. Chapman and Hall, London.

Aspinall, K., Nelson, B., Patterson, T., and Sims, A. (1997). *An extraordinary ordinary woman*. Ann's Trust Fund, Sheffield.

Audit Commission (1997). First-class delivery: improving maternity services in England and Wales. HMSO, London.

Bradshaw, M. G. and Bradshaw, P. L. (1997). Changing childbirth – the midwifery managers' tale. *Journal of Nurse Management*, 5, 143–9.

Bull, M. J. V. (1994). Selection of women for community obstetric care. In: *The future of the maternity services* (ed. G. Chamberlain and N. Patel). RCOG Press, London.

Central Midwives Board (1962) *Midwives' rules*. CMB, London.

Chadda, D. (1996). Cash shortage threatens midwife-led birth model *Health Service Journal*, **106**, 8.

Chalmers, I., Enkin, M., and Keirse, M. J. N. C. (1989). *Effective care in pregnancy and childbirth*. Oxford University Press, Oxford.

Coulter, A. and Mays, N. (1997). Deregulating primary care *British Medical Journal*, **314**, 510–12.

Cresswell, J. (1997) Delivering satisfaction *Nursing Times*, 7, 23–5.

Davies, K. (1997). Cautious welcome for primary care proposals. *Midwives*, **109**, 315.

Department of Health (1993). *Changing childbirth*. HMSO, London.

Department of Health (1996) *A service with ambitions*. HMSO, London.

Department of Health (1996). *Choice and opportunity – Primary care: delivering the future*. HMSO, London.

Department of Health (1996). *Report on confidential enquiries into maternal deaths in the United Kingdom 1991–1993* HMSO, London.

Department of Health and Social Security (1970). Standing Maternity and Midwifery Advisory Committee (Chairman J. Peel). *Domiciliary midwifery and maternity bed needs.* HMSO, London.

Department of Helath & Social Security (1972). *Management arrangements for the reorganised NHS.* HMSO, London.

Department of Health and Social Security (1987). *Health and personal social service statistics for England.* HMSO, London.

Department of Health Statistics Division 2B (1996). *Community maternity services summary information for 1995–1996.* DoH Statistics, London.

Duerden, J. M. (1995). *Audit of supervision of midwives in the North West Regional Health Authority.* Salford Royal Hospitals NHS Trust.

Duerden, J. (1997). Supervisors and midwives' morale in the NHS. *Modern Midwife,* 7, 15–19.

Enkin, M., Kierse, M., and Renfrew, M. (1995). *A guide to effective care in pregnancy and childbirth.* Oxford University Press, Oxford.

Fleissig, A. and Kroll, D. (1997). Achieving continuity of care and carer *Modern Midwife,* 7, 28–9.

Garcia, J. (1989). Getting consumers' views of maternity care. HMSO, London.

General Medical Services Committee (1997). General practitioners and intrapartum care: interim guidance. British Medical Association, London.

Green, J., Curtis, P., Price, H., and Renfrew, M. J. (1998). *Continuing to care: the organization of midwifery services in the UK – a structured review.* Books for Midwives Press, Cheshire.

Henderson, C. (1997). *Changing Childbirth and the West Midlands Region.* Royal College of Midwives, London.

House of Commons Health Select Committee (1992). *Second report on the maternity services.* HMSO, London.

Hunt, S. C. and Symonds, A. (1995). *The social meaning of midwifery.* Macmillan Press Ltd, Hampshire.

Hunt, S. C. and Symonds, A. (1996). *The midwife and society.* Macmillan Press Ltd, Hampshire.

Kirkham, M. (1989). Midwives and information-giving during labour. In: *Midwives, research, and childbirth.* Vol. 1. (ed. S. Robinson and A. M. Thomson.) Chapman and Hall, London.

Kirkham, M. (1993). Communication in midwifery. In: *Midwifery practice – a researched-based approach* (ed. J. Alexander, V. Levy, and S. Roch). Macmillan Press Ltd, Hampshire.

Kroll, D. (1994). Tunafanya nini – what business are we in? In: *The future of the maternity services* (ed. G. Chamberlain and N. Patel*).* RCOG Press, London.

Leap, N. and Hunter, B. (1993). *The midwife's tale* Scarlet Press, London.

McCourt, C. and Page, L. (ed.) (1996). *Report on the evaluation of one-to-one midwifery.* Thames Valley University, London.

Marland, H. (1993). *The art of midwifery: early modern midwives in Europe.* Routledge, London.

Murphy-Black, T. (1994). Care in the community during the postnatal period. In: *Midwives, research, and childbirth.* Vol. 3. (ed. S. Robinson and A. M. Thomson.) Chapman and Hall, London.

Nunnerley, R. (1990). Quality assurance in postnatal care. In: *Postnatal care – a researched-based approach* (ed. J. Alexander, V. Levy, and S. Roch). Macmillan Press Ltd, Hampshire.

Nursing Times (1997). Community midwives win insurance promise [editorial]. *Nursing Times,* **93**, 6.

Page, L. (1995). *Effective group practice in midwifery.* Blackwell Science, Oxford.

Royal College of Midwives (1997). *End insurance discrimination for community midwives plea.* RCM, London.

Royal College of Midwives (1997). Staking a place for midwifery in the primary care team. *Women-Centred Care,* RCM Supplement, **August 1997**, 5.

Sandall, J. (1997). Midwives' burn-out and continuity of care *British Journal of Midwifery,* **5**, 106–11.

Silverton, L. (1997). Primary care-led health services and midwifery *British Journal of Midwifery,* **5**, 525-7.

Smith, M. (1997). The demise of the traditional community midwife *British Journal of Midwifery,* **5**, 252–4.

Stewart, M. (1995). Do you have to know your midwife? *British Journal of Midwifery,* **3**, 19–22.

United Kingdom Central Council for Nursing, Midwifery, and Health Visiting (1986). *Midwives' rules* UKCC, London.

United Kingdom Central Council for Nursing, Midwifery, and Health Visiting (1993). *Midwives' rules.* UKCC, London.

Walker, J. (1996). Interim evaluation of a Midwifery Development Unit, *Midwives,* **109**, 366–70.

Walton, I. and Hamilton, M. (1995). *Midwives and Changing Childbirth.* Books for Midwives Press, Cheshire.

Warwick, C. (1997). Can continuity of care be the only answer? *British Journal of Midwifery,* **5**, 6.

Weig, M. (1993). *Audit of independent midwifery 1980–1991.* Royal College of Midwives, London.

Wraight, A. B. J., Secombe, I. and Stock, J. (1993). *Mapping team midwifery.* IMS Report 242 to the Department of Health, Institute of Manpower Studies, Brighton.

Young, D. and Lees, A. (1997). The costs to the NHS of maternity care: midwife-managed vs shared care *British Journal of Midwifery,* **5**, 465–72.

CHAPTER FOUR

General practitioners' contributions – what's really going on?

Lindsay Smith and David Jewell

Introduction

Complete obstetric care (antenatal, intrapartum, and postnatal) used to be a normal, essential part of British general practice. The norm now is for GPs to provide only antenatal and postnatal care. The number of women giving birth under the care of their general practitioner has steadily decreased from more than 85% in 1927 (Registrar General 1929), through 50% in 1946 (Royal College of Obstetricians and Gynaecologists 1948), to about 15% in 1975 (Campbell and MacFarlane 1994). Concomitantly there has been an increase in institutional birth and in the number of GPs providing only antenatal and postnatal care, and there has been a decrease in the number of GPs providing intrapartum care (Marsh *et al.* 1985*a,b*). This decline in intrapartum care by GPs is not confined to the United Kingdom. Over the past 30 years there have been marked reductions in the provision of intrapartum care by GPs in many countries (Canadian Medical Association 1987; Hingstman and Boon 1988; Smith and Jewell 1991*b*; Treffers *et al.* 1990; Cohen 1991; Gaskins *et al.* 1991; Campbell and Macfarlane 1994).

The decline in intrapartum care is the most visible and widely reported aspect of GP obstetrics. Such a view, however, gives maternity care an extremely narrow focus. For many years, large numbers of GPs have seen themselves as making a substantial contribution to maternity care by looking after women before and after birth while leaving intrapartum care to midwives and obstetricians.

The aim of this chapter is to examine the contribution of GPs to maternity care, in the context of the diversity of general practice. The decline in GPs' contribution to intrapartum care can then be seen in context. We shall conclude by considering implications of this decline.

Scope of general practice maternity care

The 'core' part of maternity care is represented by antenatal, intrapartum, and postnatal care. But even here it is important to take an inclusive approach. For instance, antenatal care includes management of other medical problems either coexisting with, or caused by, pregnancy, and postnatal care includes management of any problem arising as a result of pregnancy and occurring any time after birth, such as postnatal depression. Around the core is a wider, less clearly defined range of activities more or less closely linked to pregnancy. It might include care related to miscarriage, stillbirth, therapeutic abortion, pre-pregnancy care, and genetic counselling. Beyond these there is activity related to infertility and contraception, as well as care of children included in neonatal care, childhood surveillance, and immunization. GPs may be involved in work such as audit or serving on Maternity Service Liaison Committees which all form part of maternity services but without direct patient contact (Smith 1996).

We would predict that most GPs would include all such activity, with the possible exception of serving on Maternity Service Liaison Committees, as within the scope of the role they see themselves fulfilling for their patients. The extent to which GPs themselves undertake the work involved will vary widely according to local patterns of service provision and self-referral (especially contraception and abortion) and their own expertise (especially infertility). The National Morbidity Survey supports the idea that all such activity is a common feature of general practice (Office of Population Censuses and Surveys 1995). Table 4.1 shows the numbers of women consulting for the relevant headings in the classification.

It is not surprising that the largest number of women consulting is for contraception. The numbers of women seen with 'normal pregnancy' in the age group 16–44 is approximately 7% in one year, and approximately 5% are seen for complications of pregnancy, although it must be assumed that these form part of the 7% seen on a different occasion for normal pregnancy. Approximately 1% are seen for miscarriage – one in seven or eight of all pregnancies. According to the data, women seen in the category of 'normal delivery and other indications for care in pregnancy, labour, and delivery' represent one in five of all women seen for normal pregnancy. Taken altogether, the consultation rates for all encounters relating to contraception and core maternity care represent one quarter of all the workload for women in this age group.

These data give a general picture of contacts and workload. Additional evidence comes from descriptive studies concerning the activity and attitudes of GPs to specific problems. However, the evidence in all areas except intrapartum care remains sparse, reflecting a preoccupation with that aspect. For instance, searching Medline has not identified any papers specifically relating to contraception or preconception advice in primary care, although there is a description of the latter in this book's predecessor (Marsh 1985). As the data from the National Morbidity Survey shows, contraception represents

Table 4.1 *Persons consulting for selected headings, for all women and those in age groups 16–24 and 25–44. Data extracted from National Morbidity Survey (OPCS 1995)*

Persons consulting per 1000 women [Tables 19–21]	All women	Aged 16–24	Aged 25–44
All causes	857.5	894.2	865.1
For complications of pregnancy, childbirth, and puerperium (630–639)	21.1	49.2	48.2
Pregnancy with abortive outcome (630–639)	4.9	13.1	10.7
Complications mainly related to pregnancy (640–648)	9.1	23.8	20.2
Normal delivery and other indications for care in pregnancy, labour, and delivery (650–659)	5.8	13.2	13.5
Complications occurring mainly in the course of labour and delivery (660–669)	2.4	4.8	5.8
Complications of the puerperium (670–676)	3.6	5.0	9.4
Normal pregnancy (V22)	28.7	68.3	66.6
Post-partum care and management (V24)	19.6	42.7	47.1
Contraceptive management (V25)	140.6	470.7	255.9

a substantial component of the work of looking after young women, and with the reduction in health authority clinics general practice is set to become the primary provider of family planning in the United Kingdom.

Preconception is a more difficult area. There are certain theoretical gains from providing preconception advice, such as folic acid supplementation in preventing neural tube defects (Chapter 16). Nevertheless, many pregnancies are unintended at conception and would never be eligible for preconception advice. However it is likely to be, at least for the foreseeable future, a form of care that is unlikely to take place outside general practice and which could supplement contraceptive advice.

Infertility is an area where the work has gradually shifted from being predominantly research-based in tertiary centres to all secondary care hospitals to its becoming available in primary care. It parallels what has happened in contraception and is a contrast to the pattern for intrapartum care. The management of infertility in a single practice over five years showed that many women had had investigations started in the practice (Wilkes and Jones 1995). Two thirds had had a serum progestogen measured, half had had prolactin and their partners' semen analysed, and one third either a serum follicle stimulating hormone (FSH) or a serum lureinizing hormone (LH) measured. However, very few women had had their treatment started by their GP. A postal questionnaire survey of women's experiences in Aberdeen similarly found that almost all women had consulted their GPs for infertility and 92% had seen a specialist later (Templeton *et al.* 1990).

Concerning the management of miscarriage there is again very little direct evidence. A postal survey of GPs in Wessex reported that 21% would be unlikely to send patients who were stable and comfortable into hospital. This figure was not validated by evidence of the doctors' behaviour, but it, and the response rate of 90%, suggest that GPs feel it is an important problem and one that they feel confident to handle (Everett *et al.* 1987). In a similar study from the Netherlands, with a lower response rate, nearly all GPs stated that they would manage imminent miscarriage by themselves (Fleuren *et al.* 1994). Concerning the longer-term consequences, GPs felt that miscarriage is psychologically damaging, that GPs were suitable professionals to counsel the women, and 95% felt that they were themselves competent to do so (Prettyman and Cordle 1992).

Core maternity care

Both antenatal and postnatal care represent areas where the contribution made by GPs is difficult to quantify. Over 90% of GPs provide routine antenatal and postnatal care (General Medical Services Committee 1992). While this represents a clear commitment to the overall package, there are no published accounts that define precisely how much of the work is done by the different groups of professionals. The increasing shift of care away from hospitals in order to make it more accessible does not necessarily represent a shift towards general practice as midwives take on more responsibility for all phases of maternity care. Midwives' anecdotal accounts suggest that there is wide variation in the extent to which GPs delegate their responsibility to midwives for routine care. Some of those who discuss these trends imply that some GPs are only interested in antenatal care for the financial rewards, but such an allegation is impossible to confirm or refute under the current contractual arrangements.

One general practitioner has been responsible for a major trial of altering the schedules of antenatal care (Sikorski *et al.* 1996). Another changed the nature of antenatal clinics by orientating it primarily to education rather than screening (Thorley, personal communication). In postnatal care, there has been some interest in the range of problems experienced by women in the short (Glazener *et al.* 1995) and long term (MacArthur *et al.* 1991). Neither of these accounts discusses the precise contribution made by different health professionals. Up till now such questions seem to have mattered little to the various groups. There may even have been a subconscious wish not to collect those data since the process would have appeared divisive.

Finally, before moving on to the well-documented area of intrapartum care, there are the non-clinical aspects of maternity care to consider. Smith and Jewell (1991*a*) found that that 10–48% of GPs were involved in auditing the care provided by maternity units, 20–60% were involved in perinatal mortality meetings, and 32–52% contributed to deciding their unit's booking policy. The guidance on the constitution of Maternity Service Liaison Committees recommends that each committee has two GP representatives, one each from a fundholding and a non-fundholding practice (Department of Health 1996).

Contribution of GPs to intrapartum care

Information about all births in England and Wales are published by the Office of Population Censuses and Surveys (now Office of National Statistics) annually (OPCS 1994), classified by type of National Health Service hospital as either isolated general practitioner hospital or other NHS hospital. This latter group is not subclassified to general practitioner or consultant unit delivery so the figures do not reveal the total number of births occurring under general practitioner care.

Several papers document the general practitioner obstetrician workload in individual units (Lowe *et al.* 1987; Young 1987; Prentice and Walton 1989; Bryce *et al.* 1990) and even in a group of isolated units (Cavenagh *et al.* 1984), but there had been no published documentation of the intrapartum workload of GPs in all units prior to 1991 when Smith and Jewell (1991*b*) published their national survey of maternity units in England and Wales (Table 4.2). This found that of 611 644 deliveries in 1988 from 277 (93%) of 297 maternity units in England and Wales, 36 043 (5.9%) were under GP care. Units working alongside consultants had significantly more bookings, antenatal transfers, intrapartum transfers, and births compared with isolated units.

Table 4.2 *Median number (per unit/per year) of bookings, transfers, and births in units which women book under sole GP care (n=228; p < 0.001 for all differences)*

Type of unit	No. of bookings	Antenatal transfer	Intrapartum transfer	Births
Isolated	185	18	16	125
Alongside consultant unit	568	69	86	387
Integrated with consultant unit	106	18	18	52

Source: Smith and Jewell (1991*b*).

A number of surveys (Table 4.3) have documented the percentage of GPs providing maternity care, particularly intrapartum care.

About 30% of GPs claim to give women an alternative to consultant care by providing intrapartum care (GMSC 1992), although in some regions up to half may claim to do so (Baker 1992; Smith 1994). A significant minority claim to provide intrapartum care at home (Brown 1994) as well as care in various hospital settings (Smith 1997; Audit Commission 1997). This picture may change in the future as women exercise choice (Campbell and Macfarlane 1994).

There are several cogent reasons for GPs personally attending women in

Table **4.3** *Percentage of GPs claiming to provide intrapartum care in various British surveys*

Date	Range	Respondents (%)	Intrapartum care (Any)	Home (%)	Authors
1983	Northern reg	620/740 (83.8)	25.6	2.0	Marsh (1985)
1990	Avon, Glos, & Somerset	287/324 (88.6)	57.1	33.3	Baker (1992)
1992	SW region of England	333/424 (78.5)	45.2	27.2	Smith (1994)
1992	United Kingdom	25,485/36,478 (70.0)	31.2	nk	GMSC (1992)
1993	Nottingham	530/694 (79.2)	23.3	23.3	Brown (1994)
1995	United Kingdom[b]	439/590 (74.4)	18.6	8.3	Smith (1997)

labour who are booked for delivery under their care. There are no national statistics available on this, nor on the range or number of practical procedures which GPs provide if they do attend. In the past, attempts have been made (Royal College of Obstetricians and Gynaecologists 1982) to set guidelines for GPs providing intrapartum care in terms of the minimum number of deliveries which they must attend annually to allow them to continue to have admitting rights, not to mention the maintenance of clinical skills. Indeed, it has been suggested that falling case-load and the assumed loss of these skills is one reason for the decline in general practitioner intrapartum care (Young 1991). A 1983 northern region survey (Marsh *et al.* 1985) found that 55% of GPs providing intrapartum care attended 10 or more women in labour annually. Thirty-five per cent attended more than 10 annually in a 1992 south western region survey (Smith 1994), but only 3% in a local 1993 survey where there were no GP units (Brown 1994). But the change in the number of general practitioner bookings must also be seen against a background of falling list sizes and smaller families. Bull (1990) found that most GPs in Oxford actually attended their own patients during labour or during delivery (80% and 60% respectively of general practitioner-booked cases), as recommended by the Royal College of Obstetricians and Gynaecologists and the Royal College of General Practitioners (RCOG and RCGP 1981; RCOG 1982). In one practice, 70% of labouring women booked with their GP are attended by their general practitioner (Smith, personal observation).

Finally, attending GPs may need to intervene in a minority of labours. However, the majority perform few practical obstetric procedures for their patients (Smith 1994; Smith 1997) (Table 4.3), much less than used to be the case (Marsh *et al.* 1985*b*). This may be because such women either have normal labours which are appropriately managed by midwives, or those that develop abnormalities are either dealt with by midwives in their extended role (Smith & Jewell 1991*b*) or are transferred to consultant care. In isolated units, procedures such as low forceps deliveries and neonatal resuscitation are still carried out by GPs. Transfers to consultant units may be dictated to GPs by unit policy to which they may have little input (Smith and Jewell 1991*b*).

GPs are now less likely to augment labour with syntocinon (16% in United Kingdom (Smith 1997),17% south western region (Smith 1994), 32% northern region (Marsh *et al.* 1985)), are less likely to perform low forceps (18%, 31%, 63% respectively) or induce labour for post-maturity (20%, 17%, 61%). More recently, Baird *et al.* (1996) found that 5% (25) of labouring women in an isolated GP unit needed a low forceps delivery (one forceps per GP every three years) and another 12% of 462 women had postnatal complications requiring emergency medical support. These included low Apgar score requiring resuscitation (14), post-partum haemorrhage (10), retained placenta (9), shoulder dystocia (1), perinatal death and stillbirth (2). Marsh (1985b) found a higher level of forceps deliveries with 63% of GPs in the northern region prepared to do them and 54 (57%) of 94 actually performing at least one annually.

Various factors have been proposed to explain the reluctance of GPs to be involved in intrapartum care. These factors have included fear of litigation (Cohen 1991; Nesbitt *et al.* 1991; Brown 1994), the high cost of medical insurance premiums (Schmittling and Tsou 1989; Gaskins *et al.* 1991), waning clinical competence (Smith 1991), lack of training (Schmittling and Tsou 1989; Baldwin *et al.* 1991; Reid and Carroll 1991; Smith 1991, 1992; Young 1991;), interference with lifestyle (Cohen 1991; Nesbitt *et al.* 1991; Brown 1994), lack of facilities (Smith and Jewell 1990; Young 1991), medico-political pressure (Social Services Committee 1980; Standing Maternity and Midwifery Advisory Committee 1980; Royal College of Obstetricians and Gynaecologists 1982; Reynolds 1991), practice type (Gaskins *et al.* 1991), small size of community served (Schmittling and Tsou 1989; Gaskins *et al.* 1991; Reid and Carroll 1991), no appropriate role model (Smith and Howard 1987; Reid and Carroll 1991; Reynolds 1991; Smith 1992), lack of time (Nesbitt *et al.* 1991), inadequate remuneration (Cohen 1991; Nesbitt *et al.* 1991; Young 1991), and lack of role definition (Young 1991; Smith 1992). It is not known which of these have most bearing on the declining provision of intrapartum care by GPs, but given the range and number of reasons it is not surprising that there has been a very major reduction.

Two studies (Smith and Reynolds 1995; Smith 1996) have emphasized the importance to GPs both in training and in practice of being involved with intrapartum care. Both found that trainees (now registrars) exposed to the role model of a general practitioner providing intrapartum care are more likely to provide such care eventually as principals. Furthermore, the more women that trainees attend in labour, the more they will attend when they are principals, provided they have a supportive partnership to provide such care. This is not surprising as the decision to provide intrapartum care is usually made by the partnership and not by the individual doctors.

Summary of the evidence

In summary, the present picture of GPs' contribution to maternity care is simultaneously less clear and more inconsistent than one would wish and there is considerable uncertainty about the future. In many areas such as infertility, preconception care, and miscarriage, it appears that the work is increasing. These are also areas where the scope of the work is likely to increase in the future and where other groups, particularly midwives, are not making explicit plans to extend their activities. In the areas of antenatal and postnatal care that have for the last few years represented the bulk of their work with pregnant mothers, GPs seem to be willing and able to maintain this contribution. However, changes in midwives' working patterns together with the move towards more continuity of care, encouraged by *Changing Childbirth* (Department of Health 1993) and other publications, may encourage more midwife involvement and correspondingly less general practitioner involvement in the future. GPs' contribution to intrapartum care has declined to a large extent over a long period of time. Rather than regarding this as odd, we should perhaps wonder that their presence persists at all. The current picture is of a small number of enthusiasts keen to continue this work if at all possible, with a larger number less committed but willing to take on responsibility of attending people in labour if called upon to do so.

Reasons for encouraging GPs' contribution

There are several reasons why GPs should be involved in maternity care. First and foremost, surveys of women's views have consistently reported that they value GPs involvement (Department of Health 1993). In its detailed examination into the working of peripheral maternity units in Essex, the National Childbirth Trust (1995) found that women attending GP surgeries for antenatal care scored them highest for explaining things to them and listening to them.

Second, we believe that there are specific attributes that GPs can bring to maternity care. These are not those skills, such as the ability to suture episiotomies and do instrumental deliveries, that traditionally GPs acquired and midwives did not. Such skills are now learnt by many midwives and there is every reason to expect that both the range of skills and numbers of midwives learning them will continue to expand. Rather they are aspects that are germane to the whole of GPs' work. General practice is 'a form of primary care in which people have a personal, continuing relationship with a doctor'. Thirdly, general practice is concerned with 'the mental and physical health of individuals, usually within the context of their families, as well as the health of the family itself, seen as a unit or as a small community of individuals'. Fourth, general practice provides 'comprehensive, continuing, coordinated, accessible, and accountable care'. GPs frequently bring to maternity care long-term knowledge of their patients. Even if this is absent they bring a commitment to continue caring for the family after the end of formal maternity care. They deal with other medical problems, both arising from pregnancy and pre-existing conditions. They deal with other members of the family whose health affects, and is affected by, the pregnancy and the baby.

Finally, there is the matter of how professionals deal with deviations from normal. Such deviations pose problems both of interpretation and subsequent management. It has been suggested that pregnant women in particular can suffer from a process in which an action on the part of the carers can make abnormality and further intervention more likely – the so-called 'cascade of intervention' (Towler 1985). The problem may partly account for the rising rates of forceps deliveries and Caesarean sections. Another factor in such rates may be a fundamental tendency in many hospital doctors to feel safer themselves when doing something rather than doing nothing. GPs bring to maternity care a perspective on health and disease that is slanted towards normality (Marsh 1982). They also have long experience of handling doubt and uncertainty without intervening. Both of these attributes are particularly appropriate in the management of low-risk pregnancy. There is no direct evidence to support these assertions. However, two studies lend at least circumstantial support. The West Berkshire Study documents a largely successful attempt to transfer the total care of low-risk women in one district to a community unit. The midwives were allowed to refer directly to a specialist when they were concerned. In the event, 58% were originally booked for delivery in the unit but subsequently 49% were transferred to consultant care (Street *et al.* 1991). This rate of transfers is appreciably higher than those reported by many GPs working in the area. The Northern Regional Home Birth Study has reported that women requesting a home birth were more likely to achieve it when the general practitioner was supportive (70%) than when the general practitioner was rated as unsupportive (54%) (Davies *et al.* 1996).

It is easy to forget that general practice can also be seen as an existing resource that makes a cost-effective and clinically effective contribution to maternity care. *Changing Childbirth* (Department of Health 1993) states as one of its cardinal principles that 'Maternity services must be readily and easily accessible to all. They should be sensitive to the needs of the local population and based primarily in the community'. The key roles of the GP within general practice are to: provide accessible care for individual patients and the defined population which they comprise; provide continuity of care (over time, place, and problem); diagnose and care for both disease and illness, managing them in context; prevent illness and disease and promote health; sort patients' ill-defined problems; coordinate care; and manage resources (Smith 1996). Taken individually they are not unique to general practice, but as a whole they are a unique set of characteristics which make general practice particularly suited for the provision of routine maternity care.

Specific reasons have been postulated for the continued involvement in intrapartum care in particular (Marsh 1982). These are that the GP will provide continuity, confirm normality with the midwife, deal with minor problems, take responsibility for specialist referral, support relatives (who are likely also to be patients at some time), encourage and assess parental bonding, provide skilled hands in an emergency, and because the GP enjoys it. Such involvement with birth is a privilege with few parallels in modern general practice.

Finally, most GPs wish to provide antenatal and postnatal care and a significant minority wish also to provide intrapartum care (GMSC 1992; Brown 1994; Smith 1997). Brown's survey of Nottinghamshire GPs has been widely reported as demonstrating that a majority (66%) were unwilling to offer intrapartum care to their patients. However, it is striking in the current climate to consider the remainder: 11% had no opinion on this question, and 23% stated that they would like to be able to offer more intrapartum care (Brown 1994).

To provide high-quality maternity care GPs will need to be adequately trained and updated (see Chapter 10), adequately remunerated, and have sufficient contractual flexibility to do so. For the foreseeable future there should remain a small minority of GPs (20–30%) who wish nominally to provide intrapartum care whilst the vast majority will wish to remain involved in antenatal and postnatal care. Neither of these groups will need special training over and above the usual three-year vocational training for general practice. Of the 20–30% providing care in labour, about a third are likely to wish to have a different training so that they can provide practical intrapartum support to women delivering under their care in hospital. All GPs providing maternity care will need to work principally with community midwives (the primary maternity care team) (Royal College of General Practitioners 1995) and thus provide care for the majority of women who will have uncomplicated pregnancies. Occasionally this team will need to be supplemented, either temporarily or permanently, when complications arise. For example, a woman may require an amniocentesis following a serum screening test for Down's syndrome; if negative, she can then return to the care of the primary maternity care team. Permanent enlargement of the team would arise in a woman with pre-existing diabetes mellitus who would need specialist nurse and medical input, even starting before conception.

The future

For some years most GPs have been able to maintain their contact with maternity care without having to attend women in labour. Two important questions loom large when considering the future, and it is impossible to give confident questions to either. First, can this continue? A major direction in current policy is to improve continuity of care. Until recently, GPs were the only group providing any degree of continuity and they could justify their contribution by this yardstick alone. However, with midwives making a substantial effort to provide such continuity, this aspect of GPs' contribution becomes relatively less valuable.

Another major policy is to provide the type of maternity care that women want – GPs can continue to do this personally. In addition, as purchasers they have to be able to justify their care and to decide from where, how much, and what type of maternity care to contract. Some GPs will not wish to provide maternity care and there will be a need to retrain and to reorganize midwives to replace them completely for the provision of low-risk, community-based care. GPs who wish to continue to provide, or perhaps enlarge their role in, maternity care will need to convince health authorities and their colleagues that they have something to offer that women want which is consistent with the indicators of success of the *Changing Childbirth* report. The introduction of practice-based contracts will raise further awareness of this debate. Alternatively, GPs may refuse to change and gradually, perhaps even quickly, be excluded from any maternity care.

The second question is: does it matter? Does maternity care represent one bead on a string that can drop off with nobody noticing, or is it the keystone in the arch of primary care whose fall brings the whole structure tumbling down? To us, comprehensive and continuing care for patients and their families becomes meaningless without maternity care. The change would represent a great loss to the discipline of general practice. We would even argue that contractual arrangements in the United Kingdom should recognize this by making maternity care part of general medical services. More importantly, if GPs become excluded from all maternity care then women will lose out. Their choice of maternity care and carer will reduce and their care will become more fragmented through the loss of skilled generalists. They will also lose the advocacy of a group of professionals who provide them with the great majority of their personal medical care throughout their lives. GPs, in turn, will lose any opportunity to influence policy in maternity care.

Maternity care in the United Kingdom has recently been saved from becoming a completely hospital-based, high-tech activity. It was the persistence of an alternative model set in the community and based on a dwindling number of home deliveries that made possible the re-examination of policy in the last 10 years, culminating in *Changing Childbirth* and the changes that have followed. The idea that one of these changes would eventually be the exclusion of GPs from all maternity care would, we believe, be a major loss for all the interested parties.

References

Audit Commission (1997). First-class delivery. Improving maternity services in England and Wales. Audit Commision, London.

Baird, A. G., Jewell, D., and Walker, J. J. (1996). Management of labour in an isolated rural maternity hospital. *British Medical Journal*, **312**, 223–6.

Baker, R. (1992). General practice in Gloucestershire, Avon, and Somerset: explaining variations in standards. *British Journal of General Practice*, **42**, 415–18.

Baldwin, L., Hart, G., and Rosenblatt, R. A. (1991). Differences in the obstetric practices of obstetricians and family physicians in Washington state. *Journal of Family Practice*, **32**, 295–9.

Brown, D. J. (1994). Opinions of GPs in Nottinghamshire about provision of intrapartum care. *British Medical Journal*, **309**, 777–9.

Bryce, F. C., Clayton, J. K., Rand, R. J., Beck, I., Farquharson, D. I. M., and Jones, S. E. (1990). General practitioner obstetrics in Bradford. *British Medical Journal*, **300**, 725–7.

Bull, M. J. V. (1990). General practice obstetrics in Bradford [letter]. *British Medical Journal*; 300: 873–4.

Campbell, R, and Macfarlane ,A. (1994). *Where to be born? The debate and the evidence.* (2nd edn).National Perinatal Epidemiology Unit, Oxford.

Canadian Medical Association (1987). Obstetrics '87. A report of the Canadian Medical Association on obstetrical care in Canada. *Canadian Medical Association Journal*, **March 15th** (Suppl.).

Cavenagh, A. J. M., Phillips, K. M., Sheridan, B., and Williams, E. M. J. (1984). Contribution of isolated general practitioner maternity units. *British Medical Journal*, **288**, 1438–40.

Cohen, L. (1991). Looming manpower shortage has Canada's obstetricians worried. *Canadian Medical Association Journal*. **144**. 478–9.

Davies, J., Hey, E., Reid, W., and Young, G. (1996). Prospective regional study of planned home birth. *British Medical Journal*, **313**, 1302–6.

Department of Health (1993). Changing childbirth: report of the Expert Maternity Group. HMSO, London.

Department of Health (1996). *Maternity service liaison committees.* HMSO, London.

Everett, C., Ashurst, H., and Chalmers, I.. (1987). Reported management of threatened miscarriage by GPs in Wessex. *British Medical Journal*, **295**, 583–6.

Fleuren, M., Grol, R., De Haan, M., and Wijkel, D. (1994). Care for the imminent miscarriage by midwives and GPs. *Family Practice*, **11**, 275–81.

Gaskins, S. E., Tietze, P. E., and Cole, C. M. (1991). Obstetric practice patterns among family practice residency graduates. *Southern Medical Journal*, **84**, 947–52.

General Medical Services Committee Report (1992). British Medical Association, London.

Glazener, C. M. A., Abdalla, M., Stroud, P., Naji, S., Templeton, A., and Russell, I. T. (1995). Postnatal maternal morbidity: extent, causes, prevention, and treatment. *British Journal of Obstetrics and Gynaecology*,102, 282–7.

Hingstman, L. and Boon, H. (1988). Obstetric care in the Netherlands: regional differentiation in home delivery. *Social Science and Medicine*, **26**, 71–8.

Lowe, S. W., House, W., and Garrett, T. (1987). Comparison of outcome of low-risk labour in an isolated general practitioner maternity unit and a specialist maternity hospital. *Journal of the Royal College of General Practitioners*, **37**, 484–7.

MacArthur, C., Lewis, M., and Knox, E. G. (1991). *Health after childbirth.* HMSO, University of Birmingham.

Marsh, G. N. (1982). The 'specialty' of general practitioner obstetrics. *Lancet*, 1, 669–72.

Marsh, G. N. (1985). *Modern obstetrics in general practice*. Oxford University Press, Oxford.

Marsh, G. N., Cashman, H. A., and Russell, I. T. (1985*a*). General practitioner obstetrics in the northern region in 1983. *British Medical Journal*, **290**, 901–3.

Marsh, G. N., Cashman, H. A., and Russell, I. T. (1985*b*). General practitioner participation in intranatal care in the northern region in 1983. *British Medical Journal*, **290**, 971–3.

National Childbirth Trust (1995). Birth choices. Women's expectations and experiences. NCT, London.

Nesbitt, T. S., Tanji, J. L., Schercer, J. E., and Kahn, N. B. (1991). Obstetric care, Medicaid, and family physicians. How policy changes affect physicians' attitudes. *Western Journal of Medicine*, **155**, 653–7.

Office of Population Censuses and Surveys (1994). *Birth statistics*. HMSO, London.

Office of Population Censuses and Surveys (1995). Morbidity statistics from general practice. Fourth national study 1991–1992. HMSO, London.

Prentice, A and Walton, S. M. (1989). Outcome of pregnancies referred to a general practitioner unit in a district general hospital. *British Medical Journal*, **299**, 1090–2.

Prettyman, R. J. and Cordle, C. (1992). Psychological aspects of miscarriage: attitudes of the primary health care team. *British Journal of General Practice*, **42**, 97–9.

Registrar General (1929). *Statistical review for 1927*. HMSO, London.

Reid, A. J. and Carroll, J. C. (1991). Choosing to practise obstetrics – what factors influence family physician residents. *Canadian Family Physician*, **37**, 1859–67.

Reynolds, J. L. (1991). Family practice obstetrics in a teaching hospital – developing a role. *Canadian Family Physician*, **37**, 1121–4.

Royal College of General Practitioners (1995). *The role of general practice in maternity care*. Occasional paper 72. RCGP, London.

Royal College of Obstetricians and Gynaecologists (1982). *Report on the Royal College of Obstetricians' working party on antenatal and intrapartum care*. RCOG, London.

Royal College of Obstetricians and Gynaecologists and the Population Investigation Committee (1948). *Maternity in Great Britain*. Oxford University Press, Oxford.

Royal College of Obstetricians and Gynaecologists and Royal College of General Practitioners (1981). *Report on training for obstetrics and gynaecology for general practice: a joint working party*. RCOG and RCGP, London.

Schmittling, G. and Tsou, C. (1989). Obstetric privileges for family physicians: a national study. *Journal of Family Practice*, **29**, 179–84.

Sikorski, J., Wilson, J., Clement, C., Das, S., and Smeeton, N. (1996). A randomized controlled trial comparing two schedules of antenatal visits: the antenatal care project. *British Medical Journal*, **312**, 546–53.

Smith, L. F. P. (1991). GP trainees' views on hospital obstetric vocational training. *British Medical Journal*, **303**, 1447–52.

Smith, L. F. P. (1992). Roles, risks, and responsibilities in maternity care: trainees' beliefs and the effects of practice obstetric training. *British Medical Journal*, **304**, 1613–15.

Smith, L. F. P. (1994). Provision of obstetric care by GPs in the south western region of England. *British Journal of General Practice*, **44**, 255–8.

Smith, L. F. P. (1996). Should general practitioners have any role in maternity care in the future? *British Journal Of General Practice*, **46**, 243–7.

Smith, L. F. P. (1997). Predictors of the provision of intrapartum care by general practitioners: a five-year cohort study. *British Journal of General Practice*, **47**, 627–30.

Smith, M. A. and Howard, K. P. (1987). Choosing to do obstetrics in practice: factors affecting the decisions of third-year family practice residents. *Family Medicine*, **19**, 191–4.

Smith, L. F. P. and Jewell, D. (1991*a*). Roles of midwives and GPs in hospital intrapartum care, England and Wales, 1988. *British Medical Journal*, **303**, 1443–4.

Smith, L. F. P. and Jewell, D. (1991*b*). Contribution of GPs to hospital intrapartum care in maternity units in England and Wales in 1988. *British Medical Journal*, **302**, 13–16.

Smith, L. F. P. and Reynolds, J. L. (1995). Factors associated with the decision of family physicians to provide intrapartum care. *Canadian Medical Association Journal*, **152**, 1189–97.

Social Services Committee (Chairman: Renee Short) (1980). Perinatal and neonatal mortality. Second report from the Social Services Committee, session 1979–80, Vol. 1. HMSO, London.

Standing Maternity and Midwifery Advisory Committee (Chairman: Sir John Peel) (1980). *Domiciliary midwifery and maternity bed needs*. HMSO, London.

Street, P., Gannon, M. J., and Holy, E. M. (1991). Community obstetric care in West Berkshire. *British Medical Journal*, **302**, 698–700.

Templeton, A., Fraser, C., and Thompson, B. (1990). The epidemiology of infertility in Aberdeen. *British Medical Journal*, **301**, 148–52.

Towler, J. (1985). In: *Modern obstetrics in general practice* (ed. G. N. Marsh). Oxford University Press, Oxford.

Treffers, P. E., Eskes, M., Kleiverda, G., and van Altenn, D. (1990). Home births and minimal medical intervention. *Journal of the American Medical Association*, **264**, 2203–8.

Wilkes, S. and Jones, K. (1995). Retrospective review of the prevalence and management of infertility in women in one practice over a five-year period. *British Journal of General Practice*, **45**, 75–7.

Young, G. (1987). Are isolated maternity units run by GPs dangerous? *British Medical Journal*, **294**, 744–6.

Young, G. L. (1991). General practice and the future of obstetric care. *British Journal of General Practice*, **41**, 266–7.

CHAPTER FIVE

Multidisciplinary teamwork in maternity care

Anthony Dowell and Helene Price

'We trained hard, but every time we were beginning to form up in teams, we would be reorganized. I was to learn later in life that we tend to meet any new situation by reorganizing, and a wonderful method it can be for creating an illusion of progress while producing confusion, inefficiency, and demoralization.'

(Petronius Arbiter AD 65)

' . . . a team is a group of people who make different contributions towards the achievement of a common goal.'

(Pritchard 1981)

Introduction

The current provision and outcomes of community-based maternity care demonstrate how effectively multidisciplinary teams of health professionals can work together. Collaboration and teamworking between midwives, GPs, obstetricians, health visitors, paediatricians, and public health professionals has provided a framework of care which has witnessed significant reductions in obstetric and perinatal morbidity and mortality over the last 30 years.

GPs and midwives as two independent professional groups have defined appropriate roles and responsibilities to suit a variety of different local working situations. Effective methods of teamworking between primary and secondary care have been devised; the use of patient-held antenatal cooperation cards are a good example.

While there are many examples of good practice there remain many challenges for primary care if effective teamwork is to become standard clinical practice. The increasing autonomy of midwifery has alienated some GPs who feel that their role in maternity care is threatened. GP fundholding and commissioning seemed to many midwives to concentrate decision-making and financial control in the hands of those with little practical obstetric and maternity care expertise. There is also continuing debate as to the most appropriate composition and configuration of community maternity care teams, and their relationship with hospital colleagues. Moreover, the move to patient-centred care, exemplified in maternity care by *Changing Childbirth* (Department of Health 1993), offers potentially new and more radical definitions of a primary care team.

This chapter outlines the development of multidisciplinary teamworking and highlights current challenges and opportunities.

Any description of teamworking in primary care is likely to lead to potential confusion in terminology. Our use of 'primary health care team' (PHCT) refers to the individuals who work together to provide care for a particular group of individuals, usually the patients registered with a general practice or practices. The 'maternity team' is the subgroup of the PHCT who provide maternity care. The team can work in a variety of different ways and with more or less integration. 'Team' midwifery refers to a much more specific situation where a number of midwives provide a rota of care for an identified case-load of women.

The development of the multidisciplinary maternity team

Women have supported each other during pregnancy and childbirth in all cultures for many thousands of years. In the United Kingdom, community nursing and midwifery services developed in the 18th and 19th centuries from the work of informal carers, religious orders, and charitable groups. By Victorian times, midwives were utilized largely by poorer communities. They charged less than a quarter of a doctor's fee, would deliver the woman at home, and often remain with the family for up to 10 days after delivery. Their skills were dependent on their past experiences and observations of others and not on any formal training.

The role of the GP first developed following divisions and differences of opinion between physicians, apothecaries, and surgeons in the 17th century. As apothecaries began to treat larger numbers of generally poorer patients, a tradition of local service to local communities developed which has remained characteristic of the work of the GP until today. By the beginning of this century the role of the GP as a non-specialist, yet fully trained and working outside hospital, had become established.

Even after the development of formal nursing and midwifery organizations, considerable distance remained between the practices of medicine, nursing, and midwifery as each group pursued their own interests and doctors retained their position at the head of a disease-based health system. Until the 1960s health professionals in the community worked independently of each other. Informal collaboration might exist, for example between GPs and the local midwife, but there was no attempt to coordinate professional roles and skills. The GP often worked from a surgery built onto his/her own home and routinely provided antenatal and intrapartum maternity care.

Following the changes introduced by the 1968 charter for general practice, a number of developments occurred, leading the way to the present patterns of multidisciplinary working (Marsh and Kaim-Caudle 1976). Firstly, doctors began to employ more nursing and other staff within their own premises. Secondly, health authorities began to build health centres which housed complete teams of health professionals on the same site, including GPs. Thirdly, as workload and patient expectations began to rise there was a need to develop more efficient ways of delivering integrated care.

The present situation

The great majority of pregnant women are cared for by a multidisciplinary team of health professionals working in a variety of different ways. This care is usually shared with midwives and obstetricians in hospital.

A number of recent events have had a major impact on the composition and dynamics of the primary care team. These include:

General practice fundholding

The 1990 contract for GPs saw the advent of fundholding with, in theory, GPs having much greater autonomy and accountability for the way services were provided in primary care. Although fundholding has been abandoned since the election of the Labour government in 1997, to be replaced by commissioning groups, it had an effect while it was in place. Although for most practices maternity care was exempt from fundholding, the overall culture within general practice was for services to be determined by GPs rather than, say, midwives. This ran counter to previous trends developing primary care on locality lines, such as those recommended by the Cumberledge report for community nursing (Department of Health and Social Security 1986).

Reduction in GP provision of maternity care

There is a trend for decreasing involvement of GPs in both antenatal and intrapartum care (see Chapter 4). This is the result of several influences, including the increasing autonomy of midwives (Chapter 3), an overall reduction in the amount of contact between patient and health professionals in the antenatal period, and a reduction in the continuity of care provided by GPs.

Changing patterns of care

During the 1970s and 1980s a number of changes were implemented in the organization of maternity care in an attempt to improve the service provided to women. Foremost among these was an overall reduction in the number and pattern of antenatal visits and the transfer of care into a community setting. This provided a real impetus for community and hospital staff to work together, producing modification to traditional 'shared care'. This approach resulted in improved accessibility and an update of services with no deterioration in pregnancy outcomes for either mother or baby (Wood 1991). The number of antenatal visits has been halved to between six or seven contacts in some instances (Chapter 19). In many places midwives are now playing a much more central role in the delivery of all care.

Changing Childbirth

The rationale for the agenda developed in *Changing Childbirth* was the finding by the expert maternity group that while some services were designed to meet local needs, others were designed to meet those of professionals rather than service users (Department of Health 1993). The aim of all the recommendations was to ensure that the woman is placed at the centre of choices regarding maternity care. Maternity care is intended to be accessible, appropriate, effective, and efficient. Women should be active partners in decisions about their care. Health professionals have to play a supportive and informative role (Chapter 2). Any changes in the composition or working of maternity teams have to be viewed in the light of these criteria.

Direct implications for teamworking so far have involved arrangements to provide greater choice of place of birth and a clearly identified 'lead professional' who will provide a substantial part of the care personally.

What do women and health professionals want?

Much of the impetus for recent changes has come from the knowledge that in many instances the care provided by teams was fragmented, reduplicated, and lacking in continuity. A National Childbirth Trust study of women in Essex (Gready 1995) highlighted the importance of continuity of care, showing that those women experiencing continuity in the antenatal period were more likely to feel involved in decision-making. Knowing the midwife well was valued at all stages of the pregnancy. There was concern at the conflicting advice offered by different professionals in the team and some women were unaware of choices and options open to them.

Three quarters of women questioned in the Essex study felt that GPs, midwives, and hospital doctors were working well together. Women valued the contribution of different professionals. In another study, women preferred a combination of the GP and midwife together and most women wanted GP involvement (Dowswell *et al.* 1994).

Obstetricians have demonstrated a wish to move towards a more multidisciplinary approach to care (Cheyne 1995) and despite recent trends towards decreased GP involvement in maternity work many wish to maintain a role as part of a community based team (Smith 1996).

Effective multidisciplinary teams in primary care

These trends have resulted in a number of different models of primary care teamworking in maternity care. This variation in team membership and function has allowed flexibility in adapting teams to different working conditions. The composition and team dynamics required to deliver effective care in an inner-city practice performing no home births will be different to that for a rural practice with its own cottage hospital.

Much has been written about the successes and failures of different models of primary care teamwork, though there is little research evidence to define best practice in any setting, particularly with regard to maternity care.

An effective multidisciplinary team in primary maternity care would have the following characteristics:

- the team will establish common objectives for the provision of care. The objectives will be accepted and understood by all members of the team

- each member of the team will have a clear understanding of her/his role, function, and responsibilities

- there will be satisfactory organization and communication systems so that optimal cooperation and communication between team members is achieved

- there is a mutual respect for the role and skill of each team member, allied to a flexible approach

- there will be a mutlidisciplinary involvement in teaching, learning, and audit (Gilmore *et al.* 1974).

These characteristics were found to be lacking in primary care in reports outlined in 1981 and 1986 (Department of Health and Social Security 1981, 1986).

Over the last 10 years there has been substantial literature to promote the advantages of teamwork (Gregson *et al.* 1991; Marsh 1991; Waine 1992) even though some research has indicated that teamwork is a contentious issue for nurses and midwives in primary care (Ovretveit 1990; Pearson 1992). A number of training initiatives have taken place with the aim of developing the effectiveness of primary care teams (Lambert *et al.* 1991). These have shown, for example, that teambuilding workshops can enhance communication, teamwork, and practice organization (Spratley 1989) though research is still needed to show whether such methods can improve overall team effectiveness.

How does the primary health care team perceive itself?

The attitudes, views, and experiences of various members of existing community maternity care teams can help to provide the context for assessment of current provision and future patterns of care. Differing views about teamworking will be held by the various members of the maternity care team. A study by Wiles and Robinson (1994), in which nurses and midwives were interviewed, identified a number of issues as important for teamworking which are summarized here:

Team identity

Forty per cent of midwives in the study did not feel they were part of a primary health care team. The different way in which many midwives worked in comparison to the rest of the team accounted for less of a team identity. Midwives who worked for example in midwifery teams had more identity with each other than the rest of the PHCT. There was often relatively little contact with the rest of the team. This was marked if and when midwives held most of their clinics in hospital rather than in a general practice. But even in a practice setting where midwife-only clinics sometimes operated and where the GP was only consulted if there was a problem, contacts could be infrequent.

Philosophy of care

Midwives identified potential conflict with GPs regarding philosophies of care. Their knowledge base and approach were felt to be different to that of the GP. They felt that GPs did not spend enough time with patients, treated pregnancy as an illness, and prescribed too frequently.

Roles and responsibilities

The potential for disagreement exists between midwives, health visitors, and GPs as to the most appropriate allocation of roles and responsibilities. Midwives and health visitors may disagree over roles with new parents and preventive work with families. Midwives may feel that GPs may be reluctant to allow them to take appropriate responsibility for patients. While acknowledging the importance of teamwork, GPs continue to promote their involvement at all stages of pregnancy and the puerperium. The rationale for this is the GP's role as provider of personal continuing and comprehensive medical care to individuals and families (Royal College of General Practitioners 1995) (Chapters 2 and 4).

Models and patterns of maternity care teamwork

For the provision of community-based maternity care, the main professionals who form the team are the midwife, the GP, and the health visitor. To this 'primary maternity care team' (Royal College of General Practitioners 1995) will be added the obstetrician for high-risk pregnancies. The pregnant woman and her baby should also now be included as partners in the maternity care team, the perspective of *Changing Childbirth* having placed them at the centre of decision-making.

The model shown in Box 5.1 represents the present most common method of multidisciplinary teamworking within the community. As with all models of teamwork there are different advantages and disadvantages apparent in different settings.

Alternative models of teamwork can be devised. Team midwifery and case-load midwifery are now fairly common, for example. The balance of benefits and difficulties may be different, as shown in Box 5.2.

Box 5.1 *Difficulties and benefits of shared care*

Difficulties

- Demarcation and boundary issues
- Reduplication and fragmentation of care
- Probably not cost-effective
- Anonymity

Benefits

- Women appreciate the multidisciplinary approach
- Continuity of care by the same group of care-givers during both low and high-risk pregnancies
- Shared responsibility
- Detection and management of illness when necessary and appropriate

---

Box 5.2 *Difficulties and benefits of team or case-load midwifery*

Difficulties

- Possible exclusion of other primary health care team members
- Possible difficulties with working rotas
- Too narrow a focus

Benefits

- Continuity of care and carer
- Good communication within the midwifery team
- Reduction in conflicting advice to women and their families

---

The multidisciplinary team should also examine its effectiveness in terms of local purchasing and financial arrangements. Whilst most maternity team care is still purchased at health authority level, fundholding and the development of private, independent midwifery services may produce considerable changes in teamworking and outcome (Box 5.3).

Although there are few examples of GP fundholders purchasing maternity care so far, it is likely that this model or a local commissioning equivalent will become more widespread. There is also the possibility of women increasingly choosing to purchase the services of independent midwives, working either alone or in teams (Box 5.4).

The degree of involvement of team members can vary within each model. Thus within the traditional models of shared care the involvement of the GP may vary from little or no antenatal contact and a single postnatal visit to regular antenatal and intrapartum care with close postnatal monitoring. Models are also not mutually exclusive. Midwives working in midwifery teams can work alongside the GP and health visitor, or can develop to virtually midwife-only led care.

Box 5.3 *Difficulties and benefits of GP fundholder-led purchasing of maternity care*

Difficulties

- Potential friction as financial control given to only one of two groups of independent arrangements
- Unclear whether fundholding leads to better health care or cost savings

Benefits

- Local financial accountability
- Integration with other funding practitioners
- Local and rapid innovation possible

Box 5.4 *Difficulties and benefits of independent midwifery care*

Difficulties

- Integration with primary health care team
- Accountability and medico-legal issues
- Too narrow a focus

Benefits

- High commitment to patient choice and satisfaction
- Continuity and personal care

Assessing the evidence for the effectiveness of different types of teamworking

Many of the evaluations of different models of multidisciplinary teamworking identify various criteria for team effectiveness. Some of these are:

- continuity of care and care-giver
- acceptability of the care-giver to the woman
- assessment of risk and outcomes in relation to previously accepted standards of care.

A number of issues and questions can provide a framework within which members of local teams can discuss and debate their most appropriate roles. Some of these are outlined here.

Which women are 'suitable' for community care?

Two of the key indicators of success in *Changing Childbirth* (Department of Health 1993) are that the woman should be able to choose the person providing the majority of her care, and that in 30% of cases it should be the midwife who provides this care and assists the woman in labour. It is important that the woman can make an informed choice about the

67

multidisciplinary team most appropriate to her needs. Following an assessment of risk status, the outcomes of different methods of multi-disciplinary teamworking can be evaluated.

The proportion of women with no identifiable risk factors for pregnancy and the puerperium and hence suitable for total community care is just under 50% (MacVicar *et al.* 1993; Kean *et al.* 1996). Almost a quarter of women who are identified as low risk from such studies encounter problems in pregnancy, requiring a change in risk status. These studies use strict criteria which may be relaxed in the light of further experience. From a large study of 4500 women (Kean *et al.* 1996), of those arriving in spontaneous labour after a problem-free pregnancy, a half of nulliparaous and over three quarters of women having their second babies progressed through labour without complications. Other studies have repeated the findings that midwife-managed care in these circumstances is as safe during labour as standard consultant-led care and is a more effective option for women at low risk (Hundley *et al.* 1994). It is thus possible to provide low-risk women with a lead professional who is community based (in these cases the midwife) and who could provide continuity of care throughout the pregnancy and during labour.

However, in the above study nearly 70% of nulliparaous women considered to be low risk at booking required hospital advice or care at some point during labour. Providing a more community-based and multidisciplinary focus will not necessarily lead to significant reductions in hospital services' workload.

What is the most effective type of team?

There are several elements in this question. Firstly, how do any or all of the various configurations now available compare with previously accepted hospital-led shared care, and how do they compare with each other? This section will examine midwife-led care and team midwifery, GP-led care and GP involvement in care, and continuing obstetric involvement.

Midwife-led care

The midwife is now perceived as holding the pivotal position within the community maternity care team. With direct access to maternity beds and the impetus of *Changing Childbirth*, new styles of relationships with fellow professionals have begun and will need to develop.

Team midwifery

The difficulty of providing continuity of carer has exercised much thought within maternity care. Traditional shared-care schemes commonly left women not knowing midwifery staff during labour. One response to this has been the development of midwifery teams, with a number of midwives providing a rota of care for a named case-load of women. An early example of this in London, the 'Know Your Midwife' scheme (Flint 1993), demonstrated in a randomized controlled trial advantages to the team system. In this scheme which studied only low-risk pregnancies, women saw fewer different care-givers and were more satisfied with antenatal care. Although in the team group women had a longer first stage of labour, they required less analgesia and had a higher chance of normal delivery.

This approach has been developed in many other sites, one recent example being the reorganization of Scunthorpe and Goole maternity services (Outram 1995). Nine community-based teams have been introduced across the district, with five to seven midwives having case-loads of between 200 and 300 women. In the pilot project the team worked alongside GPs and this has been extended to the full scheme. This project has not been evaluated. Advantages of team midwifery have been said, however, to result from this scheme, including, for women: personalization of the service, continuity of care and carers, less conflicting advice, labour assessment and care in the first stage conducted at home, reduced unnecessary hospital admissions and length of stay. Advantages for midwives are said to include: increased job satisfaction, confidence and experience, flexible working patterns, improved communication in teams.

The health authority has noted reduced bed occupancy and more evenly distributed workloads. Although disadvantages such as long working hours were noted by the midwives, they would prefer not to return to previous ways of working. Team midwifery also provided the opportunity to develop innovations and skills, such as participating in education in schools and 'grandparent' sessions.

The trend towards team midwifery has been criticized by some (Smith 1996) who cite evidence that teams sometime fail to provide good continuity of care. Recent evaluations (Garcia *et al.* 1996; Green *et al.* 1998) have not demonstrated marked advantages of continuity of carer when compared to systems which offer continuity of care.

Midwife care compared with shared care

Many studies have assessed the effectiveness of midwife-led care compared with other models. One analysis (Renfrew 1994) looked at the results of three different studies and showed no differences in induction of labour, dissatisfaction with care, or other adverse events. There were positive psychological and social outcomes in pregnancy, labour, and postnatally, and reductions in clinic waiting times.

The general practitioner in a multidisciplinary team

The GP has traditionally played a major role in maternity care, though for reasons previously listed this role is diminishing, particularly during labour.

Ninety per cent of GPs have some input into antenatal and postnatal care, and 31% claim to provide labour care, although only 10–15% participate in labour in any meaningful way (General Medical Services Committee 1992; Brown 1994). The majority of GPs, therefore, now provide little labour care and minimal postnatal care, apart from baby checks and the six-week check (Smith 1996). There are strong arguments which provide a logical rationale for GP involvement in all aspects of maternity care (Royal College of General

Practitioners 1995; Smith 1996) (Chapter 4), though there are relatively few evaluations of the GP role in maternity care other than for intrapartum care. There is evidence that women value and welcome the contributions that GPs make to all stages of pregnancy.

A major and continuing role for the GP is that of the clinician responsible for the management of intercurrent illness during pregnancy.

Preconceptional and early antenatal care

The GP is well placed to promote preconception care during both routine consultations and as part of health promotion. With intimate and long-term knowledge of patients, the GP may be the most appropriate person to give counselling and advice regarding the implications of previous pregnancies, issues surrounding genetic screening, and choice of care team and place of delivery. GPs have been shown to have some impact on changing patient behaviours with regard to smoking, alcohol intake, diet, and exercise, and though this effect is limited, it may be that pregnancy is a time when women are receptive to change.

Antenatal care

GPs are appropriately placed to provide efficient and cost-effective antenatal care by providing organizational support and services to the maternity care team or by being active in that team to a greater or lesser extent. There is thus a case for the GP as generalist to be an integral part of the antenatal team and play a leading role in the medical aspects of care. Common problems of pregnancy, intercurrent illness (Chapter 20), and long-standing medical conditions such as diabetes or epilepsy can affect the outcome of pregnancy, and benefit from early medical intervention.

Intrapartum care

The GP's role in intrapartum care has been the subject of much debate and there is some evidence around which to discuss its appropriateness (Chapter 4).

Postnatal care

The time after birth can provide a valuable opportunity to review the events of childbirth and coordinate the primary care support appropriate for the woman and her new baby. Key aspects of this care are the encouragement and maintenance of breastfeeding, the detection and management of postnatal mental health problems, and family planning. The GP is in a good position to play a key role after birth and provide continuity of care as the involvement of the midwife decreases.

In summary, there is some evidence to show that enthusiastic and skilled GPs can play an effective role in all aspects of maternity care, and work as a member within a variety of care teams. Given other options now available to women, it is harder to demonstrate that GPs always have a central or essential role in maternity care teams.

The role of the obstetrician in the multidisciplinary team

The role of the obstetrician in normal pregnancy has recently been the subject of active debate (Walker 1995). Some are unhappy that obstetricians should be exposed only to abnormal pregnancy without continuing experience of the full range of physiological and pathological patterns of pregnancy and labour. They feel it is also reassuring to women to have a prior meeting with the hospital obstetric team if complications arise and intervention is necessary.

Counter views cite evidence which shows some differences in the outcome of normal pregnancies between those seen by an obstetrician compared with those who were not. Although length of labour was longer in GP units, women received less fetal monitoring, pethidine epidurals, and interventions (Klein *et al.* 1983). Moreover, studies have shown that women with normal pregnancies do not wish to see an obstetrician. It seems likely that the trend will continue of less frequent contact with hospital obstetric teams for women undergoing normal pregnancy. Many obstetricians acknowledge the necessity for a change to traditional styles of working and the need for a more multidisciplinary approach (Cheyne *et al.* 1995).

There is clear evidence that there is little or no benefit to 'low-risk' women from routine hospital specialist input, and in general women seem more satisfied with care which involves the minimum of hospital visits (Chapter 19). Although economic analyses in this area are open to a range of interpretations (Chapter 8), it seems likely that in some instances community-based GP/midwife care will 'cost less' to both women and the health service. It seems likely, therefore, that in the future women will be referred for specialist care when and where appropriate, at defined visits rather than as part of routine practice.

The role of the health visitor

The traditional role of the health visitor in maternity care has been to fulfil the statutory obligation of visiting all newborn babies after birth. As the midwife ended her role in the immediate puerperium, so the health visitor concentrated on issues such as infant feeding and immunization schedules. Over the last few years the health visitor role in general has been subject to much debate and reappraisal.

It has been recognized that many aspects of health visitors' skills and training were being underutilized. In an effective primary care team, the health visitor may be the most appropriate person to monitor the health of families either individually or in groups. They can be an influence in the preconceptional period, giving advice to individuals and groups about beneficial changes in lifestyle and the adoption of particular measures such as folate supplementation. The health visitor should be able to identify individuals and groups of women who are most at risk during pregnancy and the postnatal period.

A challenging test of good working relationships comes perhaps after birth. There should be close communication between the health visitor and the

71

midwife to ensure an effective transition of responsibilities. There is no clear evidence as to which is the most appropriate time for that transition to occur since there are proponents of both early health visitor involvement and a continuation of the midwife role later into the puerperium.

A further important shift in the health visitor role has been a more selective targeting of those individuals and families most at risk and a move away from visiting all women and their babies for a fixed number of contacts.

Medical or obstetric complications

The presence of medical or obstetric complications in a pregnancy can have significant implications for the pregnant woman as well as for the maternity care team. There may be differences of opinion among team members over the decision to involve hospital staff, with potential complications in effective communication within the team. The involvement of obstetricians or other consultants potentially complicates communication and 'loyalties' among team members. There may be an abrogation of responsibility by the community team or a 'collusion of anonymity', leaving the woman unsure who is providing which elements of care.

The use of cooperation cards and shared records together with the growth of specialist outreach clinics has improved the overall situation a great deal, and in many instances the addition of obstetrician or hospital consultant to the team provides a boost of reassurance to both the pregnant woman and health professionals.

Teams for 'special needs'

The composition and functioning of the maternity care team should adapt to accommodate the special needs of particular individuals or groups of women. Additional 'specialists' may be required and the lead professional may change or the priorities and roles of team members may differ from usual. Chapter 12 discusses in some detail the care of women with special problems, including homeless women, women with social problems, and women using non-prescription drugs and /or overusing alcohol. This is an opportunity in such instances for the care team to involve appropriate experts or specialists. Social workers, community psychiatrists, nurses, counsellors, and drug abuse nurses can all be included. Indeed, such professionals are found increasingly as permanent members of fully developed primary health care teams (Marsh 1991). Although working with women in these difficult situations presents many challenges, there can be few greater and ultimately more rewarding opportunities for communication and teamwork within maternity care.

Maternity services for women from ethnic minorities

Chapter 11 discusses the special care required by women from ethnic minorities.

The future – towards new models of care?

Despite the present overall high quality of service delivered by multi-disciplinary teams, new ways of working may produce even greater effectiveness and efficiency. Given the trends of declining general practitioner involvement in maternity care and the importance of woman-centred initiatives such as *Changing Childbirth*, the midwives' role may well increase, requiring reorientation of the roles of other members of the team.

Midwife/women-centred care

Figure 5.1 outlines the roles and responsibilities of a community-based maternity care team in which the pivotal roles are taken by the midwife and the pregnant woman. Other features of this model could include reduced antenatal visits and selective targeted visits to women after birth.

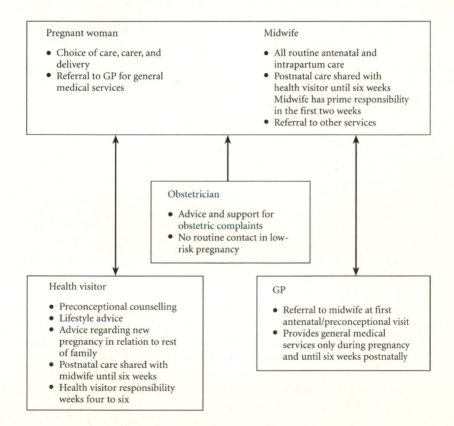

Figure 5.1 A diagramatic representation of midwife/women-centred care.

Multidisciplinary shared care – an 'equal partnership'

In many cases, the present good practice carried out by existing teams will continue. Given the available evidence and the impetus of *Changing Childbirth*, integrated teamwork might develop, as shown in Figure 5.2.

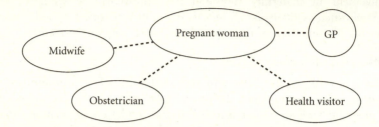

Figure 5.2 Diagramatic representation of multidisciplinary shared care.

Additional features of this method of teamwork, which most closely corresponds to current practice in many places, might include:

• greater involvement and decision-making by the pregnant woman regarding her choice of the roles played by team members

• greater awareness of the special nature of maternity care by lay team members, e.g. clerks, receptionists , secretaries, and practice managers

• reduction in antenatal visits and visits to hospital in low-risk pregnancies

• more selective targeting of women with psychological and social needs by all team members

• involvement of non-core team members such as social workers, community psychiatric nurses, and counsellors when appropriate

• clearer allocation of roles. This should occur in two ways:

  – overall policy within each general practice and local midwifery team. This will ultimately involve the development of care protocols, an exercise which requires time and sensitivity

  – policy in relation to the needs of particular women. As maternity care becomes more firmly centred in community settings, it will be appropriate to develop a method of case conferences or discussions so that care can be tailored to the needs of individual women when necessary. Although this has been an informal feature of the care offered by many practice teams, the trend towards managed care and packages of care should encourage this.

Multidisciplinary training

As maternity care changes there is a need for all those involved to share skills and ideas and to train for new ways of working together. Key elements of this multidisciplinary training are as follows:

- the acquisition of new knowledge and skills – maternity care technology is changing rapidly

- relearning previously lost skills and knowledge – the practical and 'hands on' skills of obstetrics and maternity care are very susceptible to disuse atrophy

- team-building and effective teamwork.

There are clear implications here for teachers and trainers of students and established practitioners in all of the appropriate disciplines (Chapter 10).

An enhanced role for the general practitioner

Although GPs as a whole are devoting less time to maternity care there remains an enthusiastic core who are committed to supporting women in all stages of pregnancy and birth. It is possible for them to play a more central and enhanced role in the multidisciplinary team as more care transfers to a community setting. They could develop a role as community obstetricians, becoming expert in maternal and fetal pathology and physiology.

The training and 'refreshing' of those GPs wishing to provide intrapartum care remains a subject of active debate. There must be clear agreement within the team as to who is the lead professional at a delivery, and what the appropriate response of each member of the team should be in an unexpected emergency.

General practice fundholding and the maternity care team

The implementation of the 1990 contract for GPs produced fundamental changes within primary care. The introduction of 'fundholding' aroused a strong and continuing debate with proponents claiming that general practice control over budgets resulted in improved efficiency, while critics argued that the scheme led to widening inequalities, fragmentation of services, and deterioration in relationships with patients (Coulter 1995).

Fundholding practices eventually controlled more than 2800 million of health service resources and more than 40% of the population of England were served by fundholding practices. For most of these practices the budget in real fiscal terms included prescribing, general practice-employed staff, and a core of hospital services with some exclusions, notably accident and emergency and maternity services.

For the majority of fundholding practices, maternity services were purchased by commissioning authorities, either as existing district health authorities or new joint commissioners. GPs had little or no say in this local contracting process. Following the election of the Labour Government in 1997, fundholding has been abandoned and is being replaced by commissioning groups. This has been welcomed by the great majority of health professionals as well as by the British Medical Association.

A number of issues require consideration:

- packages of care will have to be defined and costed, together with the appropriate timescales. When, for example, would midwife care begin and end?

- how will maternity services be costed?

- commissioning could, however, provide opportunities to relinquish traditional clinical roles and introduce a range of innovations in practice

- maternal and perinatal mortality and serious morbidity are currently at very low levels in the UK. It is therefore unlikely that changes brought about by commissioning will be reflected in these clinical outcomes. Appropriate evaluations and outcomes will need to be devised in these circumstances.

There is little evidence so far as to how commissioning will affect teams working in practice; but regardless of the system under which they work, teams have to address fundamental 'in house' issues.

A check-list for multidisciplinary teams

The following check-list contains questions which maternity care teams might ask themselves when considering overall effectiveness. Some are based on perceived gaps and deficiencies in current practice and some cover more general aspects of teams and team-building.

1. Who are members of your maternity care team?
Actual and potential team members should be identified and canvassed for their views. The team should consider relationships between its own members and with the local hospital obstetricians and midwives.

2. How effectively does the team communicate?
The frequency of team meetings and participation in them should be assessed. The use of guidelines and protocols should be considered.

3. What are team priorities and how are they chosen?
New developments in maternity care will lead to new priorities. Issues such as genetic counselling, the prevention of neural tube defects with folate supplements, and modification of patient lifestyles pose new challenges to teamworking. To the question 'who does what?' may be added – 'can any of us do this effectively?'.

4. Are there gaps in the care offered?
The team should always be alert to the possibility of deficiencies in the provision of care (Chapter 6). The time after birth can be considered as an example. A study of 1250 women in Scotland showed that only 13% of women were free of complaints after birth. Tiredness and depression were common and a third of women had breast problems (Glazener *et al.* 1995). This ill health was not recognized by the maternity team. It is known that professionals can easily miss mental health problems and that postnatal visits to women may be missed or are ineffective. Particular points for the team to consider are how postnatal depression is going to be recognized and by

whom, and what the relationship is between the roles of the midwife and health visitors after birth.

This check-list is not exhaustive. A useful exercise is for each team to draw up its own list of strengths and weaknesses.

Changing your team

Midwife-led care, GP commissioning, and *Changing Childbirth* all offer opportunities to provide better care for women and their babies. In order to cope with these changes, primary care teams must adapt and change too. Successful change is complex, and managing and sustaining change is not always simple. It requires motivation and commitment from the whole team together with negotiation and compromise, and an understanding of the process that is occurring. Changes within teamworking may be driven from within or without. Many of the present changes in maternity care have come from the external forces of government reports or health authority resource constraints.

The process of change involves a series of steps which often form a repeating cycle:

- identifying the need to change
- planning ways to make it happen
- making the change itself
- checking to see if the change has brought about the desired effect.

When a potential change has been identified, individuals within the team can react in different ways. Possible reactions have been described as follows:

- generate ideas to implement the change
- selling ideas to promote the change   } positive roles by team members
- sustaining the change

- accepting and passively supporting change
- obstructing the change (covert or overt) } essentially negative reactions, with no ownership by the members of the team
- ignoring the change

Successful teams include members who have the skills to be able to adopt the first three roles, though they may also view events in a negative way at times, particularly if change is rapid. Successful change will only occur if there is sufficient slack in the system, and sufficient resources in terms of time and money. Change will also only be successfully implemented if the team can define and agree common aims and goals, and if there is sufficient negotiation and consensus to ensure that all team members have an opportunity to voice their opinions.

Conclusions

- Multidisciplinary community-based maternity teams vary in their composition, philosophy of working, and effectiveness.

- Many teams provide high-quality maternity care with satisfactory outcomes for both mother and child.

- The potential for tension exists between health professionals because of a number of recent developments, including changing patterns of workload, the increasing autonomy of midwives, and the agenda generated by *Changing Childbirth*.

- There is little evidence regarding the effectiveness of particular styles of working and more research is needed.

- It is likely that the role and function of health professionals involved in maternity care will continue to change rapidly over the next few years. Reasons for this will include the growth and application of new medical and information technology, and the likely continuation of separate purchasing and providing arrangements in health care Recent changes in the philosophy and organization of maternity services aim to place the woman at the centre of choices regarding maternity care. It is appropriate and timely that community-based teams carry out their work in a way that reflects that philosophy.

- All members of existing teams will need to retain a flexible view as to their most appropriate role and function. Teams might benefit from reviewing their present effectiveness in the light of these recent and continuing developments.

- In the immediate short term, the majority of teams will no doubt continue at least in part with their historical patterns of shared care. This model, evolved from a fund of enthusiasm and goodwill, has served mothers, their babies, and health professionals well. It provides a sound and healthy basis for further change.

References

Brown, D. J. (1994). Opinions of GPs in Nottinghamshire about provision of intrapartum care. *British Medical Journal*, **309**, 777–9.

Cheyne, H., Turnbull, D., Lunan, C. B., Reid, M., and Greer, I. A. (1995).Working alongside a midwife-led care unit: what do obstetricians think? *British Journal of Obstetrics and Gynaecology*, **102**, 485–7.

Coulter, A. (1995). General practice fundholding: time for a cool appraisal. *British Journal of General Practice*, **45**, 119–20.

Department of Health (1993). *Changing childbirth: report of the Expert Maternity Group*. HMSO, London.

Department of Health and Social Security (1981). *The primary health care team. Report of a Joint Working Group of the Standing Medical Advisory Committee and The Standard Nursing and Midwifery Advisory Committee [The Harding Report]*. HMSO, London.

Department of Health and Social Security (1986). *Neighbourhood nursing: a focus for care [Cumberledge Report]*. HMSO, London.

Downe, S. (1995).GP fundholding and the maternity services. *British Journal of Midwifery*, 3, 339–40.

Dowswell, T., Hirst, J., Piercy, J., Hewison, J., Lilford, R., and Geddes, A. (1994*). Patterns of maternity care and their consequences*. Unpublished report to the Northern & Yorkshire Regional Health Authority.

Flint, C. (1993). *Midwifery teams and case-loads*. Butterworth-Heinmann Ltd, Oxford.

Garcia, J., Ness, M., MacKeith, N., Ashurst, H., Macfarlane, A., Mugford, M., *et al.* (1996). *Changing midwifery care – the scope for evaluation. Report of an NHSE-funded project evaluation of new midwifery practices* [draft]. National Perinatal Epidemiology Unit.

General Medical Services Committee (1992). Report. British Medical Association, London.

Gilmore, M., Bruce, N., and Hunt, M. (1974).*The work of the nursing team in general practice*. Central Council for Education and Training for Health Visitors, London.

Glazener, C. M. A., *et al.* (1995). Postnatal maternal morbidity: extent, causes, prevention, and treatment. *British Journal of Obstetrics and Gynaecology*, 102, 282–7.

Gready, M., Newburn, M., Dodds, R., and Grange, S. (1995*). Birth choices: women's expectations and experiences*. The National Childbirth Trust.

Green, J. M., Curtis, P., Price, H., and Renfrew, M.J. (1998). Continuing to care. The organization of midwifery services in the UK: a structured review of the evidence. University of Leeds.

Gregson, B., Cartlidge, A., and Bond, J. (1991*). Inter-professional collaboration in primary health care organizations*. Occasional Paper 51. Royal College of General Practitioners, Exeter.

Hundley, V.A., Cruickshank, F.M., Lang, G.D., Glazener, .C, Milne, J.M., Turner, M., *et al.* (1994). Midwife management delivery unit: a randomized controlled comparison with consultant-led care. *British Medical Journal*, 309,1400–4.

Kean, L., Liu, D., and Macquisten, S. (1996). Pregnancy care of the low-risk woman: the community–hospital interface. *International Journal of Health Care Quality Assurance*, 9/5, 39–44.

Klein, M., Lloyd, I., Redman, C., Bull, M., and Turnball, A.C. (1983). A comparison of low-risk pregnant women booked for delivery in two systems of care: shared-care [consultant] and integrated general practice unit. Obstetrical procedures and neonatal outcome. *British Journal of Obstetrics and Gynaecology*, 90, 118–22.

Klein, M. and Zander, L. (1989). The role of family practitioners in maternity care. In: *Effective care in pregnancy and childbirth* (ed. M. Enkin, M. Kierse, and J. Chalmers). Oxford University Press, Oxford.

Lambert, D., Spratley, J., and Killoran, A. (1991). Primary health care team workshop manual: a guide to planning and managing workshops for primary health care teams. Health Education Authority, London.

Lowe, S., House, W., and Garrett, T. (1987). Comparison of outcome of low risk labour in an isolated general practice maternity unit and a specialist maternity hospital. *Journal of the Royal College of General Practitioners*, **37**, 484–7.

MacVicar, I., Dobbie, G., Owen-Johnstone, L., Jagger, C., Hopkins, M., and Kennedy, J. (1993). Simulated home delivery in hospital: a randomized controlled trial. *British Journal of Obstetrics and Gynaecology*,**100**, 316–23.

MacVicar, J. (1990).Obsterics. In: *Healthcare for Asians* (ed. B. McAvoy and L. J. Donaldson). Oxford University Press, Oxford.

Marsh, G. N. (1991). *Efficient care in general practice.* Oxford University Press, Oxford.

Marsh, G. N. and Kaim-Caudle, P. (1976). *Team care in general practice.* Croom Helm, London.

Outram, V. (1995). Case study – the Scunthorpe way. In: *The challenge of Changing Childbirth*, section 3, p.11. Continuity of Care, English National Board, London.

Ovretveit, J. (1990).*Cooperation in primary health care.* Brunel Institute of Organisation and Social Studies, Middlesex.

Pearson, P. (1992). Defining the primary health care team. *Health Visitor*, **65**, 358–61.

Renfrew, M. J. (1994). Midwife vs medical/shared care. In: Pregnancy and Childbirth Module, Cochrane Database of Systematic Reviews (ed. M. W. Enkin, M. J. N. C. Keirse, M. J. Renfrew, *et al.*). Review no. 03295. Cochrane updates on disk, disk issue no. 1. Update Software, Oxford.

Royal College of General Practitioners (1995).*General practice in maternity care.* Occasional paper no. 72.

Smith, L.P. (1996). Should general practitioners have any role in maternity care in the future? *British Journal of General Practice*, **46**, 243–7.

Spratley, J. (1989). Disease prevention and health promotion in primary health care. Health Education Authority, London.

Waine, C. (1992). The primary care team. *British Journal of General Practice*, **42**, 498–9.

Walker, P. and James, D.K. (1995). Should obstetricians see women with normal pregnancies? *British Medical Journal*, **310**, 36–8.

Wiles, R. and Robinson J. (1994). Teamwork in primary care: the views and experiences of nurses, midwives, and health visitors. *Journal of Advanced Nursing*, **20**, 324–30.

Wood, J. (1991). A review of antenatal care initiatives in primary care settings. *British Journal of General Practice*, **41**, 26–30.

Young, G. (1987). Are isolated maternity units run by general practitioners? *British Medical Journal*, **294**, 744–6.

CHAPTER SIX

Mothers' views and experiences of care

Jo Garcia

Why do women's views of care matter?

There are many reasons why women's views and experiences matter, but perhaps the main one is that women's reactions to care around the time of birth can affect they way they care for themselves and their baby. These reactions also influence their subsequent contacts with their care-givers (Brown *et al.* 1994). Feelings of having had a good or bad experience are, of course, partly affected by the clinical events at the time, but the explanations and support they get from staff can go on mattering to them for a long time (Menage 1993; Charles 1994; Crompton 1996; Smith and Mitchell 1996). For some women, the decision about having another child may be one of the outcomes. Two comments from mothers who took part in a recent national postal survey (Garcia *et al.* 1998) help to illustrate some of these issues.

My other two children are now young adults. Antenatal and postnatal care since their births has changed considerably, and for the better. In my previous pregnancies I felt 'done-to' – having little explained, no choices, and treated with little or no respect. My age and naivety prevented me from asking questions and I therefore accepted my lot. Now I feel as if my child has been mine from conception. I've been encouraged quite rightly to take responsibility and decisions from the start, and I have felt respected. I feel this is a good start to enabling parents to take responsibility for their children.

I feel I should have had extra care after the birth of my son . . . I continually lost blood in huge clots . . . and was admitted by ambulance as I haemorrhaged . . . I felt extremely ill and exhausted. No one offered to chat through what had happened or explain things to me as to why. I'm very disappointed and it has frightened me in case it happens again.

Asking women to provide data for audit is one of the other functions fulfilled by asking women for their views. There are some aspects of care that can only be assessed by asking women directly, or are more practical to get this way. For example, if the aim is to provide women with information about local maternity services, it is sensible to ask them whether they actually received this information (Gready *et al.* 1995). Women are also the best people to provide data about the extent to which they knew the care-givers who looked after them at different stages. They are also the best informants about the pattern of care that they have received, since it is often hard to get all this information from one set of records (Hemingway *et al.* 1994; Farquhar *et al.* 1996; Fleissig *et al.* 1996; Allen *et al.* 1997). Clinical data that are not routinely collected can be obtained direct from mothers. Examples are the use of pain relief in labour (Chamberlain *et al.* 1993), or postnatal health problems such as bleeding or incontinence (Bick and MacArthur 1995).

A good example of both of these reasons for studying women who have used the maternity services is found in a recently published study of maternity and infant care in a large general practice (Mellor and Chambers 1995). This showed, among other useful findings, that most women interviewed liked having an early antenatal visit from a midwife at home to discuss plans for the birth, but a few did not. The latter felt that they were being checked up on, and one was embarrassed because she was not living in her own home. The care was changed to *offer* women a home visit rather than just arranging it. Women in this study also felt that they wanted to maintain contact with the GP even where most of the care was being given by midwives. Again, these views were taken into account in planning changes to the service.

Types of study

Studies of women's views and experiences are carried out using a range of methods – postal surveys, interviews, observation of care, and group discussions. Postal surveys are the most commonly used; samples can be drawn from women using a maternity unit, from a local population of births, or carried out at a national level. For example, the five-yearly Infant Feeding Surveys are sent to a national random sample of women at six to ten weeks, four to five months, and nine months after birth (White *et al.* 1992). The recent survey conducted for the Audit Commission (1997) was based on a random sample of women who had given birth in 1995. In 1989, the Office of Population Censuses and Surveys (OPCS) published a manual for those carrying out maternity surveys (Mason 1989). The questionnaires included in this manual have been used widely in local surveys and also adapted recently (Hemingway *et al.* 1994; Lamping *et al.* 1996). Unfortunately, many reports from local surveys are not published. A recent local study that explored some of the issues arising from *Changing Childbirth* was the Choices project, which was carried out in Essex and was a collaboration between the National Childbirth Trust and purchasers (Gready *et al.* 1995).

Studies that have used face-to-face interviews rather than self-administered questionnaires include classics in the field (Oakley 1979, 1980) and two more recent studies of the views of Asian mothers (Woollett and Dosanjh-Matwala 1990; Rudat *et al.* 1993). There are also studies that have made use of observation of care, sometimes including interviews with those observed (Kirkham 1989; Garcia and Garforth 1990; Hunt and Symonds 1995). Focus groups have been used in some cases; one reason is to provide extra information from women who may be less likely to return questionnaires (Gready *et al.* 1995).

Further examples of postal surveys and studies using other methods, and also a discussion of the advantages and disadvantages of the various methods, can be found in Garcia (1997*a*). A useful book about taking the views of service users into account is Dodds *et al.* (1996).

In the rest of this chapter I would like to pick out some key themes that arise in studies of women's views and use these to explore various methodological issues. I will cover three topics about choices:

(1) finding out from women what choices they have been given

(2) finding out what options they would like to have

(3) exploring the aspects of care that are important to them.

I will conclude by looking at the views of Asian women about maternity care. The data come from local and national studies of women who have used the maternity services.

What choices do women feel that they have been given?

A national face-to-face interview study was carried out by MORI's Health Research Unit for the Expert Maternity Group (Rudat *et al.* 1993). Women were included in the survey if they had had a baby in the UK since 1 April 1989. In the questionnaire they were asked two questions about the choice they felt that they had been given by their GP. The answers are shown in Tables 6.1 and 6.2.

Table 6.1 *How much choice did you feel you were offered by the GP in where you received your antenatal care?*

	% of women
A great deal	7
A fair amount	20
Not very much	23
Nothing at all	49
Can't remember	1

Base: all women who saw a GP in the course of their antenatal care (972 women, national sample). Source: MORI (1993).

These tables show that, at the time that this survey was carried out, few women reported that they had much choice about these aspects of their care. Other recent studies have asked similar questions. In the Choices project,

Table **6.2** *How much choice did you feel you were offered by the GP in where you could give birth?*

	% of women
A great deal	6
A fair amount	16
Not very much	23
Nothing at all	52

Base: all women who saw a GP in the course of their antenatal care (972 women, national sample). Source: MORI (1993).

which aimed to cover all women who gave birth in North Essex Health Authority in a six-week period in November and December 1994, women were asked about choices in antenatal care, and their involvement in deciding where to book for delivery (Gready *et al.* 1995). The questions used were different from those in the MORI survey. In answer to a question about where the antenatal check-ups could be, 14% of the total sample (n=787) said that they had been given a choice. There was a significant difference though between women who delivered in the three consultant maternity units serving the study population in the proportion who reported a choice in this respect. Several questions were asked in the Choices survey, for example, about decision-making about place of birth. Just over half of the whole sample (54%) said that they felt they had been fully involved in the decision about where to book for the birth. Women who delivered in a GP unit or at home were much more likely to say this than those who had delivered in a consultant unit. In answer to another question, 13% of the whole sample said that they had been offered the possibility of a home birth. In the survey carried out for the Audit Commission, a third of women reported that they had been given a choice of where their antenatal check-ups would take place.

In practice though, the answers to questions of this sort depend on the degree of choice that actually exists locally. In some places, women live near to more than one maternity unit or have access to different antenatal care options. Also, care-givers will certainly differ in the way that they present the possibilities to women. Some women may not expect choice or may take a particular form of care for granted, or they may not be interested in certain options. It may be that survey questions are not the best way to get at this sort of thing. Studies which use more qualitative methods may be more suitable. For example, a leaflet designed to give women information about the range of choices available locally might be assessed by a focus group discussion with women fairly early in the course of their antenatal care. Or one could do a study – not easy to design – which observed the first visit with a GP or midwife in pregnancy to look at sorts of questions that women ask and at the way that information is given.

What choices do women want?

The OPCS survey manual (Mason 1989) included the question:

- At the beginning of pregnancy would you like to have talked more about:
  - the choice of who you could have check-ups with?
  - whether you might have a domino delivery?
  - whether you might have a home birth?
  - the choice of hospital where you might have your baby?

The answers to this question are shown in Figure 6.1 and use data from the test surveys carried out in four districts to prepare the manual (Garcia 1989). A to D are the four districts. Up to half the women in some districts would have liked some choice about who they could have their check-ups with. A similar proportion were interested in domino delivery. Home birth was of interest to a small proportion of women. Presumably the difference between these districts in the proportions of women who are interested in having a choice about the hospital for the birth reflects differences in access to more than one hospital. The fact that over 50% replied 'no, not really' to these questions, however, gives cause for some interesting reflections!

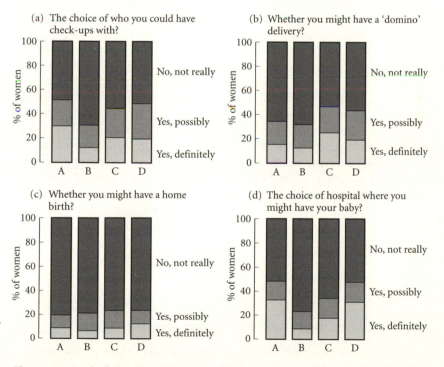

Figure 6.1 *At the beginning of pregnancy, would you like to have talked more about: (a) the choice of who you could have check-ups with? (b) whether you might have a domino delivery? (c) whether you might have a home birth? (d) the choice of hospital where you might have your baby?*

Table 6.3 *If you become pregnant again, which of these choices do you personally want to have available locally?*

	% of women
Delivery at a hospital maternity unit by hospital staff	50
Delivery in a hospital by GP/community midwife	25
Delivery in a separate GP unit	18
Domino delivery	43
Home delivery	22
Other	2
Don't know	2

Base: all women (1005 women, national sample). Source: MORI (1993).

In the MORI survey (Rudat *et al.* 1993), women were asked about their interest in choice in a different way (Table 6.3).

Women were given a list of options to look at, rather than an open question, and the wording was fuller than that in the table. It is clear that there is considerable interest in domino delivery. In addition, around a quarter of women indicated an interest in the possibility of home birth and in care from a GP or community midwife in hospital. Questions of this kind give an indication of the level of interest, but answers are likely to be affected by women's past experience of care, the sort of information that women have, and the way that services are described. Actual uptake of different forms of care cannot be directly inferred from these answers. There is, so far, only a small amount of information about which care-giver, or combinations of care-givers, women would like to see in the course of their care. In a brief report of data from a larger study, Hirst and colleagues (1996) showed that, at the first antenatal visit, women were more likely to prefer to see *combinations* of care-givers (such as GP and midwife) than to see one care giver alone. In a study carried out in the Bath district (Smith 1996), women were asked about involvement of the GP in their care. Most women indicated that they believed that the GP should have a role in routine antenatal care. Two thirds of women in this study were cared for in pregnancy by one GP whom they knew well. Several studies about the roles of different care-givers and women's preferences are in progress.

What is important to women about their care?

Some recent studies have asked women to express their preferences for different features of maternity care. Some examples are given here, focusing on women's preferences for continuity of carer in relation to some of the other aspects of care that are important. Again, it is important to note that the way in which the question is asked is likely to influence the sorts of answers that women give. Some studies have used open questions to get women's views while others have offered women lists to rank or to score in terms of how important different factors are to them.

In a study carried out in a consultant maternity hospital by Drew and colleagues (1989), women who had had a baby in the last few days were asked to score 40 aspects of maternity care on a scale from essential to irrelevant. The scale was also used to record the assessment of midwives and obstetricians about what was important to women. Only two items among the 40 referred to continuity of carer: 'being attended by the same midwife during pregnancy' and 'being attended by the same doctor during pregnancy'. These two were placed in the middle range of importance by women (and care-givers): rank 21 and 23. At the top of the list came 'the baby being healthy', and two items about communication: 'the doctors talking to you in a way you can understand' and 'having all your questions answered by staff'.

In the MORI interview survey (Rudat *et al.* 1993), women were asked: If you went through a pregnancy and birth again, what would matter most to you in terms of the care you were given? The question was an open one with no pre-set categories for women to choose from. The most common themes are listed in Table 6.4.

Table 6.4 *Women's priorities for care*

	% of women
Continuity/seeing same midwife or doctor	19
More information/explain what is involved	13
More caring/understanding/support	13
More reassurance	8
Listen to your views/treated as a person	8
More personal attention	8
More/regular checks/tests	7
Making sure baby is alright	7
None/no problems/satisfied	8
Don't know	7

Base: 1005 women. Source: MORI (1993).

Nineteen per cent of women mentioned some aspect of continuity of carer, and 13% more information or explanation. The next two categories are about their need for caring and reassurance – 13% and 8%. Two other aspects of personal care were each mentioned by about 8% of women. Making sure that the baby is alright was mentioned spontaneously by only 7% of women – in contrast to the ranking it got in the previous study, where it was one of the categories offered to mothers. Perhaps women took it for granted as one of the main features of care.

In another recent study (Garcia 1997*b*), women in three areas were asked to

Table 6.5 *Overall, before, during, and after the birth, how important do you think it is to have care?*

Percentage indicating that this is *very* important	Service		
	A	B	C
	%	%	%
That is from skilled doctors and midwives	98	94	90
That gives you the information you want	93	92	96
Where you are treated kindly	91	87	90
Where you are treated respectfully	88	82	85
That is convenient	66	65	76
That lets *you* make the decisions	76	71	68
That is from someone you know	45	37	36
Total number of women	231	185	123

complete a postal questionnaire about their experiences of maternity care. At the end of the questionnaire they were given a list of options and asked to choose which aspects of maternity care were important to them. Table 6.5 shows the results.

This question only asked women to record the importance they gave to the different aspects of care. This means that all the items that they were offered appeared to be very important for at least 36% of women – none were of no importance. This question did not ask them to choose between different aspects of care, or imply that the items in the list might be in conflict. For example, it did not allow for the possibility that having more convenient care might mean that it was less likely to be from a known caregiver.

Although studies of this type do come up with some different answers, there seem to be some common themes. If the issue of safety is raised, women are likely to indicate that it is very important for them. Women place a high value on good information and communication with staff and on being treated kindly. Concern about having known carers is important but probably not for as many women as the other items mentioned. Studies of this kind will continue to produce varying results. One way forward is to evaluate different ways of providing care in randomized trials which include women's views alongside clinical outcomes (Hundley *et al.* 1994, 1995a; Sikorski *et al.* 1996; Tucker *et al.* 1996; Turnbull *et al.* 1996).

Maternity care for women of Asian backgrounds

There is a range of studies in this area, including evaluations of linkworker and advocacy schemes (Parsons and Day 1992; Warrier and Goodman 1996). The MORI study included a special survey of women from ethnic minorities carried out by bilingual interviewers (Rudat *et al.*, 1993). Three hundred Asian women were included and they were asked some specific questions. For example, they were asked if they agreed with three statements about maternity care. Table 6.6 shows the number who agreed (either *strongly agreed* or *tended to agree*) with each of the statements.

Table 6.6 *Percentage of women agreeing with three statements about maternity care*

	% of women agreeing
Overall, maternity services in England fail to meet the needs of Asian women	52
The health professionals . . . were understanding of my cultural needs	55
I would have liked more explanation . . . in my own language	58

Base: all Asian women (300). Source: MORI (1993).

Table 6.7 *Thinking about your last pregnancy and birth, is there anything the health service could do to improve maternity services for Asian women?*

	% of women
Employ staff who speak Asian languages	17
Interpreters for all languages	22
Choice of/appropriate food	11
More care towards Asian women	9

Base: all Asian women (300). Source: MORI (1993).

Table 6.7 shows some of the suggestions that women made about ways of improving maternity care.

The question was an open one and a large number of answers were given. These are the ones most commonly mentioned. There is clearly great scope for improvement in the care given to these mothers, and audit of any changes in care presents some challenges.

Another example from the MORI survey (1993) shows up an important methodological issue for surveys of care. Information from the survey of women from Asian backgrounds can be used together with the results from the national sample. The researchers asked whether women felt that they had received plenty of useful advice throughout their pregnancy (Table 6.8).

Table 6.8 shows the proportions of women agreeing with the statement from the national sample and from an Indian, Pakistani, or Bangladeshi

Table 6.8 *I received plenty of useful advice throughout my pregnancy (from the different health professionals)*

	National sample	Indian background	Pakistani background	Bangladeshi background
% agreeing	66	55	54	78

Source: MORI (1993).

background. This looks very good for women of Bangladeshi origin. At another point in the interview, however, women were asked whether they had discussed specific items with health professionals (Table 6.9).

Table 6.9 *Percentage of women discussing specific items with health professionals*

	% of women from:			
	National sample	Indian background	Pakistani background	Bangladeshi background
Events during labour and birth	38	15	14	6
Pain relief	50	7	15	5
Breastfeeding	40	31	23	0

Source: MORI (1993).

Overall, women reported very limited discussion of these important aspects of care and comparing these two tables we can say that it is very unlikely that 95 % of women of Bangladeshi origin had no wish for information of this sort. These findings show the need for far better information for women from different ethnic backgrounds, and reveal the difficulty of drawing conclusions on the basis of rather general 'satisfaction-type' questions. Questionnaires should be as specific as possible about aspects of care that are of concern.

The MORI data came from a large interview study carried out by bilingual interviewers. Self-completion questionnaires are not generally useful for studies of women in minority ethnic groups (Brown *et al.* 1994; McIver 1994). Focus groups have been used, but recruitment is often quite difficult and the method can be more time-consuming than expected (Garcia 1997*a*).

Resources

Because there are some pitfalls to be avoided in getting women's views of care, it is worth using existing questionnaires if possible, and seeking advice from someone who has used them (Campbell and Garcia 1997). A new guide to methods for getting women's views in maternity care is being produced by the College of Health (for further information contact the College of Health on 0181 983 1225). Some of the more general issues, such as the choice of appropriate methods and sample size calculations for surveys, are discussed in health services research textbooks such as Crombie and Davies (1996). Qualitative methods are covered in a recent compilation of material reprinted from the *British Medical Journal* (Mays and Pope 1996).

References

Allen, I., Bourke Dowling, S., and Williams, S. (1997). *A leading role for midwives? Evaluation of midwifery group practice development projects.* Policy Studies Institute, London.

Audit Commission (1997). *First class delivery: improving maternity services in England and Wales.* Audit Commission, London.

Bick, D. and MacArthur, C. (1995). The extent, severity and effects of health problems after childbirth. *British Journal of Midwifery*, 3, 27–31.

Brown, S., Lumley, J., Small, R., and Astbury, J. (1994). *Missing voices: the experience of motherhood.* Oxford University Press, Oxford.

Campbell, R. and Garcia, J. (1997). *The organization of maternity care: a guide to evaluation.* Hochland and Hochland, Hale, Cheshire.

Chamberlain, G., Wraight, A., and Steer, P. (19930. *Pain and its relief in childbirth.* Churchill Livingstone, Edinburgh.

Charles, J. (1994). Birth afterthoughts: a postnatal listening service for women. *British Journal of Midwifery*, 2, 331–4.

Crombie, I. K. and Davies, H. T. O. (1996). *Research in health care: design, conduct, and interpretation of health services research.* John Wiley, Chichester.

Crompton, J. (1996). Post-traumatic stress disorder and childbirth. *British Journal of Midwifery*, 4, 290–4, 354–6, 373.

Dodds, R., Goodman, M., and Tyler, S. (eds.) (1996). *Listen with mother: consulting users of maternity services.* Books for Midwives Press, Hale.

Drew, N. C., Salmon, P., and Webb, L. (1989). Mothers', midwives' and obstetricians' views on the features of obstetric care which influence satisfaction with childbirth. *British Journal of Obstetrics and Gynaecology*, 96, 1084–88.

Farquhar, M., Camilleri-Ferrante, C., and Todd, C. (1996). *An evaluation of midwifery teams in West Essex.* Public Health Resources Unit and Health Services Research Group, Institute of Public Health, University of Cambridge.

Fleissig, A., Kroll, D., and McCarthy, M. (1996). Is community-led maternity care a feasible option for women assessed at low risk and those with complicated pregnancies? Results of a population-based study in South Camden, London. *Midwifery*, 12, 191–7.

Garcia, J. (1989). *Getting consumers' views of maternity care: examples of how the OPCS survey manual can help.* Department of Health, London.

Garcia, J. (1997*a*). Finding out what women and their families think of the service. In: *The organization of maternity care: a guide to evaluation* (ed. R. Campbell and J. Garcia). Hochland and Hochland, Hale, Cheshire.

Garcia, J. (1997*b*). *Changing midwifery care – the scope for evaluation: report of an NHSE-funded project 'Evaluation of New Midwifery Practices'.* National Perinatal Epidemiology Unit, Oxford.

Garcia, J. and Garforth, S. (1990). Parents and newborn babies in the labour ward. In: *The politics of maternity care* (ed. J. Garcia, M. Richards, and R. Kilpatrick). Oxford University Press, Oxford.

Garcia, J., Redshaw, M., Fitzsimons, B., and Keene, J. (1998). *First class delivery: a national survey of women's views of maternity care.* Audit Commission, London.

Gready, M., Newburn, M., Dodds, R., and Gauge, S. (1995). *Birth choices: women's expectations and experiences.* National Childbirth Trust, London.

Hemingway, H., Saunders, D., and Parsons, L. (1994). *Women's experiences of maternity services in east London: an evaluation.* East London and City Health Authority, London.

Hirst, J., Dowswell, T., Hewison, J., and Lilford, R.J. (1996). Women's views of their first antenatal visit [letter]. *British Journal of General Practice,* **46**, 319.

Hundley, V., Cruickshank, F., Lang, G., *et al.* (1994). Midwife-managed delivery unit: a randomized controlled comparison with consultant-led care. *British Medical Journal,* **309**, 1400–4.

Hunt, S. and Symonds, A. (1995). *The social meaning of midwifery.* Macmillan, London.

Kirkham, M. (1989). Midwives and information-giving in labour. In: *Midwives, research, and childbirth.* Vol. I. (ed. S. Robinson and A Thomson.) Chapman and Hall, London.

Lamping, D. and Rowe, P. (1996). *Surveys of women's experiences of maternity services (short form). Users' manual for purchasers and providers.* London School of Hygiene and Tropical Medicine, London.

McIver, C. (1994). *Obtaining the views of black users of the health services.* King's Fund, London. (Copies from BEBC; for information freephone 0800 262260.)

Mason, V. (1989). *Women's experience of maternity care – a survey manual.* HMSO, London.

Mays, N. and Pope, C. (1996). *Qualitative research in health care.* British Medical Journal Publishing Group, London.

Mellor, J. and Chambers, N. (1995). Addressing the patient's agenda in the reorganization of antenatal and infant health care: experience in one general practice. *British Journal of General Practice,* 45, 423–5.

Menage, J. (1993). Post-traumatic stress disorder in women who have undergone obstetric and/or gynaecological procedures. *Journal of Reproductive and Infant Psychology,* 11, 221–8.

Oakley, A. (1979). *Becoming a mother.* Martin Robertson, Oxford.

Oakley, A. (1980). *Women confined: towards a sociology of childbirth.* Martin Robertson, Oxford.

Parsons, L. and Day, S. (1992). Improving obstetric outcomes in ethnic minorities: an evaluation of health advocacy in Hackney. *Journal of Public Health Medicine*, **14**, 183–91.

Rudat, K., Roberts, C., and Chowdhury, R. (1993). *Maternity services: a comparative survey of Afro-Caribbean, Asian, and white women commissioned by the Expert Maternity Group*. MORI Health Research, London.

Sikorski, J., Wilson, J., Clement, S., *et al.* (1996). A randomized trial comparing two schedules of antenatal visits: the antenatal care project. *British Medical Journal*, **312**, 546–53.

Smith, J.A. and Mitchell, S. (1996). Debriefing after childbirth: a tool for effective risk management. *British Journal of Midwifery*, **4**, 581–6.

Smith, L. (1996). Views of pregnant women on the involvement of general practitioners in maternity care. *British Journal of General Practice*, **46**, 101–4.

Tucker, J. S., Hall, M. H., Howie P. W., *et al.* (1996). Should obstetricians see women with normal pregnancies? A multicentre, randomized controlled trial of routine antenatal care by general practitioners and midwives compared with shared care led by obstetricians. *British Medical Journal*, **312**, 554–9.

Turnbull, D., Holmes, A., *et al.* (1996). Randomized controlled trial of efficacy of midwife-managed care. *Lancet*, **348**, 213–18.

Warrier, S. and Goodman, M. (1996). *Consumer empowerment: a qualitative study of linkworker and advocacy services for non-English speaking users of maternity services*. Maternity Alliance, London.

White, A., Freeth, S., and O'Brien, M. (1992). *Infant feeding 1990*. Social Survey Division, Office of Population Censuses and Surveys, London.

Woollett, A. and Dosanjh-Matwala, N. (1990). Postnatal care: the attitudes and experiences of Asian women in east London. *Midwifery*, **6**, 178–84.

SECTION TWO

CONTEMPORARY ISSUES

CHAPTER SEVEN

The social context of maternity care

Peter Selman and Erica Haimes

Introduction

The social context of childbirth has been constantly changing over the past hundred years. In the mid nineteenth century the average family size was over six and 63% of married women had five or more live births before the end of their reproductive period (Table 7.1). Pregnancies were largely unplanned and family limitation practised on only a very limited scale. Many children died before reaching maturity.

Within two generations the world had changed so that women marrying in the 1930s were the first cohort to barely reach replacement fertility (2.1 live

Table 7.1 *Distribution of family size in Great Britain: births occurring to first marriages, 1860–1960*

Number of children live born in marriage	Women married in period:				
	c.1860	1900–09	1920–24	1935–39	1955–59
0	9	10	16	15	9
1	5	14	24	26	18
2	6	18	24	29	34
3	8	16	14	15	20
4	9	12	8	7	11
5+	63	30	14	8	8
	100	100	100	100	100
Average number of live births	6.16	3.53	2.38	2.07	2.38

Sources: *Royal Commission on Population Report (1949)*. p. 26. HMSO, London; *Report of the Population Panel (1973)*. p. 40. HMSO, London.

births) and less than 10% had more than four births. Although fertility rose briefly in the post-war period, total fertility rates in most European countries have been below 2.1 for 20 years. At the same time, infant mortality has fallen from over 150 per 1000 births to less than 10.

The story behind these dry statistics is one of dramatic change in the situation of women – the number of years spent in nursing and pregnancy falling from 15 in the 1890s to four by the 1930s (Lewis 1991). The low birth rates of the 1930s concealed a wide variation between social classes, with the fertility of manual workers about 40% higher than non-manual groups (Selman 1977). Today, class differences are much smaller. Fifty per cent of women born since the First World War have had only one or two children. The number remaining childless has fluctuated between 9 and 20%, and the proportion of live births to women with four or more living children has fallen from 8% in 1956 and 1961 to under 3% since the mid 1970s.

Other dramatic changes are occurring in the knowledge base of maternity issues, with assisted conception and issues surrounding the 'new genetics' being the likely source of new challenges for the 21st century.

The changing demographic structure of post-war Britain

The decline in family size from 1870 to 1955 involved little change in patterns of marriage – most births occurred within first marriages and second marriages became less common as fewer women were widowed. Since then, the most significant changes in family demography have been in the context of childbearing rather than the level:

- people are less likely to marry
- more marriages end in divorce
- more children are growing up in stepfamilies
- more couples live together in a non-marital union
- women are having their children later in marriage
- a rising number of births occur outside marriage
- there are more single-parent families
- more women, including mothers, are in paid employment
- one in five pregnancies end in legal abortion.

Just as the falling birth rate of the 1930s led to gloomy prognostications about the 'twilight of parenthood' (Charles 1934) and a 'parents' revolt' (Titmuss and Titmuss 1942), so the current changes have been seen as a 'farewell to the family' (Morgan 1995) and leading to 'families without fatherhood' (Dennis and Erdos 1992). However, it is clear that the social context of pregnancy and childbirth today is very different than 30 years ago, and that all those working with women through this process must be attuned to these changes.

Changes in marriage

The number of marriages in England and Wales peaked at 415 000 in 1970, but by 1993 had fallen to 299 000, the lowest level since 1944. The first marriage rate, which had risen from 55 in 1931 to over 100 in 1970, fell in 1993 to 45, the lowest rate ever recorded. After the First World War, age at marriage fell from 25.8 years for spinsters and 27.5 for bachelors to 22.5 and 24.6 in 1970 (Office of Population Censuses and Surveys [OPCS] 1987a), since when the mean age has risen to 26.9 and 28.9 in 1995 (Table 7.2). Thirty years ago, 40% of young brides were pregnant, whereas today 'shotgun' marriages are less common and over 88% of under-20 births are to unmarried teenagers (Table 7.3).

Table 7.2 *First marriages: England and Wales, 1951–1995*

	First marriages – for women (1000s)	First marriage rate (per 1000 single women aged 16+)	Mean age at first marriage (spinsters)
1951	293	76	24.4
1961	312	83	23.1
1971	347	97	22.6
1981	263	64	23.1
1991	225	47	25.5
1993	215	45	26.2
1995	199	40	26.9

Sources: *Marriage & Divorce Statistics - Series FM2*, OPCS 1974–93; *Population Trends* no. 90, Winter 1997, Table 22

Table 7.3 *Live births to women under age 20: England and Wales, 1961–1996*

Year	Total births	Births outside marriage	Percentage outside marriage
1961	59 786	11 896	19.9
1966	86 746	20 582	23.7
1971	82 641	21 555	26.1
1981	56 570	26 430	40.6
1991	52 396	43 448	82.9
1995	41 938	36 315	86.6
1996	44 700	39 300	87.9

Sources: *Birth Statistics – Series FM1*, OPCS 1974–1994; *Population Trends* no. 90, Winter 1997, Tables 9–11.

Increase in divorce

During the past 40 years there has been a significant rise in divorce in Britain and most other developed countries. Since 1961, the annual number of divorces in England and Wales has risen from 25 000 to 145 000 in 1981 and 165 000 in 1993. Haskey (1983, 1989, 1992) has estimated that 40% of today's marriages will end in divorce and that almost a quarter of the children born in the 1980s will experience their parents' divorce by the age of 16. Since 1993, the number of divorces has been falling, in part a reflection of the declining number of marriages, but the number of cohabitation breakdowns seems to be rising.

Remarriage

The increase in divorce has led to a rise in the number of remarriages and to a situation in which the bulk of these involved divorced rather than widowed persons. Between 1961 and 1981, the number of women remarrying rose from 35 000 to 89 000, and the proportion of these second marriages involving divorced women rose from 52% to 85%. By 1993 less than 10% of second marriages involved widows. Remarriage rates (per 1000 divorced or widowed) have fallen sharply, from 227 to 56 per 1000 for divorced men and from 134 to 45 per 1000 for divorced women, between 1971 and 1995 (OPCS 1996). The rates of remarriage of widowed persons fell similarly.

Stepfamilies

One consequence of the rising number of remarriages has been an increase in the number of stepfamilies. Haskey (1994*a*) has estimated that 8% of children now live in *step* or *reconstituted* families, but that in nearly a third of these the birth mother has not married her new partner. We know very little about what it means for children to grow up in a stepfamily but the limited research suggests that many experience difficulties (Ferri 1984).

Cohabitation

The decline in marriage has been accompanied by an increase in the number of couples living together without marrying. The proportion of single women cohabiting rose from 9% in 1981 to 24% in 1994–95. A majority of couples now live together before marriage and cohabitation has become an accepted part of the mating process. 'Post-marital cohabitation' has also become more common (Kiernan and Estaugh 1993).

Most younger respondents in the British Social Attitudes Survey said they would advise young people to live together before marriage, and only 6% said cohabitation was always wrong. We may, therefore, be witnessing a move from cohabitation being perceived as deviant behaviour to its acceptance not only as a prelude to marriage but increasingly as a socially acceptable alternative (Kiernan 1995).

The decision to cohabit rather than marry seems to be influenced by a number of factors. A few couples are opposed to marriage in principle; some say they are afraid of marriage breakdown, often having experienced their own parents' divorce; others say they can see no advantages in marrying or cite the high costs of a wedding; most say they expect to marry eventually (McRae 1993).

Cohabiting unions tend to be short-lived (Kiernan and Estaugh 1993), ending in either marriage or break up. The decision to marry is often linked to a decision to have children or pressure from families (Selman 1996a). Concern has been expressed over the apparent instability of non-marital relationships. Many premarital, childless cohabitations are not seen as carrying lasting commitment, but it is clear that cohabitation breakdown increasingly involves children and is one reason for the increase in single-parent families.

Conclusion

The changes described above are associated with the control women have gained over reproduction and the new opportunities and changing roles associated with this. Whether they reflect the growth of individualism (van de Kaa 1987; Dennis and Erdos 1992), reduced complementarity between men and women (Burns 1995), or a rejection of traditional values, they are developments which fundamentally change the family context of children born in the 1990s.

Changing patterns of pregnancy and birth

The relationship revolution described in the previous section has been accompanied by further changes in patterns of pregnancy and birth within and outside marriage. Since the baby boom of the 1960s there has been a shift downwards in period fertility so that by the 1980s all countries of Western Europe had sub-replacement fertility. More recently there has been a rise in fertility to replacement level in Sweden, while in Italy and Spain the total fertility rate (TFR) has fallen further – to 1.3 and 1.2 respectively. Other key changes have been later childbearing and an increase in births outside marriage.

Deferred childbearing

Women today are having fewer children and they are having them at older ages. The mean age of mothers at first birth in England and Wales, which had fallen steadily from 26.7 between 1938 and 1946 to 23.9 in the period 1967 to1970, has been rising again from the early 1970s to 26.5 in 1994. Between 1964 and 1977, birth rates fell at all ages as the TFR declined from 2.95 to 1.69. Since then the TFR has fluctuated around 1.8, but age-specific fertility rates have been falling for women under 30 and rising for older women.

The changes can also be seen in the falling proportion of births to teenagers. In 1966, 10.2% of all births were to women under age 20; by 1989 this had fallen to 8.1%, and by 1995 to 6.4% (Babb 1993). Despite this, teenage pregnancy and births are attracting more concern and condemnation than ever before (Selman 1996b), partly because most teenage births and an even higher proportion of teenage pregnancies now occur outside marriage (Table 7.3).

By 1990, teenage birth rates were very low in Sweden and most other Western European countries, although still high in the USA and central Europe (David 1990; Selman and Glendinning 1996). British levels are between those found in America and Northern Europe and rates remained unchanged throughout the 1980s when the number of teenage births was falling sharply in Denmark and France (Table 7.4).

Changing patterns and outcomes of extramarital pregnancy

One of the major changes in fertility over the last 30 years has been the growth in the number and proportion of births occurring outside marriage. Throughout the period of major fertility decline in Britain from 1870 to 1955, the proportion of births occurring outside marriage remained below 5%, except for the two periods of world war. Since then the proportion of births outside marriage in England and Wales has risen – from 6% to 12% between 1961 and 1981, and to 34% in 1995, when 77% were registered jointly by both mother and father and half of these gave the same address. In Sweden, over 50% of births now occur outside marriage (Table 7.5). A clear

Table 7.4 *Teenage fertility rates: USA, England and Wales, and other European countries, selected years 1971–1993*

	1971	**1977**	**1983**	**1990**	**1993**
USA	66.1	52.8	51.7	59.4	63.5
England and Wales	**50.8**	**29.8**	**26.9**	**33.3**	**28.9**
Sweden	34.6	22.1	11.7	12.7	11.2
Denmark	29.3	22.1	10.6	9.8	9.9
France	27.7	22.1	13.9	9.1	9.1
Netherlands	22.2	10.1	7.7	6.4	7.2

Sources: UN Demographic Year Book; Eurostat Demographic Statistics; Selman and Glendinning (1996).

Table 7.5 *Non-marital births as percentage of total births: selected European countries, 1970–1993*

Country	**1970**	**1980**	**1993**
Sweden	18.4	39.7	50.4
United Kingdom	8.0	11.5	31.8
France	6.8	11.4	34.9
Ireland	2.7	5.0	19.5
Italy	2.2	4.3	7.3

Source: *Council of Europe (1995).*

majority of such births are to women who are cohabiting (Hoem and Hoem 1988).

The increase in non-marital births has occurred despite the introduction of legal abortion. In 1969, 86% of pregnancies resulted in a birth within marriage, of which 9% were conceived before marriage, and only 7% were legally terminated. By 1992 the proportion terminated had risen to 19%, the proportion ending in a birth outside marriage had risen to 26%, and under 50% resulted in a birth within their mother's first marriage (see Table 7.6).

This growth of childbearing outside marriage in Britain was acknowledged in 1987 with the passing of the Family Law Reform Act, which 'removed the separate and disadvantageous treatment which had been accorded to children born outside marriage under previous legislation' (Cooper 1991). The Act also put an end to the use of the terms *legitimate* and *illegitimate* in Government publications after 1988.

Illegitimacy, stigma, and adoption

Thirty years ago, one major outcome of an extramarital pregnancy was the adoption of the child, usually when very young, by strangers. It has been estimated (Selman 1976) that over one in five of children born outside wedlock were placed for adoption in the 1960s. Adoption was seen as a 'neat and sensible solution' (Benet 1976) to the problems of birth parents, childless couples, and the child in need of a stable family in which to grow up. Following the passing of the 1967 Abortion Act, progressively fewer mothers relinquished their babies for adoption, and now the adoption of babies has become very rare.

We once forced unmarried mothers into mother and baby homes, persuaded them to give their babies up for adoption, and stigmatized those who kept their children; now we recognize that children must come first, have sought to provide support for lone mothers, and yet increasingly take older

Table 7.6 *Distribution of conceptions by outcome, 1969–1992*

	1969 %	1971 %	1975 %	1982 %	1992 %
Abortion	6.5	11.8	15.0	17.0	19.3
Marital births conceived	85.7	80.7	76.1	70.1	54.8
– *inside first marriage*	74.9	70.7	67.3	60.3	47.6
– *2nd or later marriage*	1.8	1.9	2.8	4.3	3.6
– *outside marriage*	9.0	8.1	6.0	5.5	3.6
Non-marital births	7.8	7.6	9.8	12.8	25.9
– *sole registration*	N/A	4.1	4.9	5.2	5.9
– *jointly registered*	N/A	3.5	4.9	7.6	20.0
Total (1000s) = 100%	832.8	835.5	693.3	755.3	828.0

Source: OPCS *conception monitors* FM1 84/6; FM1 95/2.

children away from their families, often against the wishes of their birth parents (Mason and Selman 1997). For most women today the choice is between abortion and keeping the child they give birth to. Earlier assumptions that 'illegitimate' children were unwanted are no longer appropriate when most are born to cohabiting couples.

In her classic study, *Single and pregnant*, MacIntyre (1977) noted that most single women were involved in a complex negotiation as to how they were perceived by friends, relatives, and professionals. The outcome of pregnancy was partly determined by such negotiations and often doctors made oversimplified assumptions about whether a pregnancy was wanted. With the growth in cohabitation described above, the situation of the single, pregnant woman has become even more open to wrong assumptions.

Lone parents

One outcome of the increase in births outside marriage and the rising divorce rates outlined earlier is a growth in the number of single-parent families (Table 7.7) from 570 000 in 1971 to 1.27 million in 1991 (Bradshaw and Millar 1991; Burghes 1993, 1994, 1995). In the past, such families were largely the result of the death of a parent. Late marriage and high death rates amongst men meant that even in the 19th century a clear majority of such families were mother-headed (Dormor 1992).

In the 1970s the growth in one-parent families was gradual and largely a consequence of increased marriage breakdown. More recently, the rise has been more rapid and the largest increase has been in families headed by women who have never married. This is partly due to the rise in non-marital births to single women, but also to the breakdown of cohabitations (Haskey 1994*b*). Most of these mothers are dependent on state benefits so that it is perhaps not surprising that governments have targeted them for criticism (Selman and Glendinning 1995, 1996). The Labour Government is

Table 7.7 *Households with dependent children: Great Britain, 1971–1993*

Household type	1971 %	1981 %	1986 %	1993 %
Two parent	91	88	86	78
Lone mothers	8	11	13	20
– single	−1	−2	−3	−8
– divorced	−2	−4	−6	−7
– separated	−3	−2	−3	−4
– widowed	−2	−2	−1	−1
Lone fathers	1	1	1	2
All lone parents	9	12	14	22

Sources: *General Household Survey 1993*, Series GHS no. 24, Table 2.23.

continuing with the curb in lone-parent benefit proposed by its predecessor, despite widespread concern from its backbenchers.

Conclusion: changes in family circumstances of children

The outcome of all the changes described above is that the family circumstances of children are ever more diverse, with some children experiencing many shifts within their lifetime. Table 7.8 shows the current living arrangements of children aged under 16 (Clarke 1996). Most children still live with their married birth parents, but the proportion has fallen by 15% in a decade and by 1991 more than 25% of children were in stepfamilies or single-parent families.

It is equally true that the family circumstances of children at birth have become more diverse. For most of this century until the early 1960s over 90% of births were to women in their first marriage – 30 years later only 62% of births are to such couples.

The impact of fertility control

The decline in births described earlier has clearly been the result of decisions to limit family size. The agent has been fertility control through contraception, abortion and, more recently, sterilization. However, the initial decline was achieved without modern contraceptive technology (pill; IUCD; surgical sterilization) and long before abortion was legalized.

So what has been the impact since the 1960s of the widespread use of oral contraception and IUDs, the legalization of abortion in 1967, and the growing use of both male and female sterilization? Hall and White (1995) have argued that the changing attitudes to sex and marriage described earlier were a

Table 7.8 *Children aged under 16 according to living arrangements: Great Britain, 1979–1991*

Current living arrangements of child	1979	1984	1991
Living in household with:			
Both natural parents currently			
– married	83	78	68
– cohabiting	1	1	3
Natural mother and stepfather			
– married	4	7	7
– cohabiting	1	2	3
Lone mother	9	10	17
Total	98	98	98
Living apart from mother	2	2	2

Sources: *General Household Survey Report 1979*, Table 8-23, OPCS, London; Clarke, L. (1996); Haskey, J. (1996) – using General Household survey data..

response to innovations in contraceptive technology. Likewise, van de Kaa (1987) argues that it is the advent of highly reliable contraception – with the backup of safe, legal abortion – which triggered the *second* demographic transition, by finally enabling the separation of sex from reproduction.

Contraceptive use

Oral contraception was not widely available in Britain until the 1960s; but by 1967 the proportion of married women using the Pill had risen to 20% and by 1970 40% reported ever use (Cartwright 1970). By 1976 the Pill was the most popular method of birth control used by 29% of *all* women aged 16–49.

Since then the proportion of women currently using some form of contraception has been steady at around 70%, varying by age from one in five teenagers to nearly one in four of those aged 35–44. For married or cohabiting women the figure rises to 80% overall, with less age variation.

The most striking change in contraceptive behaviour in recent years has been the growth of both male and female sterilization. In 1976, 13% of women recorded male or female sterilization as their method of birth control. By 1991, 28% of all women and one in three of married/cohabiting women had been sterilized (or had partners who were sterilized), a figure which rises to over 50% of those aged over 40. At younger ages the Pill continues to be the most popular method of reversible contraception, followed by the condom.

Little is known about how couples make the decision as to who should be sterilized. Vasectomy remains the marginally preferred method for married/cohabiting women. Arguments in terms of the lower risk of the male operation are less compelling today and most choices are probably made on other grounds, including who wants to be 'in control'.

Contraceptive services

The fall in fertility during the first demographic transition was achieved with little help from organized family planning services. Indeed, it was only in 1967 that contraception was tentatively brought into the NHS (though, in practice, largely provided by family planning associations) and only after 1974 that a free service for all women was introduced into the NHS with GP involvement.

Today, GPs are the main provider and a growing number of community family planning clinics are being closed. This move has been encouraged by both GPs and district health authorities (DHAs) on grounds of continuity of medical care, but both also have strong financial interests in such a move, and there is evidence that many women prefer clinics (Selman and Calder 1994).

The main unmet need lies in contraception for teenagers and especially those aged under 18. Research has shown that most pregnancies at this age are unplanned and result from risk-taking (Francome 1995; Selman 1996b), in which one factor is distrust of the confidentiality of existing services. Where contraceptive and sexual health advice are offered to young people outside medical premises, as in the Streetwise project in central Newcastle (Young and Selman 1996), demand tends to outstrip supply, suggesting that the problem of non-use is not primarily one of motivation. In recent years, emergency (post-coital) contraception has emerged as the most likely means of tackling continued risk-taking and reducing the number of abortions and unwanted births.

Advice on effective contraception when sexual activity recommences after a pregnancy, whatever its outcome, is vital if women are to have effective control over their lives. Abortion and maternity services need to embrace contraceptive advice and provision in a positive sense as an older tradition of post-partum and post-abortion sterilization gives way to a system of choice.

Abortion

Although continuously surrounded by controversy, the impact of the 1967 Abortion Act in removing illegal abortion, reducing maternal mortality, and enabling women to avoid unwanted births is clear. In most parts of Britain, pregnant women are now offered choices when their pregnancy is unwanted, although abortion remains illegal in Northern Ireland. The number of abortions in England and Wales rose steadily in the first two decades of the Abortion Act, rising from 91 000 in 1971 to 128 000 in 1981 and a peak of 174 000 in 1990, since when the numbers have fallen slightly (Filakti 1997).

There have been major changes in abortion since 1968:

- only a minority (21%) of abortions now involve married women

- terminations are performed earlier in pregnancy

- vacuum aspiration has replaced dilatation and curettage (D&C) as the most common procedure

- a majority of abortions are now performed as planned day cases.

It is now very rare for a woman to die from legal abortion. Since 1982 there has been one death a year on average and two years in which there were none, compared with 10 a year between 1969 and 1972. In 1960 there were 60 abortion deaths, most of which were attributable to illegal abortions.

Although the proportion of abortions performed outside the NHS has been falling in recent years, there continue to be major regional variations in access to NHS termination. In 1995, the proportion of women having NHS operations in the area where they lived ranged from 93% in Newcastle and North Tyneside District Health Authority to 18% in West Midlands Regional Health Authority, although a further 48% had NHS-funded ('agency') operations in the private sector.

The advent of legal abortion – and the availability of an ever-increasing range of tests – has made the pregnant woman's first contact with antenatal services crucial. If an abortion is agreed, it is vital that women have both pre- and post-abortion counselling and that the termination is taken as an opportunity to ensure that effective contraception is used in the future.

Summary

The availability of male and female sterilization, together with a range of highly effective reversible methods of contraception and the backup of legal abortion, should mean that unwanted births are a thing of the past, but it still seems to be the case that most adolescent pregnancies are unplanned and that the need for improved contraceptive advice for this group continues.

The growing control that women have gained over reproduction has had a number of consequences. Women are more likely to have planned their pregnancy and to have lived independent lives before becoming mothers (Boyd 1985); they are increasingly making choices about when to have their children, whether to have children outside marriage, and whether to work as well as being a mother.

Childbirth – home or hospital

Although living conditions have continued to improve for most people, home births have become increasingly uncommon over the last 30 years. In 1954, over a third of all births took place in the home; by 1970 this had fallen to 13% and by 1981 to just over 1% (Table 7.9). In 1993, 98.34% of all births took place in hospitals, the proportion ranging from 99.5% for women under 20 to 97.44% for those aged 35–39.

The rapid decline in the number and proportion of home births after 1964 was partly a response to the falling birth rate which led to the availability of hospital beds to a growing number of women. In 1970, the Peel report recommended that facilities should be improved to enable all mothers to have their baby in hospital, and this policy initiative linked to further declines in the number of births so that by 1981 the proportion of home births had fallen to an all-time low of 1.1%.

However, growing opposition to what was regarded as a depersonalizing experience (the experience of childbirth in hospital under 'medical management') led to the publication of *Changing Childbirth* (Department of Health 1993). This report recommended changes both in the philosophy and the practice of childbirth, including giving women greater opportunities to give

Table 7.9 *Number and proportion of home births, 1954–1991*

Year	Number of home births	Proportion of all births %
1954	234 000	34.0
1962	274 000	32.0
1964	253 000	28.0
1970	102 970	13.0
1976	14 667	2.5
1981	6 790	1.1
1991	7 800	1.6

Source: MacFarland and Mugford (1984).

birth at home. The report placed greater emphasis on the role of midwives, especially for the majority of low-risk 'normal' pregnancies and births.

October 1996 saw the launch of a campaign to give women more choices in maternity, including more say in where she wants to have her baby. An important part of the campaign is distribution by the Department of Health of a leaflet entitled *How to get the best from maternity services.*

However, choice of place of delivery is not simply home or hospital – a compromise for those disliking the impersonal nature of many hospital wards is a midwife-led or GP unit, or use of the 'domino' system where a midwife who has cared for a woman during pregnancy accompanies her into hospital to deliver the baby.

The debate continues as to the risks of home births. Advocates argue that the evidence is that home births are at least as safe as hospital delivery for low-risk women. Mary Newburn, Head of Policy Research at the National Childbirth Trust, has pointed out that 'when women ask about a home birth, the possible risks are spelt out very clearly to them. But they are never warned about risks of hospital delivery'.

Caring for children

Working women

The proportion of married women who work increased from 10% in the first quarter of this century to 62% in 1980 and 72% in 1991. There has also been a growth in the number of working mothers: in 1992, 59% of married women with dependent children were working in comparison with 47% in 1973; for married women with children under the age of five, the proportion has risen from 25% to 43%.

Lone parents with preschool children are less likely to work. In 1992, the labour force participation was about half that of married women – only 8% worked full time and 14% part time – less than in late 1970s. In many other countries single parents are *more* likely to work and this has led to much debate about the impact of benefits on motivation, but also on the desirability of women with young children entering the workforce. New Labour's policies for 'welfare into work' have resulted in proposals (from Social Security Minister, Harriet Harman) to require all single parents with children aged five and over to discuss plans for employment.

Schoolgirl pregnancies

For the small group of women who have children under 16, the question of future schooling becomes crucial. It is important to ensure that an interrupted education can be resumed and that an early birth does not determine the rest of a girl's life. The American response of making benefit dependent on a return to school indicates one possible response; less punitive and probably more successful is the development of schools for pregnant teenagers where they can continue their studies and receive professional and peer support in pregnancy.

Child care

If women are to resume work after having a child, alternative child care must be arranged. This can range from care by relatives through use of childminders to formal nurseries. When the child is under three, substitute day care is mainly provided by relatives, but parent and toddler groups are also used. By age three and four, playgroups and nursery classes become more important. The number of under-fives in school in the UK rose from 280 000 in 1965 to 850 000 in 1993. Other day-care places – playgroups, nurseries, and childminders – also increased, from 400 000 in 1971 to 985 000 in 1993. In April 1997, a nursery voucher scheme came into operation for all four-year-olds. The new Labour Government announced the abolition of the scheme from September 1997: all four-year-olds whose parents wish it should have free nursery places for September 1998 (Bennett 1998)

Morgan (1996) has argued that the quality of much substitute care in Britain and the USA is very poor, and that children who spend their early years with childminders or in nurseries are disadvantaged compared with those cared for at home. Her arguments challenge the claim that children benefit from 'third-party' child care and support a return to a traditional family with a working father and a caring mother. The evidence could, however, also be used to argue the need for higher quality child care, as developed in other European countries.

Overall, the UK has less publicly funded day care than any other EU country, although this may change as increased provision for single parents is developed as part of the previously mentioned 'welfare into work' policy. Sweden has gone furthest in the development of child care provision to mesh in with their very high female labour force participation. This has been necessitated by the late starting age for formal schooling – seven years. The generous maternity leave described later has meant that Swedish mothers are more able to remain in the workforce in the knowledge that they can take time off as necessary to balance their roles as mother and worker. The quality of their child care provision is also very good. This may be a key factor in Sweden now having the highest birth rate in the EU.

Support systems at home

For most women, support during and after pregnancy must come from their family as well as from the formal systems described above. Although Britain has no system of paternity leave, partners will play a major role and this will increasingly mean unmarried partners as well as husbands. With growing male unemployment and self-employment, the male role may increase. Just under 50% of working mothers of all ages report using their husband or a grandparent as a source of child care. For the youngest mothers, their own mothers will be likely to be the most important source of support; it has been noted that a cycle of teenage parenthood appears to exist, leading to grandmothers in their early and mid thirties caring for their teenage daughter's offspring. None of this should detract from the urgent need for Britain to address the shortage of high-quality child care to meet the needs of working mothers rather than seeking greater dependence on care in the home.

Legitimacy, inheritance, and the rights of unmarried fathers

With one in three children born to single mothers or to couples not legally married, questions of inheritance and the rights of unmarried fathers affect many more children than ever before. Adoption and assisted conception add further complications to the situation facing children from the moment of birth.

The need for law reform was recognized by the early 1980s when the proportion of births outside marriage had risen to over 15%. The Law Commission issued a report in 1982 which argued that the law should not discriminate against those born outside marriage and outlined one solution as the complete abolition of 'illegitimacy'.

An important aim of the 1987 Family Law Reform Act was to remove from the *child* any legal disadvantage arising from the marital status of his parents. The inheritance rights of children of unmarried parents were extended beyond those granted by the earlier 1969 Family Law Reform Act to include grandparents and siblings. However, a child of unmarried parents is still not entitled to British citizenship through the status of his father (Kiernan and Estaugh 1993).

While the rights of a child born outside marriage are now more or less the same as those of the child of married parents, the law has been less willing to grant equal rights to the unmarried father, although he may now apply to the court to hold parental rights and duties jointly with the mother. The growth in cohabitation has made it increasingly important and appropriate to encourage and acknowledge the unmarried father's parental role.

The 1991 Child Support Act has highlighted many of these issues – and indeed those raised earlier in this chapter – by seeking to establish financial responsibility on 'absent parents', defined as the biological parent of a child who does not live in the same household as the child (Clarke *et al.* 1995). An exception to this is where a married woman conceives her child by artificial insemination when her husband is taken to be the parent. An *unmarried* woman must either prove evidence that insemination was by an anonymous donor or name the donor. If a divorced birth father agrees to the adoption of his child by his wife's new husband, he would seem to ensure that no further claim for financial assistance can be made.

Maternity rights

Statutory maternity rights in Britain cover four main areas:

(1) maternity leave and maternity absence

(2) maternity benefits

(3) time off for antenatal care

(4) protection against unfair dismissal.

But within the Patient's Charter, the pregnant woman is also seen as having wider rights and expectations. *The Patient's Charter for Maternity Services* sets out the standards a pregnant woman can expect from maternity services; from a clear choice about where to have a baby and who is to be present at the birth to a right to pain relief, emergency services, and special help for a baby's needs.

Maternity/paternity leave and absence

In Britain, the statutory maternity *leave* period, to which all pregnant employees are entitled regardless of length of service, generally lasts for 14 weeks and is normally takeable from the 11th week before birth. For women with longer periods of continuous employment, additional maternity absence may be available up to the end of the 28th week after birth (Callender *et al.* 1997).

Elsewhere in Europe the right to maternity leave/absence is more clearly established and extends over a longer potential period. In Sweden, father and mother have equal rights to take time off work after the birth and for periods of need throughout a child's first five years. From January 1995, leave of absence with parental benefit is provided for a total of 15 months, to be shared by mother and father and reduced to 14 months if only one takes it. Forty-four per cent of those taking maternity leave are fathers, taking on average 45 days leave.

All pregnant women in employment have a right to time off for antenatal care and are also protected by law against dismissal or unfair treatment for any reason connected with pregnancy, child-rearing, or maternity leave.

Financial payments

Although Beveridge's universal maternity grant has now been phased out, there remain a number of financial payments available to women in relation to childbirth. Most pregnant employees are entitled to 18 weeks of **statutory maternity pay (SMP)**, which is usually 90% of salary for the first six weeks and a flat-rate payment (£57.70 from April 1998) for the remaining 12 weeks. Women not entitled to SMP are entitled to 18 weeks of **maternity** *allowance*, an insurance benefit, payable at the flat rate of SMP for employees and a lower rate for self-employed or unemployed women. Both benefits are normally payable from the 11th week before the expected week of childbirth but only for weeks in which the woman is not working. Women entitled to neither may be able to claim income support or job-seekers allowance from the Benefits Agency. In Sweden, the compensation level is higher – 90% for the first 30 days, 80% for a further 10 months, and a flat-rate payment for the remaining three months.

Mother and baby homes

As a contrast to maternity *rights*, we can look back to alternative support offered in the past to unmarried mothers. For many years such women were sent to 'mother and baby homes', to which as many as 1500 women were admitted in 1978, the last year in which statistics were recorded. The memories of those who experienced such places, especially where they had ended by relinquishing their children for adoption (Howe *et al*. 1992), are a reminder of the very real advances we have made in respecting women no matter what the context of their pregnancy and motherhood. However, recent debates over single mothers have included calls for more adoption and a speech in 1994 by Virginia Bottomley suggesting hostel care for pregnant teenagers.

Conclusion

Most women giving birth have a right to maternity leave and some form of financial support, but the rules of eligibility are complex. Many of the rights described above are rooted in a woman's employment situation. For those not in the labour force, rights are limited to means-tested benefits. Women under 16 face particular difficulties: they are not employees; not eligible for income support; assumed to be the responsibility of families; and facing a future that will all too easily be determined by their early motherhood.

For all women, the availability of informed advice is crucial, whether this is through referral to external agencies such as social workers, the Citizens' Advice Bureau (CAB), or through welfare rights workers located in hospitals or via GPs and midwives. What is, however, especially important is that those in contact with women through pregnancy and beyond – whether doctors or midwives – are knowledgeable enough to be able to direct their patients to such sources.

Further information on maternity rights (Maternity Alliance 1996*a*,*b*) can be obtained from the Maternity Alliance, 45 Beech St, London EC2P 2LX.

Challenges for the 21st century

Assisted conception

The range of procedures normally included under this term covers: artificial insemination using husband's sperm (AIH); donor insemination (DI); *in vitro* fertilization (IVF), using either a couple's own gametes or using donated sperm and/or donated eggs; embryo donation; and, finally, surrogacy (again possibly, though not necessarily, using donated sperm or eggs). Though two of these procedures have been used extensively in the past (surrogacy for an unknown duration and DI since the 1940s), they all received much greater publicity from 1978 with the birth of the world's first 'test-tube baby'. This was followed in the UK by the report of the Warnock Committee which had been appointed to consider the social and ethical implications of these new developments in human fertilization and embryology (Warnock 1985).

The point has been made earlier in this chapter that contraception provided the opportunity of sex without reproduction. The possibility of assisted conception provided another challenge: reproduction without sex (Snowden *et al.* 1983).

Though greeted with some concern initially for exactly that reason (such interventions were seen as unnatural and as 'going too far'), it would be fair to say that in the late 1990s these interventions have gained a widespread social acceptability. However, the greater degree of lay literacy on matters of conception and medical science has produced its own problems which GPs and midwives will need to be aware of when discussing these options with patients. One way of airing these issues is to move chronologically through the possible treatment process, from first consultation to post-treatment.

Patients referring themselves to GPs with 'fertility problems' may have unrealistic expectations of achieving pregnancy through 'natural intercourse' and may therefore be referring themselves too early. Whilst this needs careful discussion, it may be the case that they also have unrealistic expectations of assisted conception to solve their problems, if indeed such problems exist. GPs will also need to give some consideration to the amount of work they devote to avoiding fertility problems in the first place. It is worth noting that assisted conception does not cure infertility, it merely circumvents the consequences.

Another category of patient may consult with a GP: those with 'social infertility'. That is, patients who want to become parents but who need assistance either because they are single women who do not have or do not want a relationship with a man, or because they are gay or lesbian couples who need help from a third party to either donate sperm or to act as a surrogate mother for them.

Whilst all these different categories of patients could refer themselves directly to private fertility clinics (who may nonetheless refer them back to the GP for an initial screening as to the appropriateness of a fertility referral), it is also likely that GPs will have requests for help from patients who cannot afford private treatment. Such patients are likely to need a great deal of support whilst they undergo the long wait for treatment, which can be up to five years in some NHS-funded clinics (Haimes and Stark, forthcoming).

Not all patients referred to fertility clinics will be suitable for treatment and not all those who are suitable for some form of intervention will be suitable for assisted conception. Again, given the media hype of DI and IVF as the solution to fertility problems, the GP is likely to have to provide some support to those for whom treatment is not appropriate, since they are going to have to come to terms with the possibility of remaining childless. As with those patients seeking support whilst on the waiting list, the extent of work that the

GP is likely to have to provide remains relatively invisible, as there has been very little research on this topic.

Even when a patient is deemed suitable for treatment, the GP may retain some involvement, particularly in cases of IVF. This may range from providing assistance with the treatment process (such as providing a nurse to give the daily injections) to providing the cost of the drugs from the practice budget. Patients have reported some difficulties in persuading the GP to pay for these drugs (Haimes and Stark, op. cit.). One clinic has estimated that these are likely to cost £520 per treatment cycle at 1996 prices. Clearly, this is a matter for negotiation between the GP, the patient, and the clinic, but it is exactly these sorts of issues that rarely get discussed in the media coverage of assisted conception, yet they have major implications for both patients and doctors.

If treatment is successful, the GP will be involved in the usual antenatal care but in addition will have to be clear how much patients have told others about their treatment. Whilst doctor–patient confidentiality is always important, it may be that under these circumstances special precautions need to be taken as to the sharing of information with other professionals. Patients receiving DI are particularly reluctant to share this information with others, let alone with the child, so the need to retain patient control over information dissemination is vital, not just once treatment has ended but throughout the child's life if necessary. However, the GP may wish to counsel patients against absolute secrecy where donated gametes are involved since there are possible implications as to the fears of inheriting genetic diseases (see below), which may be entirely inappropriate under the circumstances since this may have been the motivation behind using DI in the first place.

If treatment fails (as it is likely to do in 75–80% of IVF attempts), it is possible that the GP will become the main source of support whilst patients work to accept the situation.

Genetics and primary care

The clinical implications of the 'new genetics' are discussed in Chapter 15. Here we shall just outline what are likely to be some of the practical implications of this work for general practitioners and for primary care as a whole. Most of these issues have been the subject of discussion in a multidisciplinary group in the north east, set up specifically to identify the research that is needed to resolve those practical difficulties (Genetics in the Community, University of Newcastle).

It is likely that developments in knowledge of the genetic components in disease will present a major challenge to primary care, particularly when identifying individuals and families at risk in the community. This requires both new techniques of conceptualizing the patient (as individual or as family?) and new techniques of patient care (how to elicit effective family histories; how to counsel individuals and families at risk; how to liaise effectively with secondary care; how to provide treatment in the community). Such problems are likely to involve practice nurses and midwives as much as general practitioners, so there will be a need to train and coordinate staff in the requisite skills.

It is likely that these developments will tie in with the developments in assisted conception since screening will increasingly involve preconceptual and prenatal techniques.

References

Armitage, B. and Babb, P. (1996). Population review: (4) Trends in fertility. *Population Trends*, 84, 7–13.

Babb, P. (1993). Teenage conceptions and fertility in England and Wales 1971–1991. *Population Trends*, 74, 12–17.

Benet, M. (1976). *The character of adoption*. Jonathan Cape, London.

Bennett, F. (1998). Social policy digest no. 105. *Journal of Social Policy*, 27, 99–121.

Block, G. and Thane, P. (1991). *Maternity and gender policies: women and the rise of the European welfare states, 1880s–1950s*. Routledge, London.

Boyd, C. (1985). Women's expectations of pregnancy. In: *Modern obstetrics in general practice* (ed. G. Marsh). Oxford University Press, Oxford.

Bradshaw, J. and Millar, J. (1991). *Lone parents in the UK*. HMSO, London.

Burghes, L. (1993). *One-parent families: policy options for the 1990s*. Family Policy Studies Centre, London.

Burghes, L. (1994). *Lone parenthood and family disruption: the outcomes for children*. Family Policy Studies Centre, London.

Burghes, L. (1995). *Single lone mothers: problems, prospects, and policies*. Family Policy Studies Centre, London.

Burns, A. (1995). Mother-headed families: here to stay? In: *Childhood and parenthood* (ed. J. Brannen and M. O'Brien). Proceedings of the ISA Committee for Family Research Conference, London, 28–30 April 1994.

Callender, C., et al. (1997). *Maternity rights and benefits in Britain 1996*. Department of Social Security research report no. 67. HMSO, London.

Cartwright, A. (1970). *Parents and family planning services*. Routledge, London.

Charles, E. (1934). *The twilight of parenthood*. Watts & Co., London.

Clarke, L. (1996). At the expense of the children? Demographic change and the family situation of children in Britain. In: *Children and families: research and policy* (ed. J. Brannen and M. O'Brien). Falmer, London.

Clarke, K., Glendinning, C., and Craig, G. (1995). The Child Support Act. In: *Childhood and parenthood* (ed. J. Brannen and M. O'Brien). Proceedings of the ISA Committee for Family Research Conference, London, 28–30 April 1994.

Cooper, J. (1991). Births outside marriage: recent trends and associated demographic and social changes. *Population Trends*, 63, 8–18.

Council of Europe (1995). *Recent demographic developments in Europe 1995*. Council of Europe, Strasbourg.

David, H. P. (1990). United States and Denmark: different approaches to health care and family planning. *Studies in Family Planning*, 21(1), 1–19.

Dennis, N. (1993). *Rising crime and the dismembered family*. IEA, London.

Dennis, N. and Erdos, G. (1992). *Families without fatherhood*. IEA, London.

Department of Health (1993). *Changing childbirth: report of the Expert Maternity Group* (Cumberledge report). HMSO, London.

Dormor, D. (1992). *The relationship revolution: cohabitation, marriage, and divorce in contemporary Europe*. One plus One, London.

Ferri, E. (1984). *Stepchildren: a national study*. NFER, London.

Filakti, H. (1997). Trends in abortion, 1990–1995. *Population Trends*, 87, 11–19.

Francome, C. (1993). *Children who have children*. Family Planning Association, London.

Haimes, E. and Stark, C. (forthcoming.) *Patients' evaluation of NHS-funded in vitro fertilization: final report*. Department of Social Policy, University of Newcastle.

Hall, R. and White, P. (1995). *Europe's population: towards the next century*. UCL Press, London.

Haskey, J. (1983). Children of divorcing parents. *Population Trends*, **31**, 20.

Haskey, J. (1989). Current projections of proportions of marriages ending in divorce. *Population Trends*, **55**.

Haskey, J. (1992). Patterns of marriage, divorce, and cohabitation in the different countries of Europe. *Population Trends*, **69**, 28–36.

Haskey, J. (1993). Trends in the numbers of one-parent families in Great Britain. *Population Trends*, **71**, 26–33.

Haskey, J. (1994a). Stepfamilies and stepchildren in Great Britain. *Population Trends*, **76**, 17–28.

Haskey, J. (1994b). Estimated numbers of one-parent families and their prevalence in Great Britain in 1991. *Population Trends*, **78**, 5–19.

Haskey, J. (1996). Population review: (6) Families and households in Great Britain. *Population Trends*, 85, 7–24.

Hoem, B. and Hoem, J. (1988). The Swedish family: aspects of contemporary developments. *Journal of Family Issues*, **9**(3).

Howe, D., et al. (1992). *Half a million women: mothers who lose their children by adoption*. Penguin, London.

Humphrey, R. (ed.) *Families behind the headlines*. Department of Social Policy, University of Newcastle.

Kiernan, K. (1995). Panel discussion at Family Policy Studies Centre seminar. *Cohabitation: a threat to family stability?* 5 July 1995.

Kiernan, K. and Estaugh, V. (1993). *Cohabitation: extramarital childbearing and social policy*. Family Policy Studies Centre, London.

Lewis, J. (1991). Models of equality for women: the case of state support for children in twentieth-century Britain. In: *Maternity and gender policies: women and the rise of the European welfare states, 1880s–1950s* (ed. G. Block and P. Thane). Routledge, London.

MacFarlane, A. and Mugford, M. (1984). *Birth counts: statistics of pregnancy and childbirth*. HMSO, London.

MacIntyre, S. (1977). *Single and pregnant*. Croom Helm, London.

Mason, K. and Selman, P. (1997). Birth parents' experience of contested adoption. *Adoption and Fostering*, **21**(1), 21–8.

McRae, S. (1993). *Cohabiting mothers: changing marriage and motherhood?* Policy Studies Institute, London.

Maternity Alliance (1996a). *Money for mothers and babies*. Maternity Alliance, London.

Maternity Alliance (1996b). *Pregnant at work*. Maternity Alliance, London.

Morgan, P. (1995). *Farewell to the family?* Institute for Economic Affairs, London.

Morgan, P. (1996). *Who needs parents? The effects of child care and early education on children in Britain and the USA*. Institute for Economic Affairs, London.

Office of Population Censuses and Surveys (1987a). *Marriage and divorce statistics, England and Wales, 1837–1983*. HMSO, London.

Office of Population Censuses and Surveys (1987b). *Birth statistics, England and Wales, 1837–1983*. HMSO, London.

Selman, P. (1976). Patterns of adoption in England and Wales since 1959. *Social Work Today*, 7(7).

Selman, P. (1977). *Differential fertility in working-class women in Newcastle upon Tyne*. Unpublished PhD Thesis, University of Newcastle.

Selman, P. (1996a). The Relationship Revolution: is the family collapsing or adjusting to a new world of equal opportunities? In: *Families behind the headlines* (ed. R. Humphrey). Department of Social Policy, University of Newcastle upon Tyne.

Selman, P. (1996b). Teenage motherhood then and now: a comparison of the pattern and outcome of teenage pregnancy in England and Wales in the 1960s and 1980s. In: *The politics of the family* (ed. H. Jones and J. Millar), pp. 103–28. Avebury, Aldershot.

Selman, P. and Calder, J. (1994). Family planning: women's choices. *Nursing Times*, **90**(40), 48–50.

Selman, P. and Glendinning, C. (1995). Teenage parenthood and social policy. *Youth and Policy*, **47**, 39–58.

Selman, P. and Glendinning, C. (1996). Teenage pregnancy: do social policies make a difference? In: *Children and families: research and social policy* (ed. J. Brannen and M. O'Brien). Falmer, London.

Snowden, R., Mitchell, D., and Snowden, E. *Artificial reproduction*. Allen and Unwin, London.

Titmuss, R. and Titmuss, K. (1942). *Parents revolt: a study of the declining birth rate in an acquisitive society*. Secker and Warburg, London.

van de Kaa, D. (1987). Europe's second demographic transition. *Population Bulletin*, **42**, 1–59.

Warnock, M. (1985). *A question of life*. Basil Blackwell, Oxford.

Young, F. and Selman, P. (1996). *An evaluation of the Streetwise project*. Department of Social Policy, University of Newcastle.

CHAPTER 8

The economics of maternity care

Sara Twaddle and Denise Young

Introduction

This chapter introduces the basic concepts of economic evaluation before discussing their particular relevance to maternity services. It begins by defining the terminology used by economists, the techniques used in economic appraisals, and briefly discussing issues in costing and the measurement and evaluation of outcomes of maternity care. The cost-effectiveness of different forms of maternity care is then reviewed. The chapter concludes by identifying areas where further work is required.

Economic evaluation

In this section, the basic principles of economic evaluation are outlined and the reader is introduced to some of the terminology.

Economic evaluation starts with the notion of scarcity of resources. This simply means that there are not, and never will be, enough resources to satisfy all of society's wants and desires. It is therefore inevitable that choices have to be made. As a result, some activities will be given up. This is the concept of 'opportunity cost'. The opportunity cost of the use of resources in a health care programme is the benefit that they could have generated in their next best alternative use. Therefore, economic evaluation involves looking at both the costs and benefits (or outcomes) of health care programmes. The opportunity cost of providing maternity care is the benefit that could have been obtained from the next best use of the resources. The objective of economic evaluation in health care is to implement programmes in which the benefit exceeds the opportunity costs of such programmes, to ensure that society maximizes benefit given scarce resources.

An economic evaluation should involve a comparison of at least two alternatives, even if the alternative is 'do nothing'. It is important to provide a full description of each alternative since this enables the reader to assess whether the appropriate alternatives have been considered and whether any appropriate alternative has been excluded (Coyle and Davies 1993).

Another important concept in economics is the margin. This refers to the fact that most decisions in health care are not about whether or not to introduce a programme but whether to expand or contract it. Therefore, it is important to estimate the marginal costs and benefits of a programme, that is, the cost or benefit of producing one more or one less unit of output.

Economic evaluation can address two levels of questions in health care – questions of technical efficiency and questions of allocative efficiency. The former are concerned with how best to achieve a given objective and are defined as either maximizing benefit for a given cost or minimizing cost for a given benefit. The latter are concerned with whether it is worth doing something at all and the objective is to maximize total benefit over total costs. In both cases economists are seeking a 'cost-effective' allocation of resources. For technical efficiency questions, a cost-effective solution exists when costs are minimized for a given outcome or outcomes are maximized for a given cost. For allocative efficiency questions, cost-effectiveness requires the value of outcomes to exceed the cost.

Types of economic evaluation

There are four types of economic evaluation: cost-minimization analysis (CMA), cost-effectiveness analysis (CEA), cost-utility analysis (CUA), and cost-benefit analysis (CBA). The first three techniques address questions of technical efficiency and cost-benefit analysis addresses allocative efficiency. The main difference between them are in the methods used to measure the benefits or outcomes of alternative programmes. The principles of costing are identical for each type of evaluation.

Cost-minimization analysis is the simplest form of analysis used by economists and is used where outcomes are known to be identical. Under CMA, only cost differences need to be analysed and the least costly alternative is chosen.

Cost-effectiveness analysis requires a comparison of both costs and outcomes. Using CEA, outcomes are measured in single dimensional natural units such as life years saved or cases successfully treated. Costs are related to outcomes by producing cost-effectiveness ratios which are simply measures of cost per unit of health outcome. The programme with the lowest cost per unit of outcome or maximum outcome for a given cost is chosen under the rules of CEA.

Cost-utility analysis is similar to CEA in many ways, the main difference being that CUA measures outcomes in healthy years. It combines both aspects of survival and health status into one measure, usually the quality-adjusted life year (QALY). The QALY simply combines the life years gained by an intervention with some judgement about the quality of those life years. Under CUA, the programme with the lowest cost per additional QALY obtained or the programme which maximizes QALYs for a given cost is selected.

Cost-benefit analysis incorporates multidimensional aspects of health outcome in the evaluation. Costs and outcomes are valued in the same units, usually in monetary terms, thus it is possible to determine whether the benefit of a programme exceeds its cost. When considering the efficiency of one programme, one should consider whether the benefits are greater than its opportunity costs. When more than one programme is involved, it is necessary to compare the costs and outcomes of each programme. If only one can be funded, then the programme that maximizes net benefit should be chosen. The combination that maximizes benefits should be chosen where more than one programme can be funded.

Costing in economic evaluation

The costs to be included in any study will depend on the objectives and context of the evaluation. If the evaluation is performed from a wide societal perspective, then three main categories should be considered: health service costs, costs borne by the service users and their families, and external costs borne by society (Robinson 1993). In practice, external costs are rarely included and this discussion will concentrate on costs to the health service and costs borne by the users of the services and their families.

There are three stages involved in costing resource use: identification of the relevant elements of resource use, measurement of resource use, and valuation of resource use.

The identification stage basically involves listing the likely effects on resource use of the introduction of a new programme or a change in an existing one. The perspective of the study is very important; for example, there is little point in identifying costs to users of the service if the viewpoint for the analysis is that of the hospital. For example, in considering a change in the pattern of antenatal care it is very likely that costs to pregnant women and their families will be affected. However, if the decision-maker is concerned only with the hospital budget there is little point in using scarce research time to measure these costs.

Health service costs usually include staff time (e.g. doctors and nurses), consumables (e.g. drugs and tests), hotel services (e.g. catering), overheads (e.g. hospital administration), and capital items (e.g. land, buildings, and equipment). The most obvious resource use in maternity services is staff time, and this often forms a large part of the total costs.

Women attending for maternity care and their families may also incur costs. These will include out-of-pocket expenses such as travel, child-care costs, and costs of caring for other dependants. It is important to consider these costs in economic evaluation since if they are high some women may not attend.

Such costs are called the direct costs of the programme. Economists are also interested in the indirect costs, such as lost paid (employed) and unpaid (housework, leisure) productive activities and any psychological stress which women and their families may experience such as anxiety awaiting results of tests.

Resource use is measured in natural units. For example, staff time would be measured in units of time and tests would be measured as the number of tests ordered. It is good practice to report quantities of resource use as well as costs to enable readers from other parts of the country to assess the relevance of the results to their practice.

Valuation involves placing a monetary value on each element of resource use. In many cases this will be market prices. Sometimes the true opportunity cost may diverge from these but in most cases market prices are used unless there is strong evidence to suggest that they diverge greatly (Robinson 1993). For example, staff time can be valued by wages and medical supplies can be valued by prices.

In the case of indirect costs, however, there may be no market price and values must be imputed; this is known as shadow pricing. For example, lost leisure time has been valued at 43% of the national average wage (Department of Transport 1987).

Measuring and valuing outcomes in the economic evaluation of maternity care

Outcome analysis involves a number of distinct stages. However, the outcomes depend crucially on the question being addressed. If, for example, the objective is to determine the most efficient way of providing analgesia during labour, the relevant outcome would be pain relief. On the other hand, a comparison of obstetrician-led care with midwife-managed care for normal healthy pregnancies would require consideration of a wide range of outcomes for both mother and baby.

Mugford and Drummond (1989) define the outcomes of perinatal care in terms of the effect on the quality of life of those receiving care and those on whom they depend. This 'corresponds very closely to the sort of measurement that would be considered in clinical evaluation'. It is, therefore, to clinical evaluation studies that economists have turned to for help for appropriate outcome measures in maternity services.

The general response to the question of 'what outcome measure is appropriate to use in studies of maternity services?' is invariably 'the health of the mother and baby'. Thus there are a minimum of four potential outcomes of any intervention (Table 8.1).

There has been increasing awareness recently of the importance of psychological outcomes, thus complicating matters by moving away from

Table 8.1 *Clinical outcomes in maternity care*

	Mother: Healthy	Not healthy
Baby:		
Healthy	1	2
Not healthy	3	4

the 'healthy mother and baby' scenario to the 'healthy and satisfied mother and healthy baby' scenario. The number of potential outcomes becomes eight (Table 8.2).

The problem is defining 'healthy' and 'satisfied' and there are no 'off the shelf' measures which can be used. Clinical outcomes are often used for health and satisfaction via *ad hoc* questionnaires.

Maternal and perinatal mortality are commonly reported, but few studies are large enough to pick up significant changes. Instead, studies tend to concentrate on a small number of clinical outcomes such as gestation and fetal weight at delivery, mode of delivery, Apgar scores, and admission to special care.

Morbidity is frequently proxied by process items such as admission rates. The use of such intermediate outcomes is not a problem providing: first, they are directly related to final outcome; and second, they proxy all aspects of final outcome. In maternity services, however, such measures may not be a good proxy for final outcome since, for example, social admissions for rest are not uncommon.

Economic evaluation of maternity services

Drummond and Stoddart (1984) have argued that economic evaluation must justify itself in economics terms, and that is it is only worthwhile when the potential differences in net cost between procedures is greater than the cost of the research. They suggest that economic evaluation is most appropriate when: first, large amounts of resources are at stake; second, a decision is imminent about a new technology or technique; and third, resource indications imply a need to change existing practice. Subsequently, Mugford and Drummond (1989) have included the additional criteria, namely, where resources could be allocated to a better use by changing or abandoning existing practice.

Several factors would seem to suggest that obstetrics would score well against these criteria: first, more than 4% of NHS expenditure is spent on maternity services; second, there have been a large number of recommendations recently about the way that maternity services are organized; and third, the Cochrane Pregnancy and Childbirth Module (Neilson *et al.* 1997)

Table 8.2 *Clinical and psychological outcomes in maternity services*

	Mother: Healthy and satisfied	Healthy and not satisfied	Not healthy and satisfied	Not healthy and not satisfied
Baby:				
Healthy	1	2	3	4
Not healthy	8	7	6	5

provides accessible information about the effectiveness of interventions. This allows secondary economic evaluations using the results from published studies and applying local cost data.

However, economic analysis of maternity services has not attracted high priority, with the possible exceptions being neonatal intensive care and prenatal screening. A bibliography of economic evaluations listed only 34 studies in the field of obstetrics (Backhouse *et al.* 1992). Although this may reflect the dearth of economic evaluations in general, it could be that the issues discussed above (i.e. two agents involved and the lack of appropriate outcome measures) explains the lack of published studies about maternity services.

Given this dearth of applied economic evaluation, this chapter draws on both formal economic evaluations where they exist and on other studies containing information on costs and outcomes which allow the economic impact of changes in policy to be estimated. The rest of the chapter considers the economic implications of various aspects of antenatal care, intrapartum care, postnatal care, and total packages of maternity care.

The economic implications of antenatal care

Antenatal care offers the largest scope for economic analysis. This is largely because of the potential for: first, the involvement of different professionals; second, alternative processes; third, alternative locations; and fourth, different amounts of routine care. We consider first the economic implications of various aspects of routine antenatal care and second, the implications of caring for women with high-risk pregnancies.

Routine antenatal care

There are several aspects of routine antenatal care which raise interesting economic issues. These include the appropriate number of antenatal visits, increased use of community-based care, the role of different health care professionals, ultrasound screening, and screening for complications.

Number of antenatal visits

The optimum number of antenatal visits has been a perennial source of debate, with the main evidence for different patterns of antenatal care coming from variations in levels of provision and mortality rates (Chapter 19). However, Hall and colleagues (1980) have argued that this is not valid and the rate at which asymptomatic problems are missed, diagnosed, and over-diagnosed should be considered. Based on a study of almost 20 000 clinic attendances, they showed that the productivity of clinics in terms of predicting and/or detecting obstetric problems was very low in parous women and only greater than 1% in primiparous women after 34 weeks. They subsequently recommended a pattern of five visits for parous women and additional visits only after 34 weeks for primiparous women. The Royal College of Obstetricians and Gynaecologists adopted this policy in 1984;

however, changes in practice have been slow. For example, in 1989, pregnant women in Scotland typically received 14 visits during the antenatal period (Tucker *et al.* 1994).

Despite the obvious economic implications, only one economic evaluation explicitly addresses the relative cost-effectiveness of different numbers of antenatal visits. Artells-Herrero *et al.* (1982) showed (in a Spanish hospital) that the most cost-effective allocation of resources would be achieved by reallocating resources from women receiving more than nine visits to women receiving less than five.

In the UK, only one study addresses this issue but without formal economic evaluation. Sikorski *et al.* (1996) compared the traditional pattern of antenatal visits with a pattern of reduced visits in a randomized controlled trial and found that clinical effectiveness was similar, psychological outcomes were poorer, and resource use, and hence cost, was reduced. The question of interest to policy-makers is therefore: 'Is the reduction in cost worth the reduction in psychological outcomes?'

Increased community-based antenatal care

In Scotland, a recently completed randomized controlled trial compared the traditional pattern of shared antenatal care between the obstetrician, GP, and the midwife with a new pattern of combined GP and midwife antenatal care in the community (Tucker *et al.* 1996). The conclusion of the study was that GP and midwife-based community antenatal care was more cost-effective than standard shared care for selected women.

This supports previous costing work from Aberdeen which suggested that costs to the NHS of antenatal clinics in the community are less than hospital clinics (Meldrum 1989). The lowest cost option from the point of view of the NHS was health centre antenatal clinics and the highest cost option was the hospital. However, it is important to note that if the pattern of antenatal care was changed so that the majority of visits were held in health centres, only a modest cost saving would result to the NHS since most hospital costs are fixed or semi-fixed. The more dramatic effect would be in terms of the reduced costs to women of attending.

Role of different health professionals

Staff mix in antenatal care has attracted some attention. The main issue has been whether midwives can carry out standard antenatal care as efficiently as obstetricians and/or GPs. Unsurprisingly, the few 'costing' studies in this area have concluded that midwife-only services are associated with lower costs than antenatal clinics staffed by obstetricians and/or GPs (Seiner and Lairson 1985; Giles *et al.* 1992; Graveley and Littlefield 1992). However, these results were based purely on comparisons of salary costs per hour or on the total operating cost of the clinic and did not consider the process of care or outcomes.

Ultrasound screening

This has attracted much debate (Lilford and Chard 1985). In particular, there has been controversy over whether it should be offered to all women or only to certain high-risk groups. The economic argument against blanket screening policies is that it might lead to higher resource use; however, better outcomes for scanned babies may result.

The evidence on the potential for increased resource use is ambiguous; Bakketeig *et al.* (1984) reported increased hospital admissions and length of stay in the scanned group, Eik-Nes *et al.* (1984) reported significantly reduced admission rates and Waldenstrom *et al.* (1988) reported no difference.

However, the clinical evidence on ultrasound screening is less ambiguous with no evidence of significant improvement. A meta-analysis by Bucher and Schmidt (1993) of almost 16 000 pregnancies concluded that routine ultrasound screening does not improve the number of live births nor reduce perinatal mortality.

Only one economic evaluation explicitly compares the cost-effectiveness of routine first trimester scans with a selective approach (Temmerman and Buekens 1991). It concludes that limiting scans to certain specific indications would save $22 000 per 1000 women screened and result in 10 multiple pregnancies, six missed abortions, one congenital malformation, and one tubal pregnancy being detected later. The question of interest to the policy-maker therefore becomes: 'Is the reduction in cost worth the later detection of these conditions?'

Screening for complications

The majority of screening tests for complications (rubella status, blood grouping, and full blood counts) are uncontroversial and are rarely debated. However, screening for gestational diabetes, urinary tract infections, and hypertension have attracted some attention.

Most women are routinely tested for the presence of diabetes and urinary tract infections at every visit. However, concerns about the sensitivity and specificity of the dipstick urine test have redirected attention towards alternatives targeted at higher-risk groups (Bachman *et al.* 1993). One secondary economic evaluation concluded that 'the available data do not clearly demonstrate a favourable cost-benefit ratio in universal screening for gestational diabetes' (Everett 1989).

Hypertension affects between one third and one fifth of first, and between one fifth and one tenth of subsequent pregnancies (Hall and Campbell 1987). Hence blood pressure is measured routinely at each visit. Since primiparous women are at higher risk than parous women, it has been recommended that they have at least one additional blood pressure check. However, Hall and Campbell (1992) demonstrated that 37 174 primiparous women would have to be screened to prevent one maternal death. They concluded that since the number of women potentially affected are so large and the productivity of checks so low, there may be gains from targeting high-risk groups. This study has interesting economic implications, in effect implying that the cost of 37 174 blood pressure checks are worth less than the chance of saving one life.

Management of high-risk pregnancies

Given the high risks to the health of the mother and fetus and the intensive resource use aimed at minimizing complications, this is an interesting area for economists. Traditionally, the majority of antenatal care for women with high-risk pregnancies took place in hospital, however in the last 20 years alternatives have been proposed. Monitoring of high-risk pregnancies, hypertension, multiple pregnancies, and the prevention of preterm labour have all attracted considerable attention.

Monitoring of high-risk pregnancies

There are alternatives to in-patient care for women with high-risk pregnancies: first, day-care units where they are monitored intensively over a short period and then go home; and second, home monitoring, either by hospital staff visiting women in their homes, or by self-monitoring or electronic monitoring by telephone. To inform decision-making, economic evaluations must consider the number of out-patient visits, day-care attendances, or home monitoring episodes required to reduce in-patient resource use, as well as any extra costs to women which may affect participation. In practice, however, these factors are rarely reported fully.

Day-care units have been shown to reduce in-patient stay significantly for women with bleeding and pain in early pregnancy (Bigrigg and Read 1991) and for many pregnancy complications (Soothill *et al.* 1991). Domiciliary management of high-risk pregnancy, using telephone monitoring, was found to reduce in-patient stay compared to routine care, with no significant difference in perinatal mortality (Dawson *et al.* 1989). Home-administered monitoring by means of non-stress tests was also found to be safe and associated with significantly lower costs when compared to hospital care (Reece *et al.* 1992).

Hypertension in pregnancy

The management of hypertension in pregnancy is of particular importance since it is common and has potentially fatal consequences. From an economic perspective, several studies have demonstrated reduced resource use associated with new methods of care; however, most of these have concentrated on reduced in-patient bed days.

Traditionally, care has relied on admission and bed rest, with early delivery if required. This has been challenged in recent years (Mathews 1977; Crowther *et al.* 1992) and alternative care has been introduced for less severe hypertension.

Day care has attracted the most attention since it is assumed that it will reduce in-patient care, although few studies have addressed this formally. Research shows that the introduction of day facilities changes the process of care – in-patient care reduced but out-patient care increased (Tuffnell *et al.*

1992; McGregor 1987). The threshold for treatment may also fall, with more intervention in milder disease (McGregor 1987). Consequently, total costs to the NHS might be expected to increase rather than decrease.

One economic evaluation of day care for hypertension in pregnancy (Twaddle and Harper 1992) showed that it was more cost-effective than in-patient care only if prior selection of women took place to screen out those with transient hypertension. Prior selection, it was argued, could involve an additional clinic, or visit by a GP or midwife.

The use of alternatives outside the hospital, such as domiciliary visits by community midwives and home-based monitoring schemes, have been shown to reduce the number of hospital admissions considerably (Feeney 1984; Helewa *et al.* 1993). Ambulatory blood pressure measurement is currently being investigated.

For women with hypertension, an automated blood pressure profile has been shown to reliably predict which of them are most likely to develop severe disease. This would allow most to return home, leading to potential 'massive savings in hospital beds' (Mooney and Dalton 1990).

Multiple pregnancies

Compared with singleton pregnancies, multiple pregnancies (one in eight) are associated with higher levels of preterm labour and delivery (Papiernik and Keith 1990). Multiple pregnancies are also more likely to develop hypertension and other serious complications.

Traditionally, hospital bed rest from around 30 weeks has been the treatment and this has obvious implications for the use of hospital in-patient resources. However, several studies have shown that hospital bed rest is no more effective at preventing preterm labour than home rest (Hartikainen-Sorri and Joupilla 1984; Saunders *et al.* 1985). Limiting bed rest may benefit certain high-risk groups, but no improvement in fetal outcome has been demonstrated (Crowther *et al.* 1989).

Prevention of preterm labour

Preterm delivery and the associated low birthweight infants place a large burden on scarce resources. Low birthweight infants are more likely to be admitted to a neonatal unit and have significantly higher morbidity and mortality compared with term babies (Morrison *et al.* 1989). Therefore, early detection of preterm labour and preventative action to avoid preterm delivery could lead to large health gains and reduced resource use.

Morrison *et al.* (1989) found that ambulatory uterine activity monitoring was effective in increasing gestation at birth and reducing neonatal hospital stay. Kosasa and colleagues (1990) subsequently demonstrated reduced hospital costs.

Korenbrot *et al.* (1984) considered the effect of using tocolytic agents at different gestations on hospital costs. They found that the increased costs of prenatal care were offset by the decreased costs of neonatal care when treatment was given before 34 weeks of gestation, whereas there was no cost saving after 34 weeks. Finally, Weiner and colleagues (1988) considered the cost-effectiveness of aggressive tocolysis compared with no therapy in cases of preterm labour where rupture of the membranes has occurred. There was no significant difference in cost per survivor under the two alternatives, except in pregnancies delivering before 28 weeks which had significantly higher costs per survivor associated with tocolysis.

Other high-risk pregnancies

Droste and Keil (1994) compared home bed rest with elective hospital care for women with complete placenta praevia. The authors showed that there were no significant differences in outcome between the two groups and the cost of care was significantly higher in the in-patient group. They conclude therefore that judicious out-patient care of selected women with complete placenta praevia can be both cost-effective and safe.

Economic implications of intrapartum care

Intrapartum care provides several issues of interest to the economist in terms of alternative locations for care, the different professionals involved in care, and the different processes of care.

Increased births in GP units

Despite some interesting economic issues, birth in GP units has not attracted much attention. These units tend to have low occupancy rates and therefore very high average costs per birth. A recent Scottish policy document (Scottish Office Home and Health Department 1993) suggested that occupancy should be increased to reduce average costs but offered no guidance as to how this should be done. Possible options might include reducing the number of beds in these units by closure or by redesignating them to other patients. In the long run, closing beds may reduce expenditure if staff are made redundant as a result, but redesignating them for other uses would not reduce total NHS expenditure. The success of policies to increase throughput in GP units would depend crucially upon the success and costs of persuading women to change from giving birth in a consultant unit to a GP unit.

Increased 'domino' and home births

An increase in the number of 'domino' births may involve higher expenditure on community services with few offsetting savings on hospital services. The extra community costs would result from the employment of additional midwives, the on-call payments to ensure 24-hour cover for women in labour, and start-up costs of training midwives to provide a new model of care. The degree to which hospital expenditure would be reduced is uncertain because: first, provision will still be required for the 50% of women who are high risk at the start of their pregnancy or who acquire risk factors during pregnancy (Cole and McIlwaine 1994); second, community-based staff may have a lower threshold for referral to in-patient or day care; and third, domino births take place in obstetric units which does not allow reduced capital costs unless the numbers are sufficient to allow closure of a postnatal ward. Hence, the overall impact of increasing domino deliveries may be to increase NHS expenditure.

Home births involve the least NHS expenditure of any type of birth during the intrapartum period (Ferster and Pethybridge 1973; Stilwell 1979). However, it is important to note that this does not imply that a shift towards more home deliveries would reduce total NHS costs. Given the very small proportion of births which currently occur in the home, the additional workload could be absorbed within the existing resources of most maternity hospitals, thus the difference in average cost between the two would not reflect any savings. In other words, the marginal cost of an additional hospital delivery is very low, whereas the marginal cost of an additional planned home birth may be high because, for example, of the need to put another midwife on call.

The role of different health professionals

As in antenatal care, the main issue here has been whether different professionals can deliver low-risk pregnancies to the same level of success. Several UK studies have demonstrated that intrapartum care led by midwives, obstetricians, and GPs have similar outcomes for low-risk women (Klein *et al.* 1983*a*, *b*; MacVicar *et al.* 1993; Hundley *et al.* 1995*a*). However, the process of care was different in each case, with obstetricians consistently having the highest intervention rate. The randomized controlled trial by Hundley and colleagues (1995*a*) also included a cost analysis which showed that the costs of the two locations of care were very sensitive to the assumptions employed in the analysis (Hundley *et al.* 1995*b*) and there was no clear superior alternative.

Induction of labour

A meta-analysis of randomized trials of routine induction at or beyond term suggests that there are no clinical advantages of this policy, other than a small reduction in meconium staining of the amniotic fluid. Two economic evaluations both showed that the additional resource use associated with a policy of early induction of labour are small (Engleman *et al.* 1979; Witter and Weitz 1987). The major impact is on night-time activity, which can be reduced by increased elective induction of labour. However, the potential for reducing staff, and hence overall costs, is limited because some women still go into spontaneous labour before induction (Engleman *et al.* 1979).

Monitoring in labour

Electronic fetal monitoring (EFM) during labour remains a perennial source of debate. Although the monitoring itself provides reassurance to both the mother and the staff involved in the delivery, its efficacy has not yet been established. In general, the additional cost associated with EFM is not the monitoring but the cost of additional care resulting from the monitoring, such as increased Caesarean section rates (Mugford 1993).

Antibiotic prophylaxis

Mugford and colleagues (1989) conducted a secondary evaluation of antibiotic prophylaxis after Caesarean section, using information from 58 randomized trials, which showed that the odds of developing infection dropped by 56–72% following antibiotic prophylaxis. Average costs were reduced in every case except where cephalosporin effectiveness was 50%. This was associated with an increase in cost of £88 per case averted. They concluded, however, that the harmful effects of routine prophylaxis were unlikely to outweigh the possible benefits.

Economic implications of postnatal care

Postnatal care has attracted less attention than the antenatal and intrapartum periods; nevertheless it offers some interesting economic issues.

Reductions in length of hospital stay

Yanover and colleagues (1976) found that early discharge with follow-up in the home was safe, economically feasible, and well accepted by women. However, a cost analysis conducted in three hospitals in Australia showed that early discharge with domiciliary visiting follow-up was limited in its ability to generate resource savings compared with the standard package of postnatal care (Scott 1994). Despite the lack of evidence, a recent policy document in Scotland suggested that a reduction in hospital postnatal stay of half a day could save around £6 million (Scottish Office Home and Health Department 1993). However, this crude analysis assumes a close correlation between the proportion of occupied bed-days for postnatal care and the proportion of total cost. The intensity of resources used in the postnatal period is very low compared to antenatal and intranatal care, so the application of an average cost per in-patient day for an obstetric unit, as used in the policy document, would hugely overestimate the potential savings.

Other alternatives to the current model of postnatal care have been described. These include cooperative care where mothers, partners, and babies stay together, either in hospital or in a patient hotel nearby. By shifting the costs of caring and support to the partner, cooperative care has been shown to be associated with lower costs per case for the hospital compared with traditional care for selected women (Woods et al. 1988). However, this has never been formally compared with home visits by community midwives.

Individualized postnatal care

The requirement for daily visiting until the tenth postnatal day of all women has been challenged with calls for care to be tailored to the individual woman's needs. Twaddle et al. (1993) compared tailored care with routine daily visiting and found that the change was likely to be cost-effective; it was associated with a higher quality of service at the same, or slightly reduced, cost.

Economic implications of total packages of care

Three randomized controlled trials have compared total midwife-managed care with the traditional model of shared care between the obstetrician, GP, and midwife (Slome *et al.* 1976; Flint *et al.* 1989; Turnbull *et al.* 1996). Each of these studies found that total care by midwives was equally safe and as efficacious as shared care and was preferred by women. There were significantly different processes of care between the two groups. Only one study explicitly addressed the economic implications of midwife-managed care compared with shared care. Preliminary indications suggest that midwife-led care is more cost-effective than shared care in the antenatal, intrapartum, and postnatal periods (Twaddle *et al.*, in preparation).

Conclusion

It is disappointing that so few economic issues in maternity care have been formally addressed by properly conducted evaluations. There is a need for more work of this type, in order that scarce NHS resources can be used to their best effect.

A number of important issues remain underevaluated in terms of their cost-effectiveness. There is a need to explicitly address the cost-effectiveness of reducing the number of clinic visits and the relative cost-effectiveness of care led by different professionals. There is a need to address the cost-effectiveness of 'domino' and home births. The cost-effectiveness of reduced postnatal stay in hospital should be formally evaluated. At the same time it is hoped that the inherent methodological difficulties of economic evaluation of maternity services, in particular the problems of measuring and valuing outcomes, will be addressed by researchers.

References

Artells-Herrero, J.J., Fordyce, I. D., and Mooney, G. H. (1982). *A cost-effectiveness analysis of antenatal care.* HERU discussion paper 09/82. University of Aberdeen.

Bachman, J. W., Heise, R. H., Naessens, J. M., and Timmerman, M. G. (1993). A study of various tests to detect asymptomatic urinary tract infections in an obstetric population. *Journal of the American Medical Association,* 270, 1971–4.

Backhouse, M. E., Backhouse, R. J., and Edey, S. A. (1992). Economic evaluation bibliography. *Health Economics,* 1(Suppl.), 1–236.

Bakketeig, L. S., Eik-Nes, S. H., Jacobson, G., *et al.* (1984). Randomized controlled trial of ultrasound screening in pregnancy. *Lancet,* 2, 207–10.

Bigrigg, M. A. and Read, M. D. (1991). Management of women referred to early pregnancy assessment units: care and cost effectiveness. *British Medical Journal,* 302, 577–9.

Bucher, H. C. and Schmidt, J. G. (1993). Does routine ultrasound scanning improve outcome in pregnancy? Meta-analysis of various outcome measures. *British Medical Journal*, **307**, 13–17.

Cole, S. K. and McIlwaine, G. M. (1994). The use of risk factors in predicting possible consequences of changing patterns of care in pregnancy. In: *The future of maternity services* (ed. G. Chamberlain and N. Patel). Royal College of Obstetricians and Gynaecologists Press, London.

Coyle, D. and Davies, L. (1993). How to assess cost-effectiveness: elements of a sound economic evaluation. In: *Purchasing and providing cost-effective health care* (ed. M. F. Drummond and A. Maynard), pp. 66–79. Churchill Livingstone, London.

Crowther, C. A., Neilson, J. P., Verkuyl, D. A. A., Bannerman, C., and Ashurst, H. M. (1989). Preterm labour in twin pregnancies: can it be prevented by hospital admission? *British Journal of Obstetrics and Gynaecology*, **96**, 850–3.

Crowther, C. A., Bouwmeester, A. M., and Ashurst, H. M. (1992). Does admissions to hospital for bed rest prevent disease progression or improve fetal outcome in pregnancy complicated by non-proteinuric hypertension? *British Journal of Obstetrics and Gynaecology*, **99**, 13–17.

Dawson, A. J., Middlemiss, C., Coles, E. C., Gough, N. A. J., and Jones, M. E. (1989). A randomized study of a domiciliary antenatal care scheme: the effect on hospital admissions. *British Journal of Obstetrics and Gynaecology*, **96**, 1319–22.

Department of Transport (1987). Values for journey time savings and accident prevention. DoT, London.

Droste, S. and Keil, K. (1994). Expectant management of placenta previa: Cost-benefit analysis of out-patient treatment. *American Journal of Obstetrics and Gynecology*, **170**, 1254–7.

Drummond, M. F. and Stoddart, G. L. (1984). Economic analysis and clinical trials. *Controlled Clinical Trials*, **5**, 115–28.

Eik-Nes, S. H., Okland, O., Aure, J. C., and Ulstein, M. (1984). Ultrasound screening in pregnancy: a randomized controlled trial. *Lancet*, **i**, 1347.

Engleman, S., Hilland, M. A., Howie, P., McIlwaine, G. M., and McNay, M. B. (1979). An analysis of the economic implications of elective induction of labour at term. *Community Medicine*, **1**, 191–8.

Everett, W. D. (1989). Screening for gestational diabetes: an analysis of health benefits and costs. *American Journal of Preventive Medicine*, **1**, 38–43.

Feeney, J. G. (1984). Hypertension in pregnancy managed at home by community midwives. *British Medical Journal*, Clinical Research Edition, **288**, 1046–7.

Ferster, G. and Pethybridge, R. J. (1973). Costs of a local maternity care system. *Hospital and Health Services Review*, **69**, 243–7.

Flint, C., Grant, A., and Poulengeris, P. (1989). The 'know your midwife' scheme – a randomized trial of continuity of care by a team of midwives. *Midwifery*, **5**, 11–16.

Giles, W., Collins, J., Ong, F., and MacDonald, R. (1992). Antenatal care of low-risk obstetric patients by midwives. *Medical Journal of Australia*, **157**, 158–61.

Graveley, E. A. and Littlefield, J. H. (1992). A cost-effectiveness analysis of three staffing models for the delivery of low-risk prenatal care. *American Journal of Public Health*, **82**, 180–4.

Hall, M. H., Chng, P. K., and MacGillivray, I. (1980). Is routine antenatal care worthwhile? *Lancet*, **ii**, 78–80.

Hall, M. and Campbell, D. (1987). Geographical epidemiology of hypertension in pregnancy. In: *Hypertension in pregnancy. Proceedings of the sixteenth study group of the Royal College of Obstetricians and Gynaecologists* (ed. F. Sharp and E. M. Symonds). Perinatology Press, New York.

Hall, M. and Campbell, D. (1992). Cost-effectiveness of the present programme for detection of asymptomatic hypertension in relation to the severity of hypertension and proteinuric hypertension. *International Journal of Technology Assessment in Health Care*, **8**(Suppl.), 75–81.

Hartikainen-Sorri, A. L. and Joupilla, P. (1984). Is routine hospitalization needed in antenatal care of twin pregnancy? *Journal of Perinatal Medicine*, **12**, 31–2.

Helewa, M., Heaman, M., Robinson, M. A., and Thompson, L. (1993). Community-based home-care program for the management of pre-eclampsia: an alternative. *Canadian Medical Association Journal*, **149**, 829–34.

Hundley, V. A., Cruickshank, F. M., Lang, G. D., Glazener, C. M. A., Milne, J. M., Turner, M., *et al.*(1995*a*). Midwife-managed delivery unit: a randomized controlled comparison with consultant-led care. *British Medical Journal*, **309**, 1400–4.

Hundley, V. A., Donaldson, C., Lang, G. D., Cruickshank, F. M., Glazener, C. M. A., Milne, J. M., *et al.* (1995*b*). Costs of intrapartum care in a midwife-managed delivery unit and a consultant-led labour ward. *Midwifery*, **11**, 103–9.

Klein, M., Lloyd, A., Redman, C., Bull, M., and Turnbull, A. C. (1983*a*). Comparison of low-risk pregnant women booked for delivery in two systems of care: shared care (consultant) and integrated general practice units. I. Obstetrical procedures and neonatal outcome. *British Journal of Obstetrics and Gynaecology*, **90**, 118–22.

Klein, M., Lloyd, A., Redman, C., Bull, M., and Turnbull, A. C. (1983*b*). Comparison of low-risk pregnant women booked for delivery in two systems of care: shared care (consultant) and integrated general practice units. II. Labour and delivery management and neonatal outcome. *British Journal of Obstetrics and Gynaecology*, **90**, 123–8.

Korenbrot, C. C., Aalto, L. H., and Laros, R. K. (1984). The cost-effectiveness of stopping preterm labour with beta-adrenergic treatment. *New England Journal of Medicine*, **310**, 691–6.

Kosasa,, T. S., Abou-Sayf, F. K., Li-Ma, G., and Hale, R. W. (1990). Evaluation of the cost-effectiveness of home monitoring of uterine contractions. *Obstetrics and Gynaecology*, **76**, 71S-75S.

Lilford, R. J. and Chard, T. (1985). The routine use of ultrasound [editorial]. *British Journal of Obstetrics and Gynaecology*, **92**, 434–6.

McGregor, E. (1987). Day care in the management of hypertension in pregnancy. (Unpublished.)

MacVicar, J., Dobbie, G., Owen-Johnstone, L., Jagger, C., Hopkins, M., and Kennedy, J. (1993). Simulated home delivery in hospital: a randomized controlled trial. *British Journal of Obstetrics and Gynaecology*, **100**, 316–23.

Mathews, D. D. (1977). A randomized controlled trial of bed rest and sedation or normal activity and non-sedation in the management of non-albuminuric hypertension in late pregnancy. *British Journal of Obstetrics and Gynaecology*, **84**, 108–14.

Meldrum, P. (1989). *Costing routine antenatal visits.* Health Economics Research Unit Discussion Paper 02/89. University of Aberdeen.

Mooney, P. and Dalton, K. J. (1990). An 'admission challenge test' to predict severe hypertension in pregnancy. *European Journal of Obstetrics and Gynaecology Reproductive Biology*, 35, 41–9.

Morrison, J. C., Martin, J. N., Martin, R. W., Hess, L. W., Gookin, K. S., and Wiser, W. L. (1989). Cost effectiveness of ambulatory uterine activity monitoring. *International Journal of Gynaecology and Obstetrics*, 28, 127–32.

Mugford, M. (1993). The costs of continuous electronic fetal monitoring in low-risk labour. In: *Intrapartum fetal surveillance* (ed. J. A. D. Spencer and R. H. T. Ward). Royal College of Obstetricians and Gynaecologists Press, London.

Mugford, M. and Drummond, M. F. (1989). The role of economics in the evaluation of care. In: *Effective care in pregnancy and childbirth* (ed. I. Chalmers, M. Enkin, and M. Keirse) Oxford University Press, Oxford.

Mugford, M., Kingston, J., and Chalmers, I. (1989). Reducing the incidence of infection after Caesarean section: implications of prophylaxis with antibiotics for hospital resources. *British Medical Journal*, 299, 1003–6.

Neilson, J. P., Crowther, A. C., Hodnett, E. D., Hofmeyer, G. J., and Keirse, M. J. N. C. (ed.) Cochrane Pregnancy and Childbirth Module. Cochrane Database of Systematic Reviews, Cochrane Library. Update Software, Oxford. Issued quarterly on disk.

Papiernik, E. and Keith, L. G. (1990). The cost-effectiveness of preventing preterm delivery in twin pregnancies. *Acta Genet. Med. Gemellol. Roma*, 39, 361–9.

Reece, E. A., Hagay, Z., Garofalo, J., and Hobbins, J. C. (1992). A controlled trial of self non-stress test versus assisted non-stress test in the evaluation of fetal well-being. *American Journal of Obstetrics and Gynecology*, 166, 489–92.

Robinson, R. (1993). Costs and cost-minimization analysis. *British Medical Journal*, 307, 726–8.

Saunders, M. C., Dick, J. S., Brown, I., McPherson, K., and Chalmers, I. (1985). Effects of hospital admission for bed rest on the duration of twin pregnancy: a randomized controlled trial. *Lancet*, ii, 793–5.

Scott, A. (1994). A cost analysis of early discharge and domiciliary visits versus standard hospital care for low-risk obstetric clients. *Australian Journal of Public Health*, 18, 96–100.

Scottish Office Home and Health Department (1993). *Provision of maternity services in Scotland: a policy review.* HMSO, Edinburgh.

Seiner, K. and Lairson, D. R. (1985). A cost-effectiveness analysis of prenatal care delivery. *Evaluation and the Health Professions*, 8, 93–108.

Sikorski, J., Wilson, J., Clement, S., Das, S., and Smeeton, N. (1996). A randomized controlled trial comparing two schedules of antenatal visits: the antenatal care project. *British Medical Journal*, 312, 546–53.

Slome, C., Wetherbee, H., Daly, M., Christensen, K., Meglen, M., and Thiede, H. (1976). Effectiveness of certified nurse midwives. *American Journal of Obstetrics and Gynecology*, 124, 177–82.

Soothill, P. W., Ajayi, R., Campbell, S., Gibbs, J., Chandran, R., Gibb, D., *et al.* (1991).

Effect of a fetal surveillance unit on admission of antenatal patients to hospital. *British Medical Journal*, **303**, 269–71.

Stilwell, J. A. (1979). Relative costs of home and hospital confinement. *British Medical Journal*, **279**, 257–9.

Temmerman, M. and Buekens, P. (1991). Cost-effectiveness of routine ultrasound examination in the first trimester of pregnancy. *European Journal of Obstetrics and Gynaecology Reproductive Biology*, **39**,3–6.

Terry, P. B. (1990). Routine testing and prophylaxis. *Baillieres Clinical Obstetrics and Gynaecology*, **4**, 25–43.

Tucker, J., Florey, C. du V., Howie, P., McIlwaine, G., and Hall, M. (1994). Is antenatal care apportioned according to obstetric risk? The Scottish antenatal care study. *Journal of Public Health Medicine*, **16**, 60–70.

Tucker, J. S., Hall, M. H., Howie, P. W., Reid, M. E., Barbour, R. S., Florey, C. du V., *et al.* (1996). Should obstetricians see women with normal pregnancies? A multicentre randomized controlled trial of routine antenatal care by general practitioners and midwives compared with shared care led by obstetricians. *British Medical Journal*, **312**, 554–9.

Tuffnell, D. J., Lilford, R. J., Buchan, P. C., Prendiville, V. M., Tuffnell, A. J., Holgate, M. P., *et al.* (1992). Randomized controlled trial of day care for hypertension in pregnancy. *Lancet*, **339**, 224–7.

Turnbull, D., Holmes, A., Shields, N., Cheyne, H., Twaddle, S., Gilmour, W. H., *et al.* (1996). Randomized controlled trial of efficacy of midwife-managed care. *Lancet*, **348**, 213–18.

Twaddle, S. and Harper, V. (1992). An economic evaluation of day care in the management of hypertension in pregnancy. *British Journal of Obstetrics and Gynaecology*, **99**, 459–63.

Twaddle, S., Liao, X. H., and Fyvie, H. (1993). An evaluation of postnatal care individualized to the needs of the woman. *Midwifery*, **9**, 154–60.

Twaddle, S., Young, D., Lees, A., and Major, K. The economic evaluation of midwife-managed care compared with shared care. (In preparation.)

Waldenstrom, U., Axelsson, O., Nilsson, S., Eklund, G., Fall, O., and Lindeberg, S. *et al.* (1988). Effects of routine one stage ultrasound screening in pregnancy: a randomised controlled trial. *Lancet*, **2**, 585–8.

Weiner, C. P., Renk, K., and Klugman, M. (1988). The therapeutic efficacy and cost-effectiveness of aggressive tocolysis for premature labour associated with premature rupture of membranes. *American Journal of Obstetrics and Gynecology*, **159**, 216–22.

Witter, F. R. and Weitz, C. M. (1987). A randomized trial of induction at 42 weeks' gestation versus expectant management for post-dates pregnancies. *American Journal of Perinatology*, **4**, 206–11.

Woods, J. R., Saywell, R. M., and Benson, J. T. (1988). Comparative costs of a cooperative care programme versus in-patient hospital care for obstetric patients. *Medical Care*, **26**, 596–606.

Yanover, M. J., Jones, D., and Miller, M. D. (1976). Perinatal care and low-risk mothers and infants. *New England Journal of Medicine*, **294**, 702–5.

CHAPTER NINE

Auditing care

Michael Maresh

Introduction

Before discussing precisely how maternity care can be audited it is necessary to clarify what is and is not audit. It is often claimed that audit in the maternity services has existed for many years. It has been commonplace to have local reports on clinical activity and outcome from maternity units and from those general practitioners supervising significant numbers of pregnant women. These have been supplemented by both regional and national reports such as the Confidential Enquiries into Maternal Deaths, The National Birthday Trust Surveys, and more recently the Confidential Enquiry into Stillbirths and Deaths in Infancy (CESDI). All of these exercises are to be commended as in general there will have been a high regard for data collection and thus the quality of the information. Sample size has often been large, giving a clear picture of the local, regional, or national situation. However, interpretation of the results is often difficult. What should they be compared with? What is an appropriate number of antenatal visits? What is an acceptable level of transfer from home to hospital in labour? Collecting data on such subjects may be interesting and may show trends from year to year or trends between different locations, but does it have relevance to the outcome for the woman and her baby? Clinical audit should be more than just measuring. It is about comparing practice with agreed guidelines and standards of care. If actual practice is statistically significantly different from what was agreed in advance then it will be necessary to investigate ways of bringing about change. This is the hardest part of audit. Having introduced a change in practice it is then necessary to reaudit so that the audit cycle (Figure 9.1) becomes an audit spiral with the vertical axis representing improved health care.

Clinical audit must also put the patient first and so in the maternity care audit cycle, putting the woman, the fetus, and the family in the middle of the cycle is a constant reminder of who comes first. Care should not be arranged around the professionals but should be woman centred.

A number of other terms which have already been mentioned need further

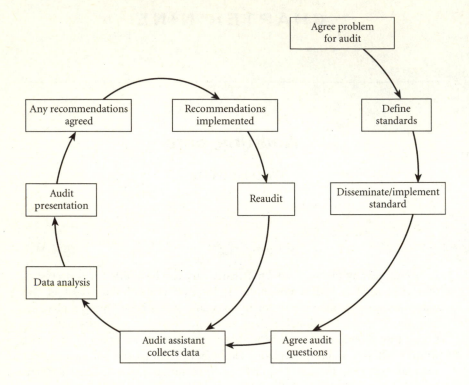

Figure 9.1

elaboration. Firstly, the word *guidelines*. An extensive academic literature has built up over the last few years. An NHS Executive publication (NHS Executive 1996) summarizes many of the points. Guidelines may be developed nationally or locally. Much work is involved in developing robust guidelines. Where national guidelines have been developed, for example with regard to biochemical screening methods for Down's syndrome (Royal College of Obstetricians and Gynaecologists 1993), it is normally advisable to rewrite them with a local perspective to give a sense of local ownership; however, reference to the national set saves a considerable amount of reinventing the wheel. Guidelines are essentially scientific statements to advise health professionals on appropriate ways to administer care. As such, they need to be developed from a careful review of the literature. If there is clear evidence from well-conducted randomized controlled trials that a particular type of management is beneficial then a guideline based on this would be classified A. An example of this would be the use of external cephalic version at term. If the management practice had not been subjected to randomized trials, but only perhaps case controlled studies, then a guideline based on this would be categorized as B. Examples of this would be in the field of rhesus disease management. If the guideline is only based on a consensus view, for example the value of antenatal thromboprophylaxis, then it would be regarded as category C evidence. These categories are summarized in Table 9.1. Unfortunately, the majority of antenatal care is given on the basis of category C or sometimes category B evidence, as little category A evidence is available.

Table 9.1 *Classification of evidence: The evidence given to this chapter has been graded following the NHS Executive classification system*

Grade A	Randomized Controlled Trials (RCTs)
Grade B	Other robust experimental or observational studies
Grade C	More limited evidence but the advice relies on expert opinion and has the endorsement of respected authorities

Another word which is frequently used is *standards*. This is often used synonymously for guidelines, but should refer to how often a guideline can be achieved. For example, the standard might be 100% for determining rhesus group status in pregnancy and recording it in the case notes. With regard to the number of *care-givers* in pregnancy, the standard may be that 80% of women should see no more than six separate *care-givers* in pregnancy (Royal College of Obstetricians and Gynaecologists 1995).

Guidelines and protocols are also often used interchangeably and this is not helped by different uses of the words between England and Scotland. A protocol is usually regarded as a local initiative which one is expected to follow unless there is clear agreement by one or more senior health professionals that it is not in the woman's interest for it to be followed. Guidelines can be used nationally, regionally, or locally and imply there is more leeway in interpretation.

Audit is increasingly being realized as being just one component of the move towards improving the *quality* of care. There are a number of dimensions to quality; clinical management should be:

- effective
- given in an efficacious way
- satisfactory for the patient
- given in an efficient manner
- be provided equitably to the whole population served by the providers (Maxwell 1984).

Quality assurance is sometimes used synonymously for clinical audit. However, while clinical audit is a key component of health care quality assurance, there are many other aspects to quality assurance such as appropriate staff training, complaints monitoring, and communication methods.

Audit of outcome

Audit is classically divided into audit of structure, process, and outcome. The ideal is to perform *outcome* audit, but in practice this is difficult to achieve. In terms of maternal mortality, the national rate is less than one in 10 000, so even in a whole hospital practice a maternal death is a rare event. Thus from a community perspective this is totally inappropriate. Maternal morbidity tends to relate to the delivery, for example with problems relating to the perineum, bladder, bowels, or a wound. Maternal problems with the perineum, particularly after a first vaginal delivery, can be used as an outcome indicator of delivery care (Glazener *et al.* 1995). However, the numbers will be small and any inference about good or poor management is unlikely to be valid. This illustrates one of the major pitfalls in clinical audit as it has been practised to date, namely a lack of statistical input into the interpretation of audit data. For these outcome indicators, even if there is an accepted standard for comparison, it is improbable in a community practice that one will be able to have large enough numbers to demonstrate whether or not there is a statistically significant difference between the practice and the standard.

An alternative method of auditing maternal morbidity is to ask the women themselves (Chapter 6). Sets of questionnaires have been developed and validated and are readily available (Mason 1989). These evaluate many aspects of pregnancy care. The woman's perspective of her pregnancy outcome may also be obtained in a qualitative manner. Whilst more complex to analyse, such data may reveal problems with service provision which may be rectifiable. A further maternal outcome which needs more research is postnatal depression, as it may be that research will demonstrate this to be dependent on measurable aspects of antenatal or intrapartum management. This is discussed further below.

Audit of structure

One of the key problems in providing high-quality care in a field where the care is provided by different health service sectors is that of *communication*. This can often be improved by having effective structures in place and, accordingly, audit of the *structure* of antenatal care may also lead to improvements in care. Examples of audit of structure would include aspects such as the design of case notes. This should be done to facilitate easy collection of relevant information and the ability to communicate information between different care-givers. The move towards a standardized national maternity record means that design deficiencies will be minimized.

More importantly, health professionals working in the community will have the same style of case notes wherever a woman is planning to deliver, and this common format should reduce the chances of errors occurring with regard to note completion, and failures to communicate using notes.

In addition to using case notes, structural audit may be performed with any communication system. If referral letters are sent to local hospitals with regard to arranging antenatal care assessments and delivery facilities, they can be audited for completeness of information. Apart from the woman's personal identifying data, referral letters would need to include details on past obstetric history, past gynaecological history, drug history, relevant family and social history, and current pregnancy details including the date of the last menstrual period which is surprisingly often omitted. Standard structured referral letters tend to decrease the frequency of omissions. A number are available and can be adapted if necessary for local use. Auditing existing communications and improving them through such approaches is a good area for fruitful, collaborative audit between hospital and community services. Similarly, discharge summaries from hospital need to be audited and modified as necessary as part of a collaborative audit.

Information leaflets need to be up to date and readily available. Whilst it is not expected that general practitioners and community midwives are going to write their own leaflets relating to specific pregnancy issues such as Down's syndrome screening, they can ensure that women have actually had this information and if necessary influence others to ensure the information is up to date.

Antenatal support groups and classes should not only be situated in convenient locations but also at varying times, including evenings, to maximize attendance. This can be easily audited by reviewing the schedules for the meetings.

Other areas of audit of structure may include the facilities available for antenatal assessment; are they appropriate, clean, private, and convenient? Furthermore, any equipment used, such as sphygmomanometers or electronic fetal heart rate detectors, needs to be regularly assessed for accuracy. Whilst some of these aspects may not readily be considered to be audit they are an essential part of the whole subject area of improving the quality of antenatal care given.

At a different level, it is necessary to ensure that there is an effective maternity services liaison committee (MSLC) on which the community staff are represented, and who see audit of local services as being on their agenda to ensure that any recommended changes in service are facilitated. Such committees can also assist in the development of clinical guidelines, for example screening for Down's syndrome. The NHS Executive have published advice on how committees can contribute to improving maternity services locally (Department of Health Maternity Services Committees 1996).

Audit of process

Process audit has been the most widely used to date. Examples of this include: whether investigations such as rhesus antibody checks are performed and, in addition, if these occurred at the appropriate times in pregnancy; whether accepted local guidelines for types of antenatal care are followed; and auditing whether those transferred from community-based to hospital-based care had been initially having an appropriate pattern of care. Whilst it is traditional to audit delivery outcome variables such as analgesia requirement, mode of delivery, and perineal damage, as mentioned before, drawing any inference from this must be done with care.

The rest of this chapter concentrates on examples of process audit drawn from various stages of pregnancy. There is limited time for health care professionals to devote to audit so it is preferable to pick topics which have all of the following characteristics:

- relevant to pregnancy outcome
- interesting to those conducting the audit
- guidelines and standards which are accepted
- feasible to collect the requisite number of cases within a reasonable time.

In addition, topics which have resource implications may be of particular relevance. Those which involve both the primary and secondary health care sectors should be studied wherever possible, as these are areas particularly prone to having problems which can almost certainly be rectified to the advantage of the women being cared for.

Audit of community prenatal care

Health professionals based in the community may have the opportunity to influence pregnancy prior to conception, and this may be audited in early pregnancy. This should involve the use of practice nurses as well as midwives, as the former have such a major role in health education and well woman screening.

Unplanned pregnancies

Care-givers may be in a position to help reduce the number of unplanned pregnancies, which in teenagers is a *Health of the Nation* priority. Difficulties with such an audit include defining the word 'unplanned', and knowing what standards to aim for in one's own community as there are differences between urban and rural settings.

Smoking

Relatively small numbers of women smoke in pregnancy and it may therefore not be possible to demonstrate significant improvements from year to year. However, since it is of such major significance with regard to fetal and childhood development, let alone subsequent maternal morbidity, it perhaps should be used as a trigger to initiate a review of whether any smoking cessation initiatives had been directed to individual women. Like unplanned pregnancies, this can be regarded as a type of adverse event audit, or occurrence screening.

Folic acid

The number of women who were taking folic acid prior to conception can be determined early in pregnancy relatively easily. Clearly, in planned pregnancies one should be aiming for a standard of 100%. However, while it is improbable that this is currently being achieved, it should not be allowed to detract from this aim. As the message gradually becomes widely known, it should be possible in an averaged-sized practice to determine on an annual basis whether the rate of folic acid usage is increasing towards this target. This is an excellent subject to audit as it fills most of the criteria mentioned above in that there is a clear guideline agreed nationally, the audit should be easily achievable, and there is a clear health benefit.

Pre-existing medical problems

Another example of an adverse event audit would be if any woman with a significant medical problem such as hypertension, diabetes, or cardiac disease had not been reviewed from a medical perspective prior to pregnancy. Similarly, the small number of women with genetic risks such as thalassaemia should have been appropriately assessed.

Time of first antenatal visit

How soon in pregnancy a woman first approaches either her general practitioner or midwife to inform them of the pregnancy might be seen as an indicator of how good community services are at promoting to women the advantages of early antenatal care, and also how accessible the services are. However, since there are many influencing factors, such as whether the woman has had previous children and ethnic and religious views, this is of less value than initially might be anticipated. For example, the advantage for a normal pregnant woman who has had previous normal pregnancies of being seen by a midwife or general practitioner at six weeks rather than waiting until 12 weeks is debatable if she does not feel in need of advice. However, for a first pregnancy this may be a useful topic if all the practitioners can agree on a standard and feel comfortable in recommending this in their routine practice.

Audit of community-based antenatal care

It must be the aim of community-based antenatal services to provide as much care as feasible close to where women live, in the community. Accordingly, any aspect of antenatal care suitable for audit could theoretically be performed within the community services. However, because of the relatively small numbers of women there is little point in auditing subjects such as the proportion of small for gestational age babies which were suspected antenatally or the incidence of undiagnosed breech presentations. Such topics are important and it would be worthwhile reviewing such cases on an individual basis – an adverse event audit – as there may be some aspects of care which were not ideal. Such a review often serves an educative process. However, any such review must clearly be performed in a non-threatening and sensitive way as there must be few practising maternity care who can honestly say that they have never missed such cases. Other relatively uncommon occurrences in community care, such as severe hypertension with significant proteinuria, may also be worth reviewing on an individual basis in this way.

Antenatal visits

Many aspects of antenatal care are of unproven value and so there are no substantial guidelines and standards to aim for. For example, is there any point in reviewing the number of antenatal visits a woman has? No doubt a consensus would say that if she had had less than three visits she would be putting herself and her baby at increased risk. Such relatively unusual cases are likely to be clear to all and be routinely reviewed as part of an occurrence audit. Perhaps of more value is to audit women with excessive numbers of antenatal visits which may represent a waste of resources and, in particular, duplication of efforts by general practitioner, midwife, and obstetrician. In a recent audit across a number of settings, the average number of visits a multiparous woman with no pregnancy complications had was 10 (Vause and Maresh, (1998 in press). On the basis of this and until better evidence is available it certainly might be worthwhile auditing the care of multiparous women who have had 12 or more visits. Those above this number may well have significant social problems and the midwife who may have being seeing the woman may well have been very effective at preventing hospital admissions by such a strategy of very frequent visits. Thus it can be seen that simple audits of such topics are fraught with problems of interpretation.

Antenatal investigations

There are a number of antenatal investigations which are performed, and if acted upon appropriately are likely to improve outcome. An example of this would be testing rhesus negative women for the development of antibodies during pregnancy. Although the appearance of rhesus antibodies is a rare event, the detection and immediate referral for action should be effective in reducing perinatal morbidity and mortality. Thus whether or not a rhesus negative woman has had her antibodies checked after 28 weeks' gestation, whilst an audit of process, could be regarded as a proxy-outcome audit. The standard should be that 100% of rhesus negative women have had it performed, and the result is in their case notes. Naturally, prevention of isoimmunization is preferable and many cases can be tracked back to inadequate prophylaxis. In a rhesus negative woman, any event which could be potentially sensitizing, such as bleeding in pregnancy, must be managed by appropriate anti-D treatment in accordance with published guidelines (National Blood Transfusion Service 1991).

Most of the rest of the blood tests which are performed in pregnancy may also be regarded as proxy-outcome measures, such as thalassaemia and sickle screening and determination of haemoglobin concentrations. Mid-stream urine testing for infection, syphilis, and hepatitis screening are not practised by all, although strong arguments can be made for this. Accordingly, one should audit adherence to the local agreed policy.

Access to hospital services

Ensuring women have had access to hospital-based services such as ultrasound scanning, and that this has been performed at appropriate times in pregnancy, can be done in retrospect although any reason for a deviation from guidelines may not be obvious at a later date. For example, the notes would need to be designed to ensure that if a choice had been offered it would be recorded.

All women should be offered the opportunity to see a consultant obstetrician in early pregnancy (Department of Health 1993), but not only is this unachievable in many parts of the United Kingdom it is also difficult to audit in retrospect whether an offer took place. However, any woman with medical problems or who had a bad obstetric history almost certainly should have seen a consultant obstetrician at an early stage and this should be auditable. Specific conditions which should prompt referral can be listed which will facilitate both appropriate referral and audit.

Transfer of community-based antenatal care to predominantly hospital-based care

Most reviews of large community-based care schemes publish data on the percentages of women who have to transfer from primarily community-based care to predominantly hospital-based. A review of 10 such studies showed a variation between 10–31% (Hall 1990). While the initial reaction might be that 31% was too high, the key point is that it almost always more convenient for the woman to have care in the community. Accordingly, as long as her care is not being jeopardized in any way it should be possible for a variable amount of care to be conducted in the community. This is essentially increasing flexibility to provide individualization of care. This is more time-consuming for the community staff as it may result in more visits and more demanding for hospital services, as it may result in direct consultant involvement.

Antenatal hospital admissions

Many emergency hospital admissions are as a result of maternal anxiety about whether or not labour has commenced. An emergency home visit by a community midwife may enable a clear diagnosis to be made. Similarly, monitoring of hypertension and proteinuria if necessary on a daily basis is a standard part of community care and again may reduce admissions.

Accordingly, effective care in the community may reduce hospital admissions and audit of admissions may reveal areas for improvement. However, it cannot be too highly stressed that admission cannot be regarded as a failure of community-based care, and that the woman's wishes and safety must come first. Whereas for one woman in a set of circumstances admission may be preferable, for another in similar circumstances care at home may be more appropriate.

Audit of care at birth

Home births

As a result of the *Changing Childbirth* initiative (Department of Health 1993), there appears to be a slight increase in women requesting home births. This increases the need for clear guidelines developed locally which can be easily audited.

Unbiased advice, preferably written, needs to be available to all women explaining the advantages and disadvantages of home birth. In the absence of good scientific data, agreement has to be reached on this between all the health professionals involved in care. The giving of this advice should be documented so that it can be audited.

Similarly, an agreed list of contraindications to home birth should have been developed so again individual cases can be audited against the agreed local guidelines.

Some community-based professionals, both midwives and doctors, may have had little recent experience in conducting home births and accordingly may have some anxieties. A statement of training requirements is needed which has to include neonatal resuscitation. In addition, the equipment which should be taken out should be defined and thus be able to be audited.

Transfers from home to hospital in labour are distressing for all concerned. Written guidelines on the criteria which should be used for agreement to transfer are relatively standard. The percentages of women being transferred may vary from area to area and is clearly somewhat dependent on the parity mix of the population. If one assumes that this is relatively constant between areas, one would expect little differences between rates. A review of published series suggests a range between 8–22% (Hall 1990). Accordingly, while individual cases of transfer should be considered, it is also possible to review overall rates over a longer period to ascertain whether the rate appears to be appropriate and whether the guidelines appear to work and indeed are being implemented.

The actual mechanics of transfer is an area where problems may occur and clear guidelines should be in existence. These must include the actual methods to be used, such as car or ambulance, staff to be involved, and what can and cannot be done at home. Although this sounds very detailed and unnecessary, the potential for problems is very real for this small number of women and the spotlight is very much on them. Litigation concerning this topic certainly occurs. With the abolition of the obstetric flying squad and the taking over of some of the responsibility for the small number of major perinatal problems which may occur at home – such as post-partum haemorrhage, eclampsia, and perinatal asphyxia – by the paramedic service, written guidelines are essential. These should have been developed by both community and hospital-based carers in conjunction with the ambulance service. A typical guideline has been produced, for example in the north west region (NHS Executive, north west region 1996). Such guidelines must make it explicit; for example, who is responsible for which components of care and what drugs can be given. With any new development such as this it is important that the paramedic service audit their results in conjunction with all the other health care professionals – this is a good example of multiprofessional and multisector audit.

Deliveries in non-consultant maternity units

Much of the above applies to deliveries which occur in non-consultant-led maternity units. The conditions under which women can be looked after in such units, the procedures that can be performed there, and the conditions for transfer must all be clearly written and a consensus view reached. Once the guidelines are clear and agreed they may be subsequently audited.

General intrapartum audit

Wherever a woman gives birth, certain criteria need to be documented. Some of these may reflect the standard of care and thus be suitable for audit. Clearly, a healthy mother and healthy baby will almost always occur with pregnancies which are considered to be of low enough risk to remain under the care of community-based staff. Thus again one has to consider proxy-outcome measures. In the mother, damage to the perineum and genital tract is an appropriate measure since this may be associated with considerable maternal distress and subsequent problems with intercourse, micturition, and defecation. Maternal satisfaction with labour is paramount not least because dissatisfaction may affect parenting and the woman's desire to have a further child. A manual of validated questionnaires (Mason 1989) can assist with this investigation. However, if care has been given by a small number of professionals, the questionnaire will have to be completed and assessed while protecting the woman's identity.

Postnatal care

Community staff undoubtedly have the dominant role and opportunity in this area. Perhaps because in the past it may have been harder for research in the community to attract funding, it is the area with the least research performed. Accordingly, guidelines and standards suitable for audit are not extensive. However, it is clearly an area where problems exist as one study has reported that 76% of women reported at least one health problem within eight weeks of birth (Glazener et al. 1995).

Breastfeeding

Successful uptake and continuation of breastfeeding confers specific advantages on the baby (Chapter 24). What is achievable and how it can be achieved is not clear from research. Guidelines to assist in the successful implementation of breastfeeding have been published (Royal College of Midwives 1993). Whilst an actual standard may not be meaningful between different communities, rates of uptake and continuation at six weeks should be audited and staff adherence to guidelines audited if rates appear to be lower than anticipated. Reasons for discontinuation should also be monitored.

Postnatal depression

Postnatal depression can be very debilitating and a real cause of post-partum morbidity. It has been stated that 10–15% of all newly delivered mothers are affected by a non-psychotic illness (Kumar and Robson 1984). Although postnatal, and antenatal, depression is a complex condition it is not necessarily difficult to recognize. However, identification of depression may prove to be problematic as many women are reluctant to reveal that they feel depressed. This can be further compounded when health professionals do not think to look for it. The use of a screening tool, such as the Edinburgh Postnatal Depression Scale (Cox *et al.* 1987), whilst not intended as a diagnostic tool, can be very useful in identifying depression in the antenatal and postnatal period, but is only of value if effective care is offered to mothers identified as scoring highly. The complexity of depression during pregnancy and the postnatal period makes it a difficult area to audit. However, health care professionals in the community are well placed to identify and initiate management in this area. A multiprofessional audit can identify issues such as the existence of guidelines and standards, acceptance by the multiprofessional team and the women involved, and assessment of the level of compliance with the recommendations. Sound development of the guidelines and standards in this area will not only assist in a reliable audit process but also highlight changes in prevalence, identification, and management over time.

Other issues

Subjects such as the adherence to guidelines for rhesus negative mothers and the offering of rubella vaccination to all susceptible mothers are simple topics to audit. It is also important that a discussion about contraception is initiated and advice documented. It should be recognized that advice apparently accepted in the immediate puerperium is frequently not taken up. While part of this may relate to non-compliance, a factor often apparently present is that conflicting advice has been given, for example with the timing of starting the combined contraceptive pill. Review of this subject again at the traditional six-week postnatal check is essential.

What has audit achieved?

When the Government started its drive towards implementing audit in 1989 (Secretaries of State 1989), those involved in providing maternity services frequently claimed that they had always audited their work. While that may have been true, they often did not manage to introduce the changes necessary to address the problems demonstrated by the audit. This is the hardest part and without it audit it is of limited value. When asked to justify with concrete examples what has so far been achieved in improving care through the vast expenditure on audit there is often a struggle for good responses. However, the initial concentration on setting up audit mechanisms without in parallel investigating methods of bringing about change and linking audit closely with education, meant initially audit was unlikely to bring about change. Now, however, as these problems are being at least partially addressed and the guideline initiative is developing, the overall culture is slowly changing and clear improvements in care may gradually become apparent. It was surely somewhat naive to expect rapid changes from an organization of different professional groups, not structured like an industry, and dealing with health and disease which is a relatively impure science.

Apart from the changes in culture towards audit and effective practice there are examples from maternity care where specific changes in practice have occurred. One of the reasons that this is already demonstrable is because of the Cochrane Pregnancy and Childbirth Module (Neilson *et al.* 1997) and the key publication *Effective care in pregnancy and childbirth* (Chalmers *et al.* 1989). Thus effective procedures have been well documented for many years on maternity topics. This has been further encouraged by the Royal College of Obstetricians and Gynaecologists' publications on effective procedures (Benbow *et al.* 1997). For instance, for instrumental delivery the ventouse has increased in popularity at the expense of forceps as the ventouse has been shown to reduce maternal trauma without increasing fetal damage. The administration of maternal corticosteroids prior to anticipated preterm delivery has also increased as this has been shown to improve perinatal outcome. Other practices which have changed include perineal suturing techniques. Many other beneficial changes are likely to have occurred in the maternity services through the various quality initiatives, but demonstrating rigorously that there have been improvements takes time and money.

Practical problems with audit

Whilst maternity research needs independent ethics approval, audit generally does not as it is conducting studies to check that accepted practice is being carried out. The only exception probably relates to patient questionnaires. If these are standard published ones then this should be acceptable. If designing them oneself, independent checking is advisable before finding that women are upset by the questions.

There is clearly not enough time to audit everything; furthermore, it is probable that considerable work will be needed initially to develop and update guidelines so that well-designed audits can be conducted. Starting with topics which are relevant, interesting, and feasible to audit will help to generate support. Sharing out the lead role for each individual audit will ensure that as many people as possible are actively involved. It is preferable that one individual takes a lead in the running of the overall audit programme, and this person will need to have the leadership qualities necessary to ensure that all members of the group become involved in the process. Ideally, the audit lead should change at fairly regular intervals, perhaps two-yearly, and this role should rotate between the different disciplines. Audit can become boring, but practical involvement is likely to fire the enthusiasm of individuals when they realize that the maternity care offered by the group can be improved still further.

Practical involvement in actual audits by as many people as possible will help to ensure that the process is not regarded as threatening by individuals. If problems are discovered with the care given by an individual health care professional, perhaps with an adverse event audit, then this clearly will need sensitive handling by the lead audit person. Usually it is not the individual who is to blame but the system of providing care which is at fault, an aspect which is emphasized in approaches such as total quality management (Berwick 1992). Examples of this could be: that the individual lacks knowledge and has not the opportunity for updating; that when incidents occurred the individual had clearly been overworking and not functioning efficiently; that there were problems in communicating between different individuals which could be addressed by general changes in the system; or that guidelines being used were deficient in detail. As long as the overall philosophy of the audit programme is constantly reflecting the collective ownership of all those providing health care, then hopefully individuals will not feel threatened and will be able to provide care in a manner they find satisfying. Having unhappy staff is a recipe for disaster for the patient.

Acknowledgements

I am most grateful for the suggestions of two midwifery colleagues, Julie Wray and Angie Benbow, when writing this chapter.

References

Benbow, A., Semple, D., and Maresh, M. (1997). *Effective procedures in maternity care suitable for audit*. Royal College of Obstetricians and Gynaecologists, London.

Berwick, D. M. (1992). Heal thyself or heal thy system: can doctors help to improve medical care? *Quality Health Care*, 1(Suppl.), S2–S8.

Chalmers, I., Enkin, M. and Keirse, M. J. N. C. (1989). *Effective care in pregnancy and childbirth.* Oxford University Press, Oxford.

Cox, J. L., *et al.* (1987) Detection of posnatal depression of the 10-item postnatal depression scale. *British Journal of Psychiatry,* 150, 782–86.

Department of Health (1993). *Changing childbirth. Report of the Expert Maternity Group (The Cumberlege Report).*HMSO, London.

Department of Health (1993*). Report of the Chief Medical Officer's Expert Group on the Sleeping Position of Infants and Cot Death.* HMSO, London.

Department of Health Maternity Services Committees (1996). *Guidelines for working effectively.* NHS Executive, Leeds.

Glazener, C. M. A., *et al.* (1995). Postnatal maternal morbidity: extent causes, prevention, and treatment. *British Journal of Obstetrics and Gynaecology,* 102, 282–7.

Hall, M. H. (1990). Identification of high risk and low risk. In: *Antenatal care* (ed. M. H Hall). *Bailliere's Clinical Obstetrics and Gynaecology,* 4(1), 65–76.

Kumar, R. and Robson, K. M. (1984). A prospective study of emotional disorders in childbearing women. *British Journal of Psychiatry,* 144, 453–62.

Mason, V. (1989). Women's experience of maternity care – a survey manual. OPCS, London.

Maxwell, R. J. (1984). Quality assessment in health. *British Medical Journal,* 288, 1470–3.

National Blood Transfusion Service Immunoglobulin Working Party (1991). Recommendations for the use of anti-D immunoglobulin. *Prescribers Journal,* 31, 137–45.

Neilson, J. P., Crowther, C. A., Hodnett, G. J., and Keirse, M. J. N. C.(ed.) (1997). Pregnancy and Childbirth Module of the Cochrane Database of Systematic Reviews. The Cochrane Collaboration, Issue 2. Update Software, Oxford. Issued quarterly on disk.

NHS Executive (1996). *Clinical guidelines. Using clinical guidelines to improve patient care within the NHS.* NHS Executive, Leeds.

Royal College of Midwives (1993). *Successful breastfeeding* (2nd edn). Churchill Livingstone, London.

Royal College of Obstetricians and Gynaecologists (1993). *Report of the Royal College of Obstetricians and Gynaecologists' Working Party on Biochemical Markers and the Detection of Down's Syndrome.* RCOG, London.

Royal College of Obstetricians and Gynaecologists (1995). *Organizational standards for maternity services. Report of a Joint Working Group.* RCOG, London.

Secretaries of State for Health, Wales, Northern Ireland, and Scotland (1989). *Working for patients.* HMSO, London.

Vause, S. and Maresh, M. (1998). Developing methods of auditing the quality of antenatal care. *British Journal of Obstetrics and Gynaecology.* In press.

Further reading

Hopkins, A. (1996). Clinical audit: time for a reappraisal? *Journal of the Royal College of Physicians of London*, **30**(5), 415–25.

Maresh, M. (1994). *Audit in obstetrics and gynaecology*. Blackwell Scientific Publications, Oxford.

Neilson, J.P., Crowther, C.A., Hodnett, E.D., Hofmeyr, G.J., and Keirse, M.J.N.C. (ed.) Cochrane Pregnancy and Childbirth Module in the Cochrane Database of Systematic Reviews. Cochrane Library. Update Software, Oxford. Issued quarterly on disc.

Perinatal audit: a report produced for the European Association of Perinatal Medicine. Parthenon Publishing.

Royal College of Obstetricians and Gynaecologists (1995). Report of a Joint Working Group on Organizational Standards for Maternity Services. RCOG, London.

Royal College of Obstetricians and Gynaecologists (1995). Report of the Audit Committee's Working Group on Communication Standards: obstetrics. RCOG, London.

Royal College of Obstetricians and Gynaecologists (1997). *Effective procedures in maternity care* (2nd edn). RCOG, London.

CHAPTER TEN

Educating the carers

Lindsay Smith and Jo Alexander

Introduction

The education and training of midwives and doctors (whether obstetricians or GPs) providing maternity care must ensure that they are competent to provide women with continuity and choice (Taylor 1986; Flint *et al.* 1989; Ford *et al.* 1991; House of Commons 1992; Department of Health 1993; Campbell and MacFarlane 1994). This includes choice of care, carer, and of place of delivery. Such knowledge, attitudes, and skills which are required to achieve competence (Newble 1992) may be acquired as an undergraduate and/or during postgraduate education and training. The acquisition of appropriate knowledge and skills is not sufficient. It is also vital for both groups to believe that they have important complementary roles in maternity care.

There are three important differences between the education and training of GPs who provide maternity care and the education of midwives. The content of midwifery education is closely prescribed centrally by the United Kingdom Central Council for Nursing, Midwifery, and Health Visiting and the related National Boards. In contrast, the content of both undergraduate and vocational GP training is very loosely determined and devolved to the universities and postgraduate GP vocational training schemes. Post-qualification, the requirements are that midwives must update professionally every three to five years and the system is fairly carefully regulated; in contrast there is no statutory requirement for GPs who provide obstetric care ever to update. Finally, midwives undergo an initial preparation (its length depending on whether they are already registered nurses) and are then fully qualified to practise as independent professionals. GPs must first qualify as a doctor (six years) and then spend another three years undergoing vocational training to become a GP. General practice is unfortunately unique in being the only medical discipline where the majority of vocational training takes place outside of the discipline, being in various secondary care junior doctor posts. These differences between doctors and midwives are crucial considerations if one is to change from the present uniprofessional system to some form of interprofessional education and training of the two disciplines. The desirability of initiatives of this type is beginning to be acknowledged (NHS Executive 1997).

Control of the involvement of GPs and midwives in maternity care is also different. Most practising midwives in the community provide antenatal and postnatal care, with many also providing intrapartum care. Except for midwives working independently, it is largely their employers (NHS managers) who determine if and where midwives provide intrapartum care. In contrast, GPs, as independent contractors, can choose to provide antenatal, intrapartum, and/or postnatal care to women registered with them for maternity services. Most (90%) have continued to provide antenatal and postnatal care but there is no doubt that few GPs now provide complete obstetric care for their own patients (Marsh *et al.* 1985; Chapter 4).

In this chapter we describe the history and present state of the education and training in the United Kingdom of midwives and of GPs who choose to provide maternity care. We conclude by suggesting how their future education and training could be improved.

Midwifery

History

Midwifery has a long history, statutory recognition first being given to the role and function of the midwife by the Midwives Act of 1902. During the last 40 years the midwifery role in the community first began to diminish as the number of home births fell, but subsequently increased again as the length of postnatal stay in hospital became ever shorter.

Government targets for an increasingly woman-centred service make it just as important now as it has ever been for midwives to be able to provide comprehensive care for women throughout their pregnancy, labour, birth, and puerperium until 28 days after delivery. They must provide and be accountable for individualized care for the mother, baby, and her family within their chosen environment and must be ready to assume this responsibility immediately on registration.

Present education and training

The United Kingdom has a long tradition of two separate routes to registration as a midwife. The programme for non-nurses is now entitled pre-registration midwifery (it was previously known as direct entry) and is a minimum of three years in duration. The programme for those who are already nurses registered on parts 1 and 12 of the professional register is now entitled pre-registration midwifery (shortened) and is a minimum of 18 months in duration; it was previously known as post-registration midwifery. Content of these programmes is prescribed by the English National Board for Nursing, Midwifery, and Health Visiting (ENB 1994).

Whichever programme they are undertaking, student midwives must have achieved the following clinical experience as a minimum:

- advised pregnant women and carried out 100 prenatal examinations
- supervised and cared for 40 women in labour
- carried out 40 births
- participated in breech deliveries at least in a simulated situation
- performed episiotomy and been initiated into suturing
- supervised and cared for 40 women at high risk
- supervised and cared for 100 postnatal women and healthy newborn infants
- observed and cared for newborns requiring special care
- cared for women with pathological conditions in the fields of gynaecology and obstetrics.

Throughout the programmes leading to registration, theory and practice are closely integrated and students undertake ongoing assessment in both.

All midwifery programmes in the UK, whether pre-registration or pre-registration (shortened), must now be at the minimum level of a diploma in higher education so that on completion the student will have gained 240 points in the higher education credit accumulation and transfer scheme (CATS). To put this in context, an honours degree requires 360 CATS points, 120 points usually being required at levels 1,2, and 3, and each taking the equivalent of a full-time year of study to attain. Some pre-registration and pre-registration (shortened) programmes are at undergraduate level and may take longer than the minimum period required.

The curricula of programmes leading to registration as a midwife must be developed in harmony with a number of regulations, for example: European Community Midwives Directive 89/594/EEC; United Kingdom Central Council (UKCC) Midwives' Rules (1993); UKCC Midwife's Code of Practice (1994a); UKCC Requirements for the Content of Pre- and Post-Registration Midwifery Programmes of Education (1994b). This ensures, as far as possible, equality of standards across the country. The ENB is also keen to encourage consumer involvement in curriculum development, implementation, and evaluation (ENB 1996a).

Whatever the academic level of the programme undertaken, the midwife must develop analytical skills which can be applied to practice and be clinically competent on registration. Whether those who have completed an undergraduate programme have better developed clinical skills on registration than those who have not is a matter for debate, but it seems reasonable to assume that the intention of such courses must be that they should result in enhanced clinical care at least in the longer term (Alexander 1995).

On registration, midwives are qualified to work both in hospital and in the community. However, it is usual for them to practise in hospital initially.

Given the current move towards greater continuity of midwifery care, this may change. The advantage of an initial period of practice in hospital should be the increase in confidence which comes from the opportunity for consolidation, but there is also the danger that the midwives may become socialized into a 'high-tech' and interventionist model of care which they then try to apply in the community setting. Their practice may be considerably more influenced by concepts of abnormality than by recognizing their role as facilitators and guardians of the normal. Many courses leading to registration now place students with community midwives for their first clinical experience in order to emphasize the predominance of normality.

Professional updating and the maintenance of clinical standards

Requirements relating to the professional updating of midwives are carefully regulated. The system is in the process of change but all midwives are required to undertake a minimum roughly equivalent to five days updating every three years. In addition, they must maintain a professional portfolio which includes reflection on clinical practice and what has been learnt as a result of it – this document is the personal property of the midwife. Undergraduate and Masters' level courses in midwifery also exist for those who are already registered as midwives; clearly their content is different from that described above but they are beyond the scope of this chapter.

All midwives have a supervisor of midwives who is there to act as their professional advisor and mentor. Supervisors, who are experienced midwives who have undergone specific preparation for this role, are also responsible for ensuring that satisfactory standards of midwifery practice are maintained. Supervisors have the right to inspect a midwife's practice and usually meet with each midwife yearly on an individual basis to help them to evaluate their practice and agree how their expertise can be maintained and developed (ENB 1996b).

The requirements outlined above apply equally to midwives employed within the National Health Service and those practising outside it. All midwives who are going to practise are required to notify their local supervisor of their intention to do so before the end of March each year. All those who have not practised for at least 12 working weeks in the preceding five years are required to undertake a structured course before doing so again.

It can be seen from the above that considerable efforts are made to ensure that those in clinical practice are up to date, but how easy it is to ensure that midwives are able to remain both competent and confident in any clinical skills which they use only rarely is debatable.

The education of student nurses contains only very limited coverage of issues related to maternity care and this is insufficient to prepare them to take an active part in the provision of related clinical care after registration. A recent position statement from the UKCC (1996) about practice nurses and antenatal care indicates that the Council expects such care to be provided by a practising midwife who is supervised by the local supervisor of midwives.

General practice

Undergraduate training

All future GPs receive education as a medical student for five (rarely six) years, and then as a junior house officer for a further 12 months. The General Medical Council (GMC) defines the principal objective of basic medical education as providing 'the knowledge, skills, and attitudes which will provide a firm basis for future vocational training' (General Medical Council 1980).

All UK university departments of obstetrics teach medical students, usually for 8–12 weeks, and require that they perform a number of normal deliveries during this time, although the reason for this requirement is not clear (Biggs *et al.* 1991). Historically, the reason was obvious since doctors could go straight into general practice and provide intrapartum care. This has now ceased.

Medical students perform an average of eight normal vaginal births and carry out few obstetric or neonatal procedures themselves (Biggs and Humphrey 1990; Biggs *et al.* 1991; Bornsztein and Julian 1991; Smith 1995). As a result most students do not believe themselves to be competent at many practical procedures after completing their compulsory obstetric and neonatal education (Smith 1995). Interestingly, those students who had witnessed a delivery in a GP unit believed themselves to be more competent. A parallel positive effect on the intention of GP trainees to provide intrapartum care was found when they were exposed to the 'low-tech' role model of their trainers providing such care (Smith 1992).

Vocational training for general practice

Vocational training (VT) for general practice is regulated by statute: the NHS (Vocational Training) Regulations 1987 in England and Wales, with corresponding regulations in Scotland and in Northern Ireland. The Joint Committee on Postgraduate Training for General Practice (JCPTGP) is the body responsible for issuing certificates to doctors on completion of VT. These certificates are required for them to:

- become principals in general practice in the NHS
- record their training status on the medical register kept by the General Medical Council.

The VT regulations prescribe a three-year training period, of which:
- at least 12 months must, and up to 18 can, be spent as a GP registrar in an approved training practice
- a six month period must be spent in two of the following specialties: A & E or general surgery, general medicine, geriatrics, paediatrics, obstetrics or gynaecology or both, and psychiatry
- the remaining 12 months may be spent in any educationally approved post accepted by the regional postgraduate organizations as relevant to GP training.

The training can be whole or part time. If the latter, it must be at least half time and completed within seven years to obtain a certificate of prescribed experience.

Nearly all new principals have done a six-month obstetric or obstetrics and gynaecology post as a senior house officer (Royal College of Obstetricians and Gynaecologists 1993), but there is at present considerable variation in the educational experiences of registrars in hospital posts (Ronalds *et al.* 1981; Reeve and Bowman 1989; Crawley and Levin 1990; Grant *et al.* 1990; Ennis 1991; Kelly and Murray 1991; Smith 1991; Styles 1991). A 1990 confidential postal questionnaire of a random sample of all UK GP trainees found that most (67%) received less than two hours of formal teaching per week, and many (80%) wanted hospital obstetric training to be more orientated towards general practice. It concluded that such training can be more efficiently organized to benefit the GP trainee, the midwife, and the mother; and that undergoing hospital obstetric training significantly increases the reported competence of trainees at most practical obstetric procedures but discourages them from using these skills in the future as a GP obstetrician (Smith 1991).

A second study of this cohort found that in 1995 a minority (18%) provided intrapartum care (28% would ideally have wished to do so) with even fewer (8%) providing home-birth care. These ex-trainees were more likely to be now providing GP intrapartum care if their GP training practice had done so (Smith 1996*a*). This was first theoretically suggested (Young 1991) and then found to be so in a cross-sectional survey of Canadian family physicians (Smith and Reynolds 1995). In particular, attending women in labour as a GP trainee is associated with doing so in the future as a GP, and also with more positive beliefs about the role of the GP (Smith 1992, 1996*a*).

Various studies have reported adversely on the amount, type, and relevance of teaching given to GP registrars in hospital senior house officer (SHO) posts (Ronalds *et al.* 1981; Reeve and Bowman 1989; Crawley and Levin 1990; Grant *et al.* 1990; Smith 1991, 1992). In particular, Smith (1991) found that only two thirds felt that they were competent to perform a normal birth unaided, manage a severe postpartum haemorrhage, or resuscitate a newborn infant; less than half felt competent to intubate a neonate; and less than 40% believed they were competent to perform a low liftout forceps delivery. These practical skills are ones which the future GP obstetrician would need to possess. However, the majority of GPs who provide only shared antenatal and postnatal care would not. Furthermore, despite increasing the perceived competence of registrars, actually holding such a post had a significant negative effect on these beliefs: trainees who had started in post believed even more strongly that it reduced self-confidence and failed to encourage future provision of intrapartum care (Smith 1991). The conclusion of this study was that training is not appropriately focused.

Continuing medical education for GPs

Following completion of vocational training and successful summative assessment, GPs, like midwives and consultants, have an ongoing need for further education. This can be divided into continuing medical education (CME) and higher professional education (HPE). The latter is needed to complete the basic vocational learning to practice as an autonomous GP and is rarely possible at present. The former is usual for all practising GPs from qualification to retirement.

At present there is no formal requirement for GPs to update in obstetrics after they become GPs. Some do so but the content, timing, and benefits (if any) of such updating is not known. GPs can attend any form of education but usually attend only those that are approved for the postgraduate education allowance (PGEA). If a GP undergoes 30 hours of approved education per year averaged over five years, split between three areas (health promotion, disease management, service management), then they can claim the full allowance. They need not undertake any obstetric education at all.

The future

Changes could be made to how maternity care is taught to aspiring GPs and midwives (NHS Executive 1997). Least disruptive would be change to their respective uniprofessional systems and most disruptive (but most beneficial) would be change to interprofessional education and training. Several positive changes could be made to the setting (more community based), content (more emphasis on the common and normal), and teachers (joint teaching by midwives, GPs, consultants, and lay people) whilst still retaining a uniprofessional structure.

However, it is expected that interprofessional learning would have many advantages over the present systems, particularly in terms of teamworking, mutual understanding, reduction in the duplication of care (primary vs. secondary, midwifery vs. medical), and in improving the quality of maternity care that women receive. Principles of such learning and some practical examples are given.

Uniprofessional education and training of midwives

Courses leading to registration as a midwife

At first sight, the change in focus of maternity care and the need to ensure the provision of good quality care in the community do not appear to present as many challenges for the education of midwives as they do for the education of GPs. At least on paper there is a long tradition that the initial education of midwives should prepare them to work both in hospital and community settings. The practical problem, however, has been that the clinical experience gained during initial education has often been in very watertight compartments so that there is perhaps a tendency for one 'type' of care to be associated with care in hospital and another 'type' of care to be associated with community care. Given that most women with high-risk characteristics tend to deliver in hospital, it is perhaps not surprising that care in hospital tends to have followed a more medical, pathology-centred model than the holistic model espoused by many who practice predominantly in the community. There appears to be a need to move away from the 'type' of care being heavily influenced by its location, towards its being determined primarily by the needs of the individual woman wherever she might be. It is thus crucial for student midwives to gain as much experience as possible with 'integrated' midwives (Wraight et al. 1993) who care for women both in hospital and in the community.

It is also worth noting that recent work has shown that the routine 'six-week' postnatal assessment does not meet women's health needs and that its content and timing needs reconsideration (Bick and MacArthur 1995). Surely the time has come for this assessment to be carried out by a midwife previously involved with the mother? Preparation for this role would need to be included in courses leading to registration.

Ongoing education for midwives

A study to establish the current role and responsibilities of midwives and their educational needs in order to fulfil their widening role, and to develop an educational package to assist them, has recently been completed (Pope et al. 1996.) One element of the study was a postal questionnaire of a stratified random sample of 1100 midwives, every maternity unit in England being approached to assist with the sampling. In addition, a questionnaire was sent to the 'key' 205 supervisors of midwives, most of them being identified through the directory of emergency and special care units, and a questionnaire was sent to those on the register of independent midwives in England.

The continuing education needs identified by the midwives and supervisors included communication, counselling, the management of change, ethico-legal issues, and 'professionalism'. Other issues identified included the complexities of using knowledge from a variety of sources, including different research traditions, to achieve quality care. Clinical skills identified included intravenous cannulation, perineal suturing, ultrasonography, labour and delivery in water, and cardiotocograph (CTG) interpretation. The identification of CTG interpretation and, to a lesser extent, perineal suturing seems surprising given that they are included in courses leading to registration. The report also emphasized that the way in which any midwifery workforce rotation system is organized has considerable influence on whether the midwives develop the confidence and skills needed to provide an optimum service.

The educational package produced as part of the work has the development of relationships for effective practice and the context in which care is delivered as its key themes. The activities developed throughout the package are driven by the need for midwives to be able to negotiate their practice in the best interests of service users from a sound knowledge base. The researchers indicate that the need for specialist counselling skills and clinical skills is beyond the scope of the package and must be obtained from other sources.

Uniprofessional education and training of GPs

GPs need to be better educated and trained to provide high-quality maternity care. General practitioners can provide women with choice in maternity care by being available and accessible, by being advocates for women as their *personal* doctor, by facilitating informed choice, and by providing some personal clinical care (General Medical Services Committee and Royal College of General Practitioners 1997). Offering GP bookings as an alternative to consultant or midwife booking is one option that GPs could provide. Such clinical GP care provides continuity of care to women (Department of Health 1993) and thus enhances the quality of maternity care provision (Smith 1992). But GP care can best be provided in conjunction with high-quality midwifery care; together the GP and community-based midwife form the core of the primary maternity care team (Royal College of General Practitioners 1995; Smith 1996*b*; NHS Executive 1997). Future multiprofessional care should be based on interprofessional education of this team (see later).

Undergraduate

In the future, undergraduate education will be more integrated and will consist of core and elective modules. The core will contain basic obstetric education but its exact content remains undetermined. But if it is no longer one of the aims of basic core obstetric and neonatal undergraduate education to provide graduates with the skills, knowledge, and attitudes to be competent at providing safe intrapartum care, then why should they spend valuable time in an overcrowded undergraduate curriculum on a labour ward at all? At the very least the educational relevance and value of routinely expecting students to witness abnormal deliveries, and perhaps perform normal deliveries, needs to be reassessed. Such a change would also enhance the labouring woman's privacy. Additional optional or elective obstetric education (General Medical Council 1991; Lowry 1992) could be available because it is likely to enable interested students to become more competent at intrapartum care by providing more hands-on experience (Smith 1995). Alternatively, and perhaps more appropriately, interested students could experience relevant education about intrapartum practical procedures (and thus achieve competence) at the postgraduate level (Lowry 1993).

Practice

It is the Royal College of General Practitioners' intention that 18 rather than 12 months of the statutory three-year training period should be spent in a training practice (Royal College of General Practitioners 1994). There is also an expectation that in the future:

- part of hospital SHO posts should be spent learning in the community, being taught by primary care professionals in order to enhance the relevance of hospital training

- there will be a greater emphasis on the individual educational needs of SHOs.

It is the College's expectation that all GP registrars will be given the opportunity to receive relevant education and training to enable them to provide a full range of obstetric and gynaecology care for the women in their care (Royal College of Obstetricians and Gynaecologists 1993; Royal College of Obstetricians and Gynaecologists and Royal College of General Practitioners 1993). This would include adequate exposure to intrapartum care.

The majority of registrars believe that their practice obstetric training could be improved by designating as 'GP obstetrician' trainers certain GPs who are providing full obstetric care to the women on their lists (Smith 1992). Those who select GP training practices should require that at least one partner provides intrapartum care, and that registrars are encouraged to attend women in labour and at birth.

Hospital senior house officer – experience in GP training

1. *Education and training.* The great majority of GP registrars wish that their training was more orientated towards their future needs in general practice. One way to achieve this would be for those who intend providing shared care only, to be trained by GPs and community midwives who provide this care already. The significant minority who wish to become GP obstetricians could have training jointly: in practice by experienced GP obstetricians and community midwives, and in hospital obstetric posts by interested obstetricians and hospital midwives. This would mean that most GP registrars would stop doing hospital obstetric jobs, and midwives could extend their role in consultant or midwife maternity units (Towler 1984; Coupland *et al.* 1987; Smith 1989; Hare *et al.* 1990; Street *et al.* 1991), effectively taking over the role of the senior house officer.

There are various ways forward towards this ideal situation in the education and training of 'hospital' obstetrics and gynaecology SHOs who are to be GPs. These include:

- primary care professionals coming in to hospitals to teach
- sessional release of SHOs to learn in the community
- joint obstetric and general practice appointments (over a year or six months)
- joint community and hospital SHO posts over six months.
- sessional release from a training practice for educational obstetric and gynaecology sessions in hospital as part of a longer time spent training in a GP training practice.

A pilot study of sessional release (option 2) found that the attachments put registrars' hospital obstetric SHO training in perspective; enabled them to care for women with uncomplicated pregnancies; was a positive experience; they learnt about the role of community midwives; the case-load was often inadequate; more structure to sessions was requested; and they wished to see GPs providing maternity care as well as midwives (Smith 1998).

2. *Assessment.* Summative assessment was introduced in September 1996 and became legally mandatory in 1997. It consists of four modules: multiple choice questionnaire, assessment of consultation skills, written submission of practical work, and the trainer's report. The assessment does not include intrapartum clinical skills but will cover antenatal and postnatal care; it is thus a valid assessment for the majority of GP registrars who do not wish to provide intrapartum care as GPs. However, at present, admission to the GP obstetric list (which increases the remuneration that the GP receives for providing obstetric care) is dependent in nearly all cases upon the satisfactory completion of a resident six-month obstetric and gynaecology post; completing such a post is also necessary to sit the Diploma examination of the Royal College of Obstetricians and Gynaecologists. Possession of this Diploma is often regarded as a prerequisite for a new partner to join a practice. Furthermore, if obstetric training for the majority of registrars who wish to provide only shared care were practice based, assessment of competence by the membership examination at the Royal College of General Practitioners (MRCGP) would be more valid; the significant minority who wish to provide full care could sit a modified Diploma examination jointly set by the Royal College of Obstetricians and Gynaecologists and Royal College of General Practitioners. In this way, GP registrars would receive training and assessment appropriate to their future needs, uninterested registrars would not be required to do unnecessary hospital obstetric posts, midwives could extend their role and enhance their professional status, and pregnant women would receive improved care from GPs who are trained to provide care which is appropriate to their needs.

Continuing medical education

It is the Royal College of General Practitioners' view that, at the end of a three-year vocational training course, the newly qualified GP principal still has much to learn. The College suggests that provision should be made for a further two years of higher professional education to occur soon after becoming a principal. Such education would be in addition to the continuing medical education (CME) that all principals should undertake each year.

There should be a statutory requirement for time to be spent studying obstetrics if the GP is on the 'obstetric list', parallel to the requirement for midwives. This would be part of CME. In addition, it would be hoped that some young GPs will wish to undertake further obstetric training and education as part of their higher professional education. This would be voluntary.

Interprofessional education and training

Principles

'Interprofessional education' is the term used to describe a situation where people from, or preparing to enter, more than one profession are educated together. It can be argued that this is a better term than 'multiprofessional' as the stem 'inter' implies interaction and partnership between those involved rather than simply being many together (Centre for the Advancement of Interprofessional Education 1996; NHS Executive 1997).

There is a considerable amount of literature on the value of interprofessional education, some authors concentrating on education leading to a first professional qualification (Areskog 1988; Studdy *et al.* 1994; Zungolo 1994; Larson 1995), others including continuing education (Brooking 1991; Goble 1991). Whether discussing doctors, midwives, nurses, health visitors, occupational therapists, community social service supervisors, physiotherapists, or laboratory technicians, there seems to be a general consensus that health care requires collaboration and teamwork, that patients or clients can suffer when it is missing, and that joint education helps to foster it (Horder 1991).

Both the World Health Organization (Areskog 1988) and the English National Board for Nursing, Midwifery, and Health Visiting (ENB 1996*a*) have stressed the importance of the issue and there is now an organization, the Centre for the Advancement of Interprofessional Education (CAIPE), dedicated to its promotion amongst those involved with primary health and community care (Horder 1991).

CAIPE conducted an extensive literature review for its report concerning interprofessional education in mental health (CAIPE 1996). The principles and characteristics of effective interprofessional education, developed from those identified within it, are given in Box 10.1.

Box 10.1 *The principles and characteristics of effective inter-professional education*

Interprofessional education:

- works to improve the quality of care provided; the development of a shared philosophy promotes teamwork and the provision of a seamless service. Brooking (1991) considers that separation and conflict between professional groups result in fragmentation of knowledge and skills and thus in deficiencies in client care

- focuses on the needs of service users and their carers; this facilitates the development of a collaborative culture between professionals and service users

---

- involves service users and their carers, empowering all those involved so that differing views of service priorities may be aired. Contact with consumers willing to take part in developing multi-professional education might be made through Maternity Service Liaison Committees

- promotes interprofessional collaboration; because each profession comes to understand the role of the other and how it interacts with their own, trust is established and communication enhanced. Collaborative competencies are developed, the chance of misunder-standings reduced, and appropriate referral made more likely. Horder (1991) in particular believes that greater openness about uncertainties, resentments, or failures can enhance collaboration. Potential conflict situations are likely to be handled better in the future

- encourages professions to learn with, from, and about one another; by articulating what each considers to be the essence of good prac-tice, an understanding of differing professional cultures and methods of operation is developed. This does not mean that all participants need to think alike or that professional identity is threatened but Areskog (1988) believes that a common frame of reference provides a good basis for teamwork

- enhances practice within professions; through discussion each pro-fession gains a deeper understanding of its own practice. Areskog (1988) writes of the benefits of increased self-knowledge. It is not a deskilling process but there has to be recognition that profes-sional roles may need to change to meet the needs of service users

- respects the integrity and contribution of each profession; it helps to ensure that each profession will utilize fully the expertise of the other. Stereotypes are challenged and prejudice dispelled

- increases professional satisfaction; enthusiasm is maintained. This benefit is maximized if the initiative is valued by managers and professional regulatory bodies and carries educational credit.

It is also worth considering the attributes of good practice related to the provision of shared learning, as modified from the list provided by CAIPE (1996). They include:

- clarity of purpose and of intended learning outcomes
- commitment from all stakeholders
- institutional support (sufficient funding and help to synchronize curricula)
- involving all participating professions and agencies in the planning and provision

- equal status among the planners and among the participants
- developing realistic plans that fit with current operational systems and sharing information about professional education already being provided
- using participative education methods such as problem solving related to areas of mutual interest
- exploring differing and conflicting views openly, honestly, and with mutual respect
- evaluation to investigate the benefits to the practitioner, their organization, and service users.

For shared learning at continuing professional development level, it is particularly important that the initiative should build on an analysis of needs and priorities and that a method is devised for ensuring that the collaborative development process is maintained, for example by ongoing short meetings with a specific focus.

At first sight, shared learning may appear to be a method to reduce costs but in reality the complex planning and administration, the necessary preparation and support of teachers, and the use of small groups may prove expensive. In the longer term, any possible extra cost should be offset by increased clinical effectiveness. For interprofessional initiatives to succeed there has to be considerable political will behind them (Larson 1995, CAIPE 1996).

Practicalities

Various examples exist of interprofessional learning but practical constraints make such developments slow and none have been formally evaluated to date. We briefly describe four learning fora which are consistent with the principles just delineated.

1. Advanced Life Support in Obstretics (ALSO ®). The initial project was funded by the *Changing Childbirth* team and ran its first teaching weekends in 1996. It is based on, and closely follows the format of, the North American ALSO ® Program which is run by the American Academy of Family Physicians. The British version, like the American, is a two-day residential course consisting of a mixture of lectures and practical workshops and ending with a written examination and practical viva using mannequins. The syllabus comprises common obstetric problems and rare but important maternal and neonatal emergencies. The teachers and learners are multidisciplinary. General practitioners, midwives, and junior doctors learn together. It is being evaluated but results are not yet available.

2. *Joint Medical/Midwifery Postgraduate Educational Project.* This project is based at the School of Health Care in Liverpool's John Moores University and comprises a seven-month, part-time, theoretical and practical programme for midwives, SHOs, and GPs. Accreditation has been gained for Masters level credit, for PGEA purposes, and from the ENB; such multiple accreditation is

clearly highly desirable. The work was financed by *Changing Childbirth* development funds and the programme ran for the first time in 1996. Following evaluation and some modifications, it was run again in 1997.

3. *Association for Community-based Maternity Care (ACBMC)*. This is the only national United Kingdom body concerned with maternity care which is interdisciplinary, its membership comprising GPs, midwives, consultants, and lay people. It was founded to promote community-based maternity care. Since its formation in 1988 it has run biannual study days which have rotated around the UK. These days are a mixture of lectures and small-group workshops. It has two distinctions from other such CME days. First, its teachers and learners have always reflected its interdisciplinary membership; and second, consumers have also regularly taught and learnt together with the professionals.

4. *Practical Update for GPs in Intrapartum Care: An Example of Multi-professional Teaching (Stosiek et al. 1996)*. This short course, which has now ceased, was developed by the Centre for Midwifery Studies at the University of Portsmouth in collaboration with Dr Ann White, a GP tutor. Its aims were to develop knowledge, skills, and confidence to enable GPs, midwives, and consultants to work effectively as teams; to explore the roles and relationships of GPs, midwives, and consultants in light of the changing patterns of maternity care; and to facilitate women's choice. The course was of 19 hours duration, each GP spending two seven-hour shifts on the delivery suite on a one-to-one basis with a midwifery lecturer. A consultant obstetrician joined the group for the three-hour theoretical session and two hours were allowed for the completion of a reflective journal, action plan, and final evaluation. Much of the theoretical session was built around case scenarios and the evaluations were very positive.

Consumer involvement

If the maternity services are to become truly woman centred it is clearly essential that consumers are involved in the planning of the education of those who provide these services and also in the delivery of some elements of it. Some suggestions relating to this have been made earlier. When planning for such involvement it is important to consider payment, child care provision (and insurance cover), travel expenses, and other practical issues such as time of day and refreshments. It may also be important to assist these consumers to gain critical appraisal skills in order to take part in the debate concerning evidence-based practice. Critical appraisal skills workshops for a number of Maternity Service Liaison Committees have been financed by *Changing Childbirth* development funds and involved consumers, doctors, midwives, purchasers, and providers. These workshops were very positively evaluated, including the benefits of interdisciplinary learning (Critical Appraisal Skills Programme 1997). It may also be useful to provide practical workshops on the use of the Cochrane Library databases (Alexander *et al.*

1996). As with all new initiatives, evaluation is required. The representation of consumers from minority groups requires careful consideration

Summary of recommendations

We would like to see the following ways of learning together to be introduced in the near future in the UK. Our detailed reasons are given earlier in this chapter. In summary, such innovations would improve teamwork, enhance women's choice and continuity of care, and ultimately achieve the high-quality maternity care that pregnant women need and deserve:

- midwifery and medical students should learn the basics together
- hospital obstetric SHOs (including GP registrars) and senior midwifery students should learn together
- GPs, midwives, and consultant obstetricians should learn and update together
- all groups should be taught by interdisciplinary groups, including lay people
- the obstetric list should be abolished in its present form
- the present diploma examination of the RCOG should be renamed and jointly set (based on evidence where available) and examined by the three Royal Colleges (Royal College of Midwives, Royal College of Obstetricians and Gynaecologists, and Royal College of General Practitioners)
- this joint examination should only be required by those GPs providing intrapartum care
- only exceptionally should groups learn in a unidisciplinary setting or be taught by teachers of one discipline.

References

Alexander, J. (1995). Midwifery graduates in the United Kingdom. In: *Issues in midwifery* (ed. T. Murphy-Black), pp. 83-98. Churchill Livingstone, Edinburgh.

Alexander, J., Gwyer, R., and Pitman, B. (1996). Collaborating with Cochrane and disseminating the database. *British Journal of Midwifery*, 4(12), 637–9.

Areskog, N.-H. (1988). The need for multiprofessional health education in undergraduate studies. *Medical Education*, 22, 251–2.

Bick, D. E. and MacArthur, C. (1995). Attendance, content, and relevance of the six-week postnatal examination. *Midwifery*, 11, 69–73.

Biggs, J.S. and Humphrey, M.D. (1990). Undergraduate education in obstetrics and gynaecology in Australia and New Zealand, 1989. *Australian and New Zealand Journal of Obstetrics and Gynaecology*, 30, 185–90.

Biggs, J. S., Harden, R. M, and Howie, P. (1991). Undergraduate obstetrics and gynaecology in the United Kingdom and the Republic of Ireland, 1989. *British Journal of Obstetrics and Gynaecology*, **98**, 127–34.

Bornsztein, B. and Julian, T. M. (1991). Quantifying clinical activity in a multisite clerkship in obstetrics and gynaecology. *Obstetrics and Gynaecology*, **78**, 869–72.

Brooking, J. (1991). Doctors and nurses: a personal view. *Nursing Standard*, **6**(12), 4–8.

Campbell, R. and MacFarlane, A. (1994). *Where to be born? The debate and the evidence* (2nd edn). National Perinatal Epidemiology Unit, Oxford.

Centre for the Advancement of Interprofessional Education (CAIPE) (1996). Developing interprofessional education in mental health: report for the Sainsbury Centre, review of the roles, and training of mental health care staff. CAIPE, London.

Coupland, V. A., Green, J. M., Kitzinger, J. V., *et al.* (1987). Obstetricians in the labour ward: implications of medical staffing structures. *British Medical Journal*, **295**, 1077–9.

Crawley, H. S. and Levin, J. B. (1990). Training for general practice: a national survey. *British Medical Journal*, **300**, 911–15.

Critical Appraisal Skills Programme (1997). *CASP for MSLCs – a project enabling MSLCs to develop an evidence-based approach to Changing Childbirth*. Final project report. PO Box 777, Oxford OX3 7LF.

Department of Health (1993). Changing childbirth: report of the Expert Maternity Group. HMSO, London.

English National Board for Nursing, Midwifery, and Health Visiting (1994). *Creating lifelong learners – guidelines for midwifery programmes of education*. ENB, London.

English National Board for Nursing, Midwifery, and Health Visiting (1996*a*). *Corporate plan – operational objectives 1996/97*. ENB, London.

English National Board for Nursing, Midwifery, and Health Visiting (1996*b*). *Supervision of midwives – the English National Board's advice and guidance to local supervising authorities and supervisors of midwives*. ENB, London.

Ennis, M. (1991). Training and supervision of obstetric senior house officers. *British Medical Journal*, **303**, 1442–3.

European Community Midwives Directive, 89/594/EEC. Amendment to directives.

Flint, C., Poulengeris, P., and Grant, A. (1989). The 'Know your midwife' scheme – a randomized trial of continuity of care by a team of midwives. *Midwifery*, **5**, 11–16.

Ford, C., Iliffe, S., and Franklin, O. (1991). Outcome of planned home birth in an inner-city practice. *British Medical Journal*, **303**, 1517–19.

General Medical Council (1980). *Recommendations on basic medical education*. GMC, London.

General Medical Council (1991). *Undergraduate medical education*. Discussion document by the working party of the General Medical Council Education Committee. GMC, London.

General Medical Services Committee and Royal College of General Practitioners (1997). *General practitioners and intrapartum care*. BMA, London.

Goble, R. (1991). Keeping alive intellectually. *Nursing*, 4(33), 19–22.

Grant, J., Marsden, P., and King, R. (1990). Senior house officers and their training. I: Personal characteristics and professional circumstances; II: Perceptions of service and training. *British Medical Journal*, **299**, 1263–8.

Hare, M. J., Miles, R. N., Lattimore, C. R., and Southern, J. P. (1990). 'Senior house officer Report' staffing in practice: five years' experience of a consultant-based service in obstetrics and neonatal paediatrics. *British Medical Journal*, **300**, 857–9.

Horder, J. (1991). CAIPE: Striving for collaboration. *Nursing*, 4(33), 16–18.

House of Commons (1992). Maternity services : second report of the Health Select Committee. Vol. 1. HMSO, London.

Kelly, D. R. and Murray, T. S. (1991). Twenty years of vocational training in the west of Scotland: the practice component. *British Journal of General Practice*, **41**, 492–5.

Larson, E. (1995). New rules for the game: interdisciplinary education for health professionals. *Nursing Outlook*, 43(4), 180–5.

Lowry, S. (1992). Strategies for implementing curriculum change. *British Medical Journal*, **305**, 1482–5.

Lowry, S. (1993). Trends in health care and their effects on medical education. *British Medical Journal*, **306**, 255–8.

Marsh, G. N., Cashman, H. A., and Russell, I. T. (1985). General practitioner participation in intranatal care in the Northern region in 1983. *British Medical Journal*, **290**, 971–3.

Newble, D. I. (1992). Assessing clinical competence at the undergraduate level. *Medical Education*, **26**, 504–11.

NHS Exective (1997). Learning together – professional education for maternity care. DoH, London.

Pope, R., Graham, L., Cooney, M., and Holliday, M. (1996). Identification of the changing educational needs of midwives in developing new dimensions of care in a variety of settings and the development of an educational package to meet these needs. University of Greenwich.

Reeve, H. and Bowman, A. (1989). Hospital training for general practice: the views of trainees in the North Western region. *British Medical Journal*, **298**, 1432–4.

Ronalds, C., Douglas, A., Gray, D. J. P., and Selly, P. (ed.) (1981). *Fourth national trainee conference*. Occasional paper 18. Royal College of General Practitioners, London.

Royal College of General Practitioners (1994). *Education and training for general practice*. Policy statement 3. RCGP, London.

Royal College of General Practitioners (1995). *The role of general practice in maternity care*. Occasional paper 72. RCGP, London.

Royal College of Obstetricians and Gynaecologists (1993). *Report of the DRCOG working party*. RCOG, London.

Royal College of Obstetricians and Gynaecologists and Royal College of General Practitioners (1993). *General practitioner vocational training in obstetrics and gynaecology*. RCGP, London.

Smith, H. (1989). Working without registrars. *Nursing Times*, **85** (6), 75.

Smith, L. F. P. (1991). GP trainees' views on hospital obstetric vocational training. *British Medical Journal*, **303**, 1447–52.

Smith, L. F. P. (1992). Roles, risks, and responsibilities in maternity care: trainees' beliefs and the effects of practice obstetric training. *British Medical Journal*, **304**, 1613–15.

Smith, L. F. P. (1995). The effects of undergraduate education on the perceived obstetric and neonatal competence of medical students. *Medical Education*, **29**, 77–84.

Smith, L. F. P. (1996a). *Predictors of the provision of intrapartum care by GPs: five-year cohort study*. MD thesis, University of Bristol.

Smith, L. F. P. (1996b). Should GPs have any role in maternity care in the future? *British Journal of General Practice*, **46**, 243–7.

Smith, L. F. P. (1998). Community training by GPs and midwives of hospital obstetric SHOs: a pilot study. *British Journal of General Practice* (In press.)

Smith, L. F. P. and Reynolds, J. L. (1995). Factors associated with the decision of family physicians to provide intrapartum care. *Canadian Medical Association Journal*, **152**, 1789–97.

Stosiek, J., Alexander, J., and White, A. (1996). Improving choice and care for women through joint initiatives. *The Association for Community-based Maternity Care Newsletter*, **13**, 6–7.

Street, P., Gannon, M. J., and Holt, E. M. (1991). Community care in West Berkshire. *British Medical Journal*, **302**, 698–700.

Studdy, S. J., Nicol, M. J., Fox-Hiley, A. (1994). Teaching and learning clinical skills. Part 1: Development of a multidisciplinary skills centre. *Nurse Education Today*, **14**, 177–85.

Styles, W. McN. (1991). Training experience of doctors certificated for general practice in 1985–90. *British Journal of General Practice*, **41**, 488–91.

Taylor, A. (1986). Maternity services: the consumer's view. *Journal of the Royal College of General Practitioners*, 36, 157–60.

Towler, J. (1984). Midwives' units: wishful thinking or reality? *Midwives Chronicle*, **97**, 3–5.

United Kingdom Central Council for Nursing, Midwifery, and Health Visiting (1993). *Midwives' rules*. UKCC, London.

United Kingdom Central Council for Nursing, Midwifery, and Health Visiting (1994a). *The midwife's code of practice*. UKCC, London.

United Kingdom Central Council for Nursing, Midwifery, and Health Visiting (1994b). *Requirements for the content of pre- and post-registration midwifery programmes of education*. Registrar's letter 8/1994. UKCC, London.

United Kingdom Central Council for Nursing, Midwifery, and Health Visiting (1996). *Practice nurses and antenatal care – council position statement*. Registrar's letter 8/1996. UKCC, London.

Wraight, A., Ball, J., Seccombe, I., and Stock, J. (1993). *Mapping team midwifery*. IMS report series 242. Institute of Manpower Studies, Brighton.

Young, G. L. (1991). General practice and the future of obstetric care. *British Journal of General Practice*, **41**, 266–7.

Zungolo, E. (1994). Interdisciplinary education in primary care : the challenge. *Nursing and Health Care*, 15(6), 288–92.

SECTION THREE

CLINICAL
CHALLENGES

Narrowing the gap: social class, age, and ethnic differences in maternity outcomes

Janet Hirst and Maggie Eisner

This chapter focuses on inequalities in the health of pregnant women and their babies, reflecting a broader picture of social inequalities in health (Black 1980). Disappointingly, recent evidence suggests that these inequalities are not diminishing (Benzeval *et al.* 1995).

We outline what is known about the effects of social class, age, and ethnic differences on maternity outcomes and make recommendations as to how the community maternity services can help to narrow the gap.

Problems – definitions and evidence

Readers will be aware that it is not easy to define the terms used in this area, and that there are problems in collecting statistics. Although *mortality* seems to be an unambiguous term, it is difficult to differentiate between those maternal deaths directly caused by pregnancy and childbirth and those due to related or coexistent medical problems. Estimates of the annual number of maternal deaths worldwide vary between 585 000 (WHO 1995) and 1.3 million (reported by Population Action International, quoted in Dillner 1995).

What is classified as *morbidity* will depend on the expectations of both women and health professionals, and on the way data are collected.

In Britain, the most widely used measure of *social class* is the Registrar General's classification, introduced in 1911 but revised several times since. Until recently, it has been based on men's occupations, taking account of the degree of skill involved and the social position implied; married women were classified by their husband's occupation. Until there has been several years' experience of collecting data on women's occupations, its applicability to women will remain limited. It is also questionable whether someone's occupation, considered alone, is a valid measure of social class. As it is generally understood, 'class' is a complex concept which also involves economic status and level of education. In discussing the effect of 'class' on maternity outcomes, the most important factors are often poverty and poor educational level.

The measurement of *age* is uncontroversial, although there are different views of the appropriate age for motherhood.

The classification of *ethnicity* is even more problematic than social class. People may be assigned to ethnic groups according to their country of origin, their parents' country of origin, their religion, language, culture, or even skin colour. In addition, their self-defined ethnicity may be different from others' perceptions. This creates difficulties both in research and in practice.

It is also often difficult to obtain statistically valid *evidence* of the effect of differences in maternity services on the major outcomes of mortality and morbidity because very large samples are needed for statistical significance. When studies do not involve large enough populations, the results may be confused by variables which have not been accounted for. Changes in maternity services are often introduced on such a small scale that the only outcomes which can be validly measured are 'soft' (but important) ones such as user satisfaction.

Maternity outcomes

The *maternal mortality* rate in the UK declined steadily from 1952 to 1982, halving every 10 years (Chapter 7). Between 1982 and 1990, however, the rate stabilized at 10 per 100 000 maternities (mothers delivered of live or stillborn babies) (Department of Health 1994). Some authors have attributed the reduction in maternal deaths to improvements in women's health, knowledge, and behaviour, and in their social living and working conditions, while others feel that it mainly reflects improvements in the maternity services (Tew 1990; Stones *et al.* 1991; Loudon 1992). Thompson (1995) suggested that 'to keep women off the road to maternal death, women must be educated, they must be free to chose when and whether to became pregnant , and they must have access to quality care when they become pregnant'. Between 1988 and 1990, 238 women died directly or indirectly as a result of pregnancy (that is, due to obstetric complications or interventions, or to unrelated disease aggravated by the pregnancy). Half had had substandard care during their pregnancy; for others this was a feature alongside complications such as hypertensive disorders and pulmonary embolism (Keirse 1994; Macfarlane *et al.* 1995).

Antenatal and postnatal morbidity is more difficult to study and document than mortality. However, one study of 2164 maternities showed that 523 women (24%) had experienced at least one episode of morbidity in the antenatal period and the year following childbirth. Morbidity included problems such as impaired glucose tolerance, antenatal anaemia, and urinary infection, as well as 'near miss' events including severe haemorrhage, fulminating pre-eclampsia, and pulmonary embolus (Stones *et al.* 1991). The study did not include the multiple problems handled by the GP and community midwife, such as antenatal infections and postnatal depression (Chapter 20), so total morbidity would be very much higher than that reported. Several studies have revealed a high level of postnatal maternal morbidity (Sleep and Grant 1987; Rutter and Quine 1990; Glazener *et al.* 1995). Of 1249 women surveyed by Glazener *et al.*, 85% reported at least one episode of postnatal morbidity such as depression, perineal pain, excessive fatigue, anaemia, headache, and urinary symptoms. Morbidity may be even more extensive than this as non-responders in the study tended to be younger, unmarried, with lighter babies and an unrecorded social class.

Infant and perinatal mortality and morbidity are inextricably linked with the health of mothers. However, because the Registrar General's classification of social class is based on men's occupations, the statistics collected by the Office of Population Censuses and Surveys (OPCS) relate to fathers. In 1994, in England and Wales, babies born to fathers in unskilled manual occupations had infant mortality rates 40% higher than the babies of fathers in professional occupations (OPCS 1995). The statistics refer to births jointly registered by both parents, regardless of whether they are married. Rates of stillbirth and infant death increase consistently down the social scale.

Poor growth rates *in utero* and during infancy are well known to be closely related to poor nutrition during pregnancy. Pregnant women living on state benefits or other low income often cannot afford enough of the healthy food they need (Dallison and Lobstein 1995). The adverse effects of low birth weight are not confined to infancy, but may be detected in later life (Kogan 1995; Chapter 15). Postnatal depression has been shown to have adverse consequences for the infant and to affect children's development; infants of depressed mothers tend to be discontented and to withdraw from maternal contact (Murray *et al.* 1991).

Perinatal outcomes also differ according to ethnic background. In 1994, perinatal mortality rates in the UK were lowest for mothers born in Australia, Canada, or New Zealand (6.4 per 1000 births) (OPCS 1995). The rate for babies of mothers born in the UK (8.6) was exceeded for babies whose mothers were born in the Irish Republic (11.2), Pakistan (15.0), and the Caribbean (17.4). The high perinatal mortality rate for babies born to mothers from Pakistan was associated with an increase in congenital anomalies and preterm births. However, the picture is complicated by regional variations: a study of outcomes for 11 046 infants in one London borough found that the perinatal mortality of Asian infants was similar to that of white infants, although that of infants of African and West Indian mothers was higher (Lyon *et al.* 1994).

Socio-economic class

For a brief period during the 1930s, poverty had one advantage: women from the lowest social class had the lowest maternal mortality from direct causes such as severe toxaemia and puerperal sepsis, despite poor living conditions and hygiene. This has been attributed to their lower risk of iatrogenic infection because they had less contact with health carers (Tew 1990). Today, there is no doubt that living on a low income is detrimental to the health of the pregnant woman and her baby (Chrisholm 1989; Rutter and Quine 1990; Oakley 1991; Quine *et al.* 1993; Benzeval *et al.* 1995; Dallison and Lobstein 1995; Hayes 1995; Kogan 1995; Peacock *et al.* 1995; Wilcox *et al.* 1995; Godfrey *et al.* 1996). Poverty translates into a catalogue of maternity risk factors, many of them avoidable. Women on low incomes are reported to find it less easy to take up screening services and to take up and maintain antenatal care; they are also more likely to attend late for their first antenatal visit. They are more likely to smoke, to be poorly nourished, to have inadequate social support, and to experience more negative life events. They have an increased risk of preterm birth and of low birthweight, are more likely to experience either antenatal or postnatal depression, and are less likely to breastfeed. They are also more likely to feel dissatisfied with their maternity care, and have been reported to feel anxious and doubtful about taking control of what is happening to them.

Ethnicity

It is not clear why some minority ethnic groups have poor maternity outcomes. Much of the apparent effect of ethnicity is probably due to poverty, poor housing, and poor education (Proctor and Smith 1992). The cultural tradition of consanguineous marriages, particularly among Muslim families, is often cited as contributing to a high perinatal mortality rate due to congenital abnormalities caused by autosomal recessive disorders, but may have been overemphasized (Proctor and Smith 1992). People from minority ethnic groups have been found to be more likely to be unemployed, to have low-paid jobs (often well beneath their qualifications), and to do shiftwork. As Benzeval *et al.* (1995) have stated: 'A person's health cannot be divorced from the social and economic environment in which they live.'

The higher parity of minority ethnic women, and a higher proportion of older mothers, are also relevant. Differences in health behaviour may be important but some of these may, in fact, be advantageous to minority ethnic women – smoking , for example, is very rare in Pakistani-born women.

Minority ethnic women face other problems in addition to those of poverty. Access to the health service is well known to be negatively correlated with social class, but minority ethnic women may also have to face racism and stereotyping by maternity carers (Bowler 1993), as well as inadequate solutions to language and communication problems (Balarajan and Raleigh 1993; Hayes 1995). Appropriate screening tests – for example, for haemoglobinopathies – may not be systematically organized; language and communication problems may be particularly damaging in situations requiring counselling such as antenatal screening tests or the management of fetal abnormalities.

Age

Both older and younger women face disadvantages in maternity outcomes.

The teenage pregnancy rate in Britain is among the highest in Europe. In 1991 there were 9.3 conceptions per 1000 women in England and Wales under the age of 16. Of these, 51% ended in abortion (Botting 1995). In 1992, 48 000 teenagers in England and Wales had a baby (Ineichen *et al.* 1994). Some teenage pregnancies are intentional; others result from failure to use contraception, or failure to use it properly. Many, however, fall between the extremes of 'intentional' and 'accidental', and simply result from risky sexual behaviour without consideration of the consequences. The disappointing UK statistics may be related to problems with access to family planning services, and especially to the inadequacy of sex education in schools. In the Netherlands, with a teenage pregnancy rate one seventh of that in Britain, sex education is statutory from primary school onwards.

Babies born to teenage mothers have an increased risk of perinatal death, premature birth, congenital defects, and sudden infant death syndrome (Wilson 1995).

Teenage mothers tend to be from a low social class (Ineichen and Hudson 1994; Wilson 1995; Woodward 1995) and experience some of the same problems as anyone on a low income, such as being unable to afford a healthy diet for a growing mother and baby. There appears to be an undercurrent of social problems that leads teenagers to become pregnant; research has also demonstrated a clear link between poor self-esteem and risky sexual behaviour (Friedman and Phillips 1981). Despite the well-publicized views of some politicians, it is unlikely that many teenagers deliberately become pregnant as a means of jumping council housing queues and obtaining extra Social Security benefits. There are varied reasons why teenagers become pregnant or decide to continue with an unintended pregnancy. Some want to get away from home because of difficult family relationships. Some lack any other horizons and hope to improve their status and give meaning to their lives by becoming mothers. Others, especially if they have lacked love in their earlier childhood, feel that a baby will enable them to express love and will love them in return. A study by Rainey (Rainey *et al.* 1995) found that out of 200 13–18 year-old females, 40 (20%) reported sexual abuse, and that these young women were more likely to be trying to conceive, had partners pressuring them to conceive, and had fears about fertility.

Teenage mothers have been found to suffer from a higher incidence of general health problems in pregnancy, such as urinary tract infections, anaemia, and hypertension (Konje *et al.* 1992). Many pregnant teenagers also smoke and consume more alcohol than older mothers; the rapidly increasing use of illegal drugs by young people is almost certainly reflected to some extent among pregnant teenagers. They may be struggling with the psychological pressures of whether to request an abortion or adoption for their baby. They are often single (Babb 1993) or in the early stages of a relationship with a partner who is equally immature and uncertain. They may well have less support from their own parents than older mothers, although they need it even more. In addition to this, single teenage mothers are stigmatized as taking advantage of the welfare state and as being immature and unfit for parenthood.

One of the issues for older women having their first baby is lack of confidence about mothering. Many older first-time mothers, often age 35 or more, have postponed childbearing while they developed their careers. Their success at work (often in professional occupations) sometimes gives them an articulate and confident personal style which conceals their vulnerability and fears about pregnancy and adjusting to motherhood; they may also live far from their family of origin, so they have little practical support and little recent experience of babies. However, they are likely to have good health at the outset because they are often more highly educated, may feel more content with their career achievements, and come from a higher social class (Berryman and Windridge 1995).

The best known maternity problem for older women is birth anomalies, particularly Down's and Edwards' syndromes, so they are more likely to be offered and to accept screening tests. Older women, especially first-time mothers, tend to be treated as 'high risk' antenatally, although there is little modern evidence that this is true. In the past, when family planning was mostly practised by women of higher social classes, the apparent age-related risks may have been partly due to a combination of high parity and low social class. First-time older mothers can feel belittled by the old-fashioned term 'elderly primigravida'. Nevertheless, there is evidence for older mothers of an increased Caesarean section rate (Mansfield and Cohn 1986), miscarriage rate (Berryman and Windridge 1995), and stillbirth and neonatal mortality rates (Macfarlane *et al.* 1995). Mothers over 35, compared with those in their 20s, also reported more postnatal problems, including extreme tiredness and stress incontinence, although they were more likely to breastfeed (Berryman and Windridge 1995).

What can be done by the community maternity services to narrow the gap?

Those who provide maternity services have been publicly urged to do more to narrow the gap in outcomes. The *Changing Childbirth* report (Department of Health 1993) recommended that general practitioners, midwives, and obstetricians review the way in which they work. It adopted an admirably woman-centred approach, and brought about a national reconsideration of the way maternity care is provided. However, it set targets for specific changes without proposing clear, practical ways to achieve them, although some examples of good practice were included; plans for financing any changes in practice were absent. It also made many general practitioners feel marginalized, causing them to move out of maternity care (Zander 1995).

A wide range of strategies have been suggested to narrow the gap in maternity outcomes. Kogan (1995) highlighted paying more attention to the stresses in a pregnant woman's life and providing counselling and information on behavioural risks. Woodward (1995), discussing the rise in unplanned teenage pregnancies, concluded that it is not possible to propose a single, simple strategy to tackle the problem. Glazener *et al.* (1995) drew attention to the need for continued vigilance by health professionals in the postnatal period, suggesting the provision of lay and social support . Benzeval *et al.* (1995) offered broad, comprehensive strategies for tackling inequalities, suggesting that we need to find ways of strengthening individuals, strengthening communities, improving access to essential facilities, and encouraging economic and cultural changes. Keirse (1994) stated that 'it is not good enough for services to be readily available. They must be accessible, not alien, hostile, or superfluous'.

It is important to acknowledge that any health services can have only a limited effect on the inequalities caused by social factors such as poverty and poor housing. The latter need to be tackled by political and economic measures which are beyond the range of this book. We can only make suggestions about how the community services can try to counteract the effects of inequality, and at least avoid the excesses of the 'Inverse Care Law' (Tudor Hart 1971) which observes that those most in need of health care receive the least of it.

The essence of community-based maternity care is multidisciplinary teamwork (Marsh 1985; Chapter 5). There are opportunities for midwives, general practitioners, health visitors, practice nurses, social workers, dieticians, counsellors, ultrasonographers, physiotherapists, obstetricians, and others to work together to have a positive effect upon family planning, preconceptional care, maternity care, and beyond. Women need a cohesive link between hospital and community services because most will receive antenatal and postnatal care in the community and give birth in hospital, and many will, at some point in the pregnancy, need hospital-based care (Kean *et al.* 1996).

Accessibility

Where is the best place for community maternity care? It would be inappropriate to propose a completely uniform pattern – women differ both in their needs (physical, psychological, and social) and in their ability to benefit from different aspects of the service. The best way to provide services will vary between different localities and health care teams, and for different women served by the same team. Some organizational features of maternity services have been shown to benefit disadvantaged women, and we can learn from local and national examples of good practice.

In most parts of Britain, it is well established that maternity services are best provided as close to women's homes as possible, preferably in familiar and relatively informal surroundings such as health centres and general practice surgeries. 'Low-risk' pregnancies are often managed entirely within the community by midwives and general practitioners. A review of antenatal care initiatives in primary care settings has shown that maternity care in the community improves access for women, encourages a higher uptake of care, improves communication, and leads to improved user satisfaction, with no detrimental effect on maternity outcomes (Wood 1991). Continuity of carers is also greater in the community setting, although multidisciplinary care sometimes involves the woman meeting quite a large number of team members.

For women with low-risk pregnancies, it may be possible to extend continuity of community care to cover the birth itself, either through the community midwife attending her women in labour in the main hospital maternity unit through team midwifery (midwives working in groups) or through midwife-led maternity care (*Changing Childbirth Update* 1996).

In some areas, outreach consultant clinics, with on-site ultrasonography and perhaps linkworkers, mean that women with 'high-risk' pregnancies (whose psychosocial needs are often greater than those of women with low-risk pregnancies) can also benefit from friendly, accessible maternity care. This is particularly helpful for socially disadvantaged women who may feel intimidated by the hospital setting and have difficulty negotiating or affording the journey. Wood (1991) reviewed six antenatal care initiatives in primary care settings in London (Lambeth, Tower Hamlets, and Hackney), Edinburgh (Sighthill), Glasgow (Easterhouse), and Birmingham, set up between 1975 and 1985. She showed that the whole spectrum of maternity outcomes, from morbidity to user satisfaction, was at least as good as those for women receiving traditional shared care. A more recent successful example is the Ashwell Project in Bradford, based in a GP surgery in an inner-city area with a predominantly Asian Muslim community of Pakistani origin (Jones and Danby 1995). Home visits by midwives are appropriate for some women who do not attend antenatal clinics, although it is probably more cost-effective to attract them to a woman-friendly clinic.

The antenatal clinic

Several authors have suggested fewer antenatal visits (Hall *et al.* 1980; Steer 1993; Chapter 19), but if the number of visits is to be cut, their *content* also needs to be reviewed: if the visit means only three minutes with a midwife or GP and a quick 'prod', many women will not feel it is worth the effort to attend. Community maternity care involves much more than routine screening tests. The antenatal clinic setting should include access to health advice, information about support groups and about social security benefits and, above all, the opportunity to develop trusting relationships with midwives and doctors. Women must be able to raise their own concerns with the midwife or doctor – this means both allowing enough time in the system and creating an atmosphere where all women can feel confident enough to speak. *Changing Childbirth* (Department of Health 1993) cites an example of good practice from a Staffordshire GP antenatal clinic where the number of standard antenatal visits was reduced but women were encouraged to attend on as many other occasions as they wished. The clinic sessions included informal group discussions with health professionals, with refreshments provided.

Although conventional screening tests are of doubtful value (Steer 1993), specific screening tests for particular groups of women must not be overlooked. Haemoglobinopathies in some minority ethnic groups, or 'triple testing' which in some areas is offered only to older women, are examples. These tests need particularly sensitive explanation and counselling.

'Narrowing the gap' necessitates paying attention to many organizational aspects of the clinic to make it more attractive to disadvantaged women. Flexible appointment systems can give women the opportunity to attend when they feel they need advice or reassurance rather than having to wait until the next prescribed visit. Waiting areas can be made more comfortable, perhaps with refreshments available and magazines people really want to read. Health education material should be screened for readability and attractively displayed. Good play areas for accompanying children are essential. Access to all areas and security for both wheelchairs and pushchairs should be provided.

A sometimes neglected aspect of clinic organization is the training and support of administrative and clerical staff. They should be treated as team members and encouraged to develop positive, welcoming attitudes to disadvantaged women. It helps to create an accessible service if, for example, administrative staff are patient with those with language problems, recognize that the difficulty of fitting Asian names into an English filing system is a deficiency of the filing system rather than the woman, and are neither disapproving nor patronizing towards teenage mothers. This ideal will be fostered if the staff themselves are treated with respect by the health professionals.

Postnatal care

Disadvantaged women are particularly vulnerable to postnatal depression. Midwives, GPs, and health visitors are all involved in its detection and management. They need to create an atmosphere where women are able to express their feelings freely. As well as being aware of the greater prevalance of postnatal depression, this means making the time available for women to talk about their emotions, worries, and fears. The Edinburgh Postnatal Depression Scale, a simple questionnaire (Cox *et al.* 1987), has been shown to be a useful screening tool for health visitors to identify women who may benefit from counselling for postnatal depression (Holden *et al.* 1989). There is scope for developing and validating such tools in other languages.

Health education

The antenatal clinic itself is an important setting for health education (Chapters 12 and 19). Often, those who most need to adopt healthier habits are the least likely to do so, particularly when pregnancy has caused stress or additional economic hardship. Some women see the very behaviour they are advised to change (e.g. smoking or eating comforting junk food) as the main crutch that keeps them going during stressful periods. Any contact the primary health care team has with women of childbearing age can be an opportunity to reiterate healthy lifestyle messages. However, it is very important for midwives, doctors, and others to be sensitive to the meaning of habits such as smoking in these women's lives, and the barriers they see to changing their behaviour. As an example, women may know that breast milk is best for their baby but lack the confidence to breastfeed in front of others (especially male family members) and live in homes without a private space to feed. Fear of being criticized or looked down on is one of the factors which stops women attending regularly for maternity care, and makes it hard for them to trust the health professionals enough to get the best out of the service. 'Changes to women's behaviour stand more chance if the information that they are given is supplemented with personal support and sensitive individual advice' (Benzeval *et al.* 1995).

Antenatal classes and parent education sessions have traditionally been regarded as part of antenatal care and are provided by most community maternity services. However, they are often used least by the disadvantaged women who may need them most. Such classes must be thoughtfully planned for the particular groups they are aimed at, and the setting (venue, time of day, style of presentation), format (talks by 'experts', group discussions, question and answer sessions), and content reviewed. The simplest changes may be effective – uptake of antenatal education in a deprived area of Salford was greatly increased by changing the name from 'parentcraft classes' to 'pregnancy club' (Department of Health 1993). The group format may not be appropriate for all women; examples of alternative approaches are discussed below.

Midwives in Bradford observed a low uptake of traditional parent education sessions by Asian women, despite the introduction of innovations such as own-language sessions during antenatal clinic times, informal question and answer sessions, involvement of liaison officers and interpreters, and informal meetings at Asian women's centres, community centres, and women's own homes. Asking women about the reasons for this low uptake, they found that they felt that members of their extended family could support and teach them instead and that housework and childcare took priority; they felt anxious about attending classes, especially without another family member. The midwives noted that many of the women had access to video players. As a result, three educational videos were made in Urdu and Bengali, covering pregnancy and antenatal care, coping with labour, and breastfeeding. Two more, on Caesarean section and life with a new baby, are planned. Punjabi versions may be produced, and the videos marketed nationally as an educational resource (Walker and Pollard 1995).

The present political climate encourages 'partnership' between public services and private industry. There are some useful examples of support for health education from commercial organizations (Department of Health 1993). The Maternity Alliance used sponsorship from a detergent manufacturer to produce and distribute a birth plan and a postnatal support aid for use by groups of mothers. The Royal College of General Practitioners used advertising to finance 'Emma's Diary', an easily readable personalized account of pregnancy, distributed in many antenatal clinics. The nutrition helpline, a telephone advice service for pregnant women, was run by Sheffield University and funded by Birthright, a mother-and-baby research charity, together with a supermarket chain. Other supermarkets were involved, together with the Maternity Alliance and the Health Visitors' Association, in producing written information on healthy eating for women before, during, and after pregnancy.

GP and community antenatal clinics might be able to make use of local advertising or sponsorship to produce educational material, although the health professionals should vet sponsors and advertisers carefully, and retain control over anything written. Sponsors need not be in a health-related field – in fact, it may be appropriate to avoid organizations whose commercial interests might be directly served by involvement in health-related projects. Although the support of commercial organizations is valuable, it is very important not to forget that they may have vested interests.

There are several important issues in education for teenagers about pregnancy, childbirth, and motherhood. First is the prevention of unwanted pregnancy, as targeted in the Government's document *Health of the Nation* (Department of Health 1992). Contraception should be seen in the general context of sexual health promotion for young people, and involves people other than health professionals – central government, local education and social services departments, individual schools, voluntary agencies, the media. The wide-ranging recommendations made in *The sexual health of young people* (Yorkshire Regional Health Authority Working Party 1994) include the right to appropriate sex education for all young people, integrating training in the provision of sex education into professional education for teachers, and provision of appropriate sexual health services specifically aimed at young people, perhaps in non-traditional settings to improve uptake and effectiveness. Changing the setting of a family planning clinic for teenagers has been shown to have dramatic results. Ineichen (Ineichen and Hudson 1994) suggests that we could learn from the Netherlands and the USA where school-based contraceptive clinics have reduced teenage pregnancies and encouraged boys to be proactive in the choice of contraception. Peer-led sex education in schools, where older pupils are trained to lead sessions with groups of young people, have been very successful in some areas in the UK (Reid 1982).

Deciding whether to continue with an unintended pregnancy is always a painful and difficult choice, and particularly complex for teenagers. The GP may be faced with a family delegation in which the parents are sure of the right course of action but the daughter appears silent and confused, or by a distressed young woman who feels she dares not tell her family. Pregnant teenagers often present late, and are frequently uncertain of their dates. The situation can arouse strong feelings in doctors themselves, especially if they have teenage daughters. Helping the young woman to make the best choice for herself is a task which demands great sensitivity and clinical skill. The time needed for the doctor to explain the options and for the young woman to reflect on all the implications must be balanced against the urgency of the situation if termination is chosen. It is important that support, and possibly specialist counselling, are provided afterwards.

Teenagers who decide to continue with a pregnancy need to continue their general education as well as receiving specific education for pregnancy, childbirth, and motherhood. Many education departments provide special school units for pregnant pupils; because of their low pupil–teacher ratios and committed staff, they are often strikingly successful, even though such pupils may previously have felt alienated from the school system. Some teenagers may prefer to remain in their own schools and continue with their existing educational plans. This is appropriate for some young women with sufficient energy and determination; it is unfortunate that some schools strongly discourage pregnant pupils from remaining in school, and more flexible policies may be needed.

Communication

Communication is an obvious issue for women who are not fluent in English, but is important for those working with all disadvantaged women. Carers need to use complex interpersonal skills to reach out to each individual woman to ensure that she feels comfortable and empowered to ask for what she wants, and sufficiently relaxed to understand and recall what is being explained to her. Interpreters (or preferably, linkworkers – see later) are obviously essential for women with no English. The use of family members as interpreters is fraught with difficulties – their own English may be limited, and their relationship with the patient (they may be her own young children, her husband, or many others) adds complex problems, including confidentiality. Many women who are reasonably fluent in everyday conversational English will also have difficulty understanding some of the more technical language of antenatal care. Interpreters and linkworkers can have an extended role with these women.

In addition, many native speakers of English have difficulty understanding what professionals say to them, either because they are poorly educated and do not understand the words and expressions or because they are too anxious, intimidated, or preoccupied to take everything in and remember it clearly. Teenagers, in particular, are often too frightened to ask professionals to explain things they do not understand. Midwives and doctors need to be sensitive to this, and modify the way they explain things appropriately for each woman.

Written information may also be useful, but leaflets are often not written simply enough. Some women have difficulty reading and writing and may well be too embarrassed to mention it. It can be useful to offer to help a woman to write her answers to the questions in a birth plan, as well as discussing them with her. Written material in minority languages may be useful. The name of the language needs to be in English on the leaflet so that health professionals know which one to offer. It should be remembered that many women who do not speak English cannot read and write their native language. Information in different languages about health issues and services is sometimes produced on audio or videotapes (Walker and Pollard 1995). **Health advocates and linkworkers** are an important source of support for many minority ethnic women. The Asian Mother and Baby Campaign (Rocheron *et al.* 1989) was an important influence behind their introduction.

Linkworkers are usually employed by health trusts. Fluent in two or more languages, they are usually members of minority ethnic communities. They may be based in hospitals and community settings and may provide a range of services, including support, translation, interpreting, and advice about health services and social services. They can be used in family planning, antenatal and postnatal clinics, and may accompany midwives, general practitioners, and health visitors on home visits. Because they are employed by trusts but work alongside health professionals in the community, it is important that community professionals such as midwives and GPs are involved in their job specification, selection, and training rather than leaving this to hospital-based administrators.

As well as improving communication, linkworkers can also complement the community maternity service by facilitating health education and encouraging uptake of screening services. When women enjoy the company of the female linkworkers, they can also provide social support by listening, chatting, and advising them where to go for further advice or help. Their general familiarity with minority ethnic communities, and specific experience with individual women, means they may also be a valuable source of ideas for service development. When changes in maternity care for minority ethnic women are planned, it may be useful to consider including linkworkers in the process.

Health advocacy services are well established and integrated into other sectors of the health service, notably mental health and mental handicap; in some areas, they have been introduced into maternity services, usually for minority ethnic women. Their role is communication and liaison between the women and the services. Ideally, they should be 'non-aligned' rather than employed by health service providers; they may be provided by the community health council or by voluntary agencies. The latter are often funded by local councils so their service is vulnerable to financial restrictions. Where advocacy services exist, they try to supply advocates for all the languages common in the local community. Since other disadvantaged women, with fluent English, can have difficulties communicating with maternity services, a health advocacy service might be beneficial for them too.

The provision of health advocates and linkworkers, and the distinction between their roles, varies in different areas. Midwives and doctors may need to familiarize themselves with what is available locally to ask for existing advocates or linkworkers to be based at their clinics and to arrange to be involved in their selection and training, as well as campaigning for the introduction and sustainable funding of such services.

Social support

People need social support at times of change and stress, so it is not surprising that such support in pregnancy has been shown to be beneficial. There have been studies observing the effect of existing support from family and friends, and others demonstrating the effect of introducing support from health carers (O'Hara 1986; Oakley *et al.* 1990; Bryce *et al.* 1991; Benzeval *et al.* 1995; Blondel and Breat 1995). This effect is particularly marked in otherwise disadvantaged women. Social support reduced antenatal and postnatal depression, improved self-esteem, and reduced the likelihood of hospital admission. In addition, women were more likely to have a spontaneous onset of labour and delivery; it is suggested that infant outcomes, such as birthweight, breastfeeding rates, and the health of the baby, could also be improved.

In a study of single women or women with unemployed partners, a weekly telephone support programme was introduced for one group and compared with those not provided with such support. The women in the intervention group were less anxious, less depressed, had better self-esteem, used the community resources more, and were less likely to skip meals (Bullock *et al.* 1995).

A project in Hackney introduced an information pack for new mothers which aimed to provide emotional and practical support. Nearly half of the births in Hackney are to socially deprived women, minority ethnic women, and women who have a language difficulty. The information pack complemented information that was normally offered to English-reading mothers shortly after the birth. The pack offered practical advice on how to voice their needs, how to cope with the emotional changes of pregnancy, and how to set up self-help groups. Many women found it reassuring that they were going through the same problems as others and just over half the women expressed an interest in setting up antenatal support groups (Moody 1996). Social support during pregnancy can provide longer-term health promotion benefits: mothers who had taken part in a trial of social support in pregnancy (extra visits and telephone calls from a midwife) were followed up after seven years; they and their children still appeared to be in better health than the control mothers and children (Oakley *et al.* 1996).

Many disadvantaged women are isolated from the natural support networks of family or community. This results from social changes far beyond the control of health professionals, but support can be offered in various different ways. Women can be encouraged to make more use of the potential support of their friends or family. Social support may be provided by contact with professional health carers, health advocates, women with experiences of childbirth who have had some basic training in supporting others, or simply groups of other women in the same situation. It may be appropriate to offer one-to-one contacts at home or at a mutually convenient place, telephone contacts, or group support. What women need from 'social support' will vary but important elements are listening and allowing women to express their worries and fears, ask questions, and obtain advice. Support continues to be valuable during the antenatal and postnatal periods and even up to one year after childbirth. Support programmes to encourage and maintain breastfeeding among those less likely to do it have been introduced. In Glasgow, women who have breastfed are being trained to help new mothers to do the same and help promote breastfeeding as a natural choice (McInnes 1996). An example from the more privileged sector of society could perhaps be copied among disadvantaged women: members of the National Childbirth Trust's antenatal groups often continue to provide mutual support for months and even years after childbirth.

Teenagers appear to be less likely to use support groups. Many community maternity services provide teenage parenting classes, which tend to focus upon educational advice about the health of the mother and her baby. It is uncertain whether these are also effective in providing social support for the mother and addressing her own concerns. Teenagers respond well to their peers, as has been clearly demonstrated in the peer-led sex education schemes (Reid 1982). It might be very helpful to introduce one-to-one peer support within local communities and away from the medical environment – pregnant teenagers could be supported by those who had managed well in a similar situation, perhaps a year or two earlier. Setting up such a scheme might involve midwives and doctors collaborating with health visitors, and perhaps with other statutory or voluntary agencies working with young people.

Funding

Since the changes made in the NHS around 1990, funding became an increasingly complex issue (Chapter 8). On the one hand, the variety of different purchasers of health care, and the direct involvement of GPs in commissioning care (through either fundholding or commissioning groups), created scope for the development of innovative services appropriate to the local population. On the other hand, financial considerations constrained both providers (usually hospital trusts) and purchasers in the development of special services, especially if they were labour-intensive. Purchasers had to set priorities to enable them to ration health care according to the available resources, and the funding of new developments such as the introduction of appropriately trained linkworkers for minority ethnic women depended on how much priority they received. Some important pilot projects such as the Newcastle Bangladeshi midwifery project were initiated with special funding, shown to be effective, and then discontinued because sustainable mainstream funding was not available (Sen and Holmes 1996).

Fundholding has been abandoned by the new Labour Government but the above fundamental problems will still have to be addressed by commissioning groups.

Racism and stereotyping

The inbuilt racism of institutions such as hospitals, and stereotyping by individual health professionals, contribute to the creation of inequality in the maternity care experiences of minority ethnic women. It is almost inevitable that people make sense of society by stereotyping; that is, by developing sets of beliefs about the personal attributes of a group of people (Blalock and Devellis 1986). GPs and midwives like to think of themselves as open-minded and free from prejudice. However, it is distressing to read about negative stereotyping of minority ethnic women by midwives who use stereotypes to make judgements about the kind of care different women want, need, and deserve (Bowler 1993). Understanding the culture of people we perceive as different from ourselves because of their ethnicity, class, or age is essential. However, we should guard against making unsupported assumptions about individuals, for example that a Muslim woman would be unwilling to consider termination of pregnancy for fetal abnormality, or that a teenage mother would not be capable of using a diaphragm for future contraception. With a background of understanding, we should aim to treat each woman as an individual. This is a very difficult balance to strike and deserves considerable attention in the training of all health professionals.

Conclusion

The greatest challenge to maternity services stems from the problems of social inequality. To meet it will require a flexible and imaginative approach on the part of health professionals, and serious commitment on the part of politicians and health planners.

References

Babb, P. (1993). Teenage conception and fertility in England and Wales, 1971–1991. *Population Trends*, 74, 12–17.

Balarajan, R. and Raleigh, V. S. (1993). *Health of the Nation. Ethnicity and health: a guide for the NHS*. Department of Health, London.

Benzeval, M., Judge, K., and Whitehead, M. (1995). *Tackling inequalities in health*. King's Fund, London.

Berryman, J. C. and Windridge, K. C. (1995). *Motherhood after 35: a report of the Leicester motherhood project*, p.2. Leicester University and Nestle.

Black Report (1980). *Inequalities and health*. Department of Health and Social Security, London.

Blalock, S. and Devellis, B. (1986). Stereotyping: the link between theory and practice. *Patient Education and Counselling*, **8**, 17–25.

Blondel, B. and Breat, G. (1995). Home visits during pregnancy: consequences and pregnancy outcome, use of health services, and women's situation. *Seminars in Perinatology*, **19**(4), 263–71.

Botting, B. (1995). The health of our children: decennial supplement. HMSO, London.

Bowler, I. (1993). 'They're not the same as us': midwives' stereotypes of south Asian descent maternity patients. *Sociology of Health and Illness*, **15**(2), 157–8.

Bryce, R. L., Stanley, F. J., and Garner, J. B. (1991). Randomized controlled trial of antenatal social support to prevent preterm birth. *British Journal of Obstetrics and Gynaecology*, **98**, 1001–8.

Bullock, L. F. C., Wells, J. E., Duff, G. B., *et al.* (1995). Telephone support for pregnant women: outcome in late pregnancy. *New Zealand Medical Journal*, **108**, 476–8.

Changing Childbirth Update (1996). Quarterly news letter from the *Changing Childbirth* Implementation Team. Issue 6, p.10.

Chrisholm, D. K. (1989). Factors associated with late booking for antenatal care in central Manchester. *Public Health*, **103**, 459–66.

Cox, J., Holden, J., and Sagovsky, R. (1987). Detection of postnatal depression: development of the Edinburgh Postnatal Depression Scale. *British Journal of Psychiatry*, **150**, 782–6.

Dallison, J. and Lobstein, T. (1995). *Poor expectations. Poverty and undernourishment in pregnancy*. NCH Action for Children and the Maternity Alliance.

Dillner, L. (1995). Inequalities cause reproductive deaths. *British Medical Journal*, **311**, 147–8.

Department of Health (1992). The Health of the Nation – a strategy for health in England. HMSO, London.

Department of Health (1993).*Changing childbirth*. HMSO, London.

Department of Health (1994). Report on confidential enquiries into maternal deaths in the United Kingdom, 1988–1990. HMSO, London.

Friedman, S. B. and Phillips, S. (1981). Psychological risk to mother and child as a consequence of adolescent pregnancy. *Seminars in Perinatology*, **5**, 33–7.

Glazener, C. M. A., Abdalla, M., Stroud, P., Naji, S., Templeton, A., and Russell, I. T. (1995). Postnatal maternal morbidity: extent, causes, prevention, and treatment. *British Journal of Obstetrics and Gynaecology*, **102**, 282–7.

Godfrey, K., Robinson, S., Barker, D. J. P., *et al.* (1996). Maternal nutrition in early and late pregnancy in relation to placental and fetal growth. *British Medical Journal*, **312**, 410–14.

Hall, M., Chng, P. K., and MacGillivray, I. (1980). Is routine antenatal care worthwhile? *Lancet*, **July 12**, 78–81.

Hayes, L. (1995). Unequal access to midwifery care: a continuing problem? *Journal of Advanced Nursing*, **21**, 702–7.

Holden, J., Sagovsky, R., and Cox, J. (1989). Counselling in general practice setting:

controlled study of health visitor intervention in treatment of postnatal depression. *British Medical Journal*, **298**, 223–6.

Jones, S. and Danby, J. (1995). *The Ashwell Project*. Unpublished paper presented at the Association of Community-based Maternity Care Spring meeting.

Ineichen, B. and Hudson, F. (1994). *Teenage pregnancy*. National Children's Bureau, London.

Kean, L. H., Liu, D. T. Y., and Macquisten, S. (1996). Pregnancy care of the low-risk woman: the community–hospital interface. *International Journal of Health Care Quality Assurance*, **9**(5), 39–44.

Keirse, M. J. N. C. (1994). Maternal mortality: stalemate or stagnant. *British Medical Journal*, **308**, 354–5.

Kogan, M. D. (1995). Social causes of low birthweight. *Journal of the Royal Society of Medicine*, **88**(11), 611–15.

Konje, J., Palmer, A., Watson, A., Hay, D. M., and Imrie, A. (1992). Early teenage pregnancies in Hull. *British Journal of Obstetrics and Gynaecology*, **99**, 969–73.

Loudon, I. (1992). Transformation of maternal mortality. *British Medical Journal*, **305**, 1557–60.

Lyon, A. J., Clarkson, P., Jeffrey, I., and West, G. A. (1994). Effect of ethnic origin of mother on fetal outcome. *Archives of Diseases in Childhood*, **70**, 40–3.

Macfarlane, A., Mugford, M., Johnson, A., and Garcia, J. (1995). *Counting the changes in childbirth: trends and gaps in national statistics*, p.21. National Epidemiology Unit, Oxford.

McInnes, R. (1996). Promoting breastfeeding in an inner-city area. *Changing Childbirth Update*, **6**, 7.

Mansfield, P. K. and Cohn, M. D. (1986). Stress and later-life childbearing: important implications of nursing. *Maternal Child Nursing Journal*, **15**, 139–51.

Marsh, G. N. (1985). The primary health care team in obstetrics. In: *Modern obstetrics in general practice* (ed. G. N. Marsh). Oxford University Press, Oxford.

Moody, G. (1996). *Maternity Action*, **71**, 6–7.

Murray, L., Cooper, P. J., and Stein, A. (1991). Postnatal depression and infant development. *British Medical Journal*, **302**, 978–9.

Oakley, A. (1991). Using medical care: the views and experiences of high-risk mothers. *Health Services Research*, **26**, 651–69.

Oakley, A., Rajan, L., and Grant, A. (1990). Social support and pregnancy outcome. *British Journal of Obstetrics and Gynaecology*, **97**, 155–62.

Oakley, A., Hickey, D., and Rajan, L. (1996). Social support in pregnancy : does it have long-term effects? *Journal of Reproductive and Infant Psychology*, **4**(1), 7–22.

Office of Population Censuses and Surveys (1995). *Infant and perinatal mortality – social and biological factors, 1994*. OPCS monitor, DHE 95/3.

O'Hara, M. W. (1986). Social support, life events, and depression during pregnancy and the puerperium. *Archives of General Psychiatry*, **43**, 569–73.

Peacock, J. L., Bland, J. M., and Anderson, H. R. (1995). Preterm delivery: effects of socio-economic factors, psychological stress, smoking, alcohol, and caffeine. *British Medical Journal*, **311**, 531–6.

Proctor, S. R. and Smith, I. J. (1992). A reconsideration of the factors affecting birth outcome in Pakistani Muslim families in Britain. *Midwifery*, **8**, 76–81.

Quine, L., Rutter, D. R., and Gowen, S. (1993). Women's satisfaction with the quality of birth experience: a prospective study of social and psychological predictors. *Journal of Reproductive and Infant Psychology*, **11**, 107–13.

Rainey, D. Y., Stevens-Simon, C., and Kaplan, D. W. (1995). Are adolescents who report prior sexual abuse at higher risk for pregnancy? *Child Abuse and Neglect*, **19**(10), 1283–8.

Reid, D. (1982). School sex education and causes of unintended pregnancies – a review. *Health Education Journal*, **41**, 4–11.

Rocheron, Y., Khan, S., and Dickenson, R. (1989). Links across the divide. *Health Service Journal*, **90**, 951–2.

Rutter, D. R. and Quine, L. (1990). Inequalities in pregnancy outcome: a review of psychological and behavioural mediators. *Social Science Medicine*, **30**(5), 553–68.

Sen, D. and Holmes, C. (1996). Newcastle Bangledeshi midwifery project. *MIDIRS Midwifery Digest*, **6**(2), 225–9.

Sikorski, J., Wilson, J., Clement, S., Das, S., and Smeeton, N. (1996). A randomized controlled trial comparing two schedules of antenatal visits: the Antenatal Care Project. *British Medical Journal*, **312**, 546–53.

Sleep, J. and Grant, A. (1987). West Berkshire perineal management trial: three-year follow-up. *British Medical Journal*, **295**, 749–51.

Steer, P. (1993). Rituals in antenatal care – do we need them? *British Medical Journal*, **307**, 698.

Stones, W., Lim, W., Al-Azzawi, F., and Kelly, M. (1991). An investigation of maternal morbidity with identification of life-threatening, near-miss episodes. *Health Trends*, **23**(1), 13–15.

Tew, M. (1990). *Safer childbirth? A critical history of maternity care*, pp.198;209. Chapman and Hall, London.

Thompson, J. (1995). *Women of the world, from a midwife's perspective*. Report of the NGO women's forum, Beijing, 30 August -9 September. *Midwifery*, **1**, 217–19.

Tudor Hart, J. (1971). The inverse care law. *Lancet*, **I**, 405–12.

Walker, J. and Pollard, L. (1995). Parent education for Asian mothers. *Modern Midwife*, **September**, 22–3.

Wilcox, M. A., Smith, S. J., Johnson, I. R., *et al.* (1995). The effects of social deprivation on birthweight, excluding physiological and pathological effects. *British Journal of Obstetrics and Gynaecology*, **102**(11), 918–24.

Wilson, J. (1995). Caroline: a case of the pregnant teenager. *Professional Care of the Mother and Child*, **5**(5), 139–40.

Wood, J. (1991). A review of antenatal care initiatives in primary care settings. *British Journal of General Practice*, **41**, 26–30.

Woodward, V. M (1995). Psychosocial factors influencing teenage sexual activity, use of contraception, and unplanned pregnancy. *Midwifery*, 11, 210–16.

World Health Organization (1995). Maternal mortality worse than we thought. *Safe Motherhood*, 19, 1–2.

Yorkshire Regional Health Authority Working Party (1993). *The sexual health of young people*. Report.

Zander, L. (1995). *Changing Childbirth two years on*. Conference proceedings, Kensington, London.

CHAPTER TWELVE

Maternity care for women with special needs

Mary Hepburn

Introduction

It is well recognized that antenatal care should be appropriate to women's needs. In *Changing Childbirth* (Department of Health 1993), the Expert Maternity Group emphasized the importance of accessibility, service delivery in the community, provision of appropriate high-risk management when necessary, involvement of women in planning their care, and cost-effectiveness. Their recommendations referred to women without special needs and, in particular, the Expert Maternity Group specifically excluded socio-economic factors and related issues such as nutrition, smoking, and drug use as outwith their remit. However, many kinds of special needs unrelated to deprivation, such as learning difficulties, mental illness, and under-age pregnancy, may necessitate modification of both service delivery and content. Socio-economic deprivation not only exacerbates such difficulties but is also associated with a range of problems in addition to poverty, including homelessness, drug use, and prostitution, all incurring special needs and all characterized by ineffective service use (Townsend and Davidson 1982). Identification of special needs is therefore an important part of the assessment of all pregnant women.

Current trends

Provision of appropriate maternity care for women with special needs is essential. Increasing numbers of reports, either documenting specialized services or discussing the need for their development, reflect increasing awareness of this fact. Some deal with very specific groups such as the mentally ill (Levy *et al.* 1992; Miller *et al.* 1992), ethnic minorities (Thomas and Dines 1994), travellers (Vernon 1994), or adolescents (Levy *et al.* 1992; Yordan and Yordan 1993); some consider more general issues such as homelessness (Bassuk and Weinreb 1993; O'Connell 1993; Reilly 1993; Ovrebo *et al.* 1994) or poverty (Mayer *et al.* 1990; Cardale 1992; Woodard and Edouard 1992); some consider any combination of factors or circumstances which make women inaccessible to, or inappropriate for, care by standard services (Hepburn 1991; Rodriguez *et al.* 1993; Borgford-Parnell *et al.* 1994; Dickinson *et al.* 1994; Cook 1995); some discuss the use of specific interventions such as home visiting (Dineen *et al.* 1992; Bradley and Martin 1994; Marcenko and Spence 1994); while examples of services meeting specific needs are reported in *Changing Childbirth Update* (Cowl 1995; Hepburn 1995*a*).

That such reports come from many different countries demonstrates international awareness of the problem – a field change in outlook rather than individual enlightenment. Recognition of need is important but will not in itself ensure effective provision of care. Attendance at specialized services may identify women as having special needs and it can therefore be difficult to balance the need for specialized care against the risk of stigmatization. That the inaccessibility of services to those with greatest need documented more than a decade ago (Townsend and Davidson 1982) still exists (Benzeval *et al.* 1995) suggests a depressing lack of progress. Nevertheless, awareness of the existence of special needs is an essential first step in providing the appropriate care which all women need and to which they are entitled.

Special needs

What are special needs?

Women and their carers may not agree on what constitutes a problem. Women may have special needs without having problems as in the case of travelling women, while young age may be considered a problem by carers but not necessarily by the woman herself. Some women, such as those with learning difficulties, may have special needs but by the nature of their problem be unaware that this is the case. Special needs may be multiple and this is especially true of deprivation-related problems. For example, drug use in pregnancy may be accompanied by homelessness, social isolation, extreme poverty, prostitution, risk of sexually transmitted diseases including HIV, legal problems, and/or a custodial sentence for the woman. In addition, poverty will not only cause difficulties *per se* but may exacerbate other problems involving special needs.

How do special needs present?

Some problems, such as severe learning difficulties, may be apparent without questioning. Some factors may seem apparent but it is important not to draw inaccurate conclusions as, for example, on the question of age. Similarly, associations between race, religion, and culture are not necessarily predictable and ethnic origin does not always accurately reflect service requirements (Chapter 11). Some problems may be less obvious but will be volunteered by women seeking help. Some will only be identified by specific enquiry but women may not be asked about them or may choose not to reveal them.

How are special needs identified?

Unless volunteered by either the pregnant woman or her referrer some problems, such as drug or alcohol use, may only be identified by specific questioning. Problem drug and alcohol use are both underreported but since alcohol use is legal it may be the level of use which is underestimated.

The design of case records is often unhelpful in identifying special needs. Most contain a list of questions to be asked at booking and while many contain some questions about consumption of cigarettes, alcohol, or illegal drugs, inclusion of all of these questions in the routine history is by no means routine. Staff may not ask about special needs through lack of awareness, lack of the necessary skills, or embarrassment. Specific questioning about behavioural problems is much more likely to cause offence if perceived to be selectively applied rather than part of a routine history. Since accurate prediction is not possible, routine enquiry is essential. The way the question is asked is also important. While staff are often reluctant to ask questions which they think are 'judgemental', they should realize that it is rarely the question *per se* but more commonly the way it is asked which is perceived as judgemental. Prefacing the question by 'I know this probably doesn't apply to you but. . . ' or even 'I hope you're not offended but we ask all women this question' indicates clearly the 'correct' response and discourages disclosure. Use of euphemistic language is similarly unhelpful so, for example, asking women if they use any 'unprescribed medicines' – a necessary routine question in its own right – should not be expected to elicit a history of illegal drug use. Often problems in turn cause other problems. For example, where there is a history of problem drug or alcohol use, sources of finance should be established to identify possible health and social problems due to criminal activity and/or prostitution. In addition, while the examples of special needs discussed in this chapter are considered individually, it is important to remember that many coexist.

When should questions be asked?

It is important to have some time alone with the woman in case there is information she would not want to discuss in front of a companion. It is also important to talk to her on her own to find out whether she is happy to be pregnant, whether she wants to continue with the pregnancy, and to establish her wider views about her pregnancy. Speaking to the woman on her own is the only way to be sure the views she expresses are truly her own. Ensuring the woman has the opportunity to be accompanied by a supportive advocate is equally important and reconciling these rights may prove difficult. She may not appear keen for her companion to leave, or her companion may be unwilling to leave (suggesting an abnormally controlling and possibly abusive relationship), and in such situations staff may hesitate to insist. However, she may not realize questioning might prove embarrassing or, if given the choice in front of a partner or other companion, she may feel unable to ask them to leave. All women should be given the opportunity for one-to-one discussion without needing to ask for it and this can usually be achieved unobtrusively and unthreateningly.

Domestic circumstances

All pregnant women should be considered in the context of their families, with care not only medically but also socially appropriate. Women should be asked about their partner and other people with whom they live, including other children. While the past obstetric history and health of previous children is important, it is also essential to establish whether the woman herself is their principal carer and, if there were previous child-care problems, whether circumstances have changed in the interim.

Attendance at an antenatal clinic does not indicate that a pregnancy is either planned, intended, or wanted nor indicate the circumstances in which a pregnancy occurred. Assumptions should not be made about a woman's domestic circumstances, including her relationship with the baby's father, whether her partner is this baby's father, the paternity of other children, and the gender of her regular partner. The individuals who provide the woman with support should be identified. Questions should be sufficiently open to allow these issues to be explored. It should also be remembered that women may be in an abusive relationship or suffer domestic violence and appropriate direct questions should be asked routinely.

Accommodation

In addition to recording an address for all women, it may also be relevant to establish the security of their accommodation. If owned or rented by a partner or other person with whom they have an unstable relationship, or if they are in temporary accommodation, they may have to move or may even become homeless during the course of their pregnancy. The condition of their housing may be important in terms of its suitability for a young baby. While home visiting may often be a routine part of antenatal care, in the case of many women with special needs it also provides an opportunity to assess both their accommodation and also other family members or residents. Realizing this, women may not tell the truth about where or with whom they are living, and unannounced home visits may then provide valuable information. Women, for various reasons, may also spend considerable amounts of time at addresses other than their 'official' address and such information would be important should it prove necessary to contact them. They therefore need to be reassured that such information would be treated in confidence and be for health care workers only.

Service delivery

Geographical/physical accessibility

While community care close to the women's homes is ideal, those with high-risk pregnancies (theoretically including all those with deprivation-related problems by virtue of the associated increase in perinatal mortality and morbidity) may have to receive some care centrally. Problems which require dedicated service provision (whether medical or social) may affect too few women to justify multiple community outlets. If only a few specialized community clinics are established in areas of maximum need they may not be easily accessible to women other than those in their immediate vicinity and, paradoxically, a centrally sited clinic may then be more accessible. Similarly, women who do not have a fixed long-term address, such as those who are homeless, live in temporary accommodation, or belong to travelling families, may find a peripheral community clinic unsuitable. In Glasgow, the Women's Reproductive Health Service (WRHS) for women with special needs provides care through a citywide network of community clinics (Hepburn 1997), so women moving around the city can attend any of them depending on where they are staying at any given time. However, women sometimes attend different community sites either to avoid detection of a problem or because that problem is making their lifestyle chaotic. While continuity of staff or good communications between staff will be helpful, attendance at a centrally sited clinic may be a more effective alternative. All health service buildings should be accessible to disabled people but this may not apply where care is delivered from other settings.

Financial costs of attending are also important. Hospitals may reimburse travelling expenses but this will not help women with insufficient money to attend in the first place. Attendance at community-based services may still incur expenses but reimbursement may be impossible since many small community health centres do not have facilities for keeping money on site.

Administrative accessibility

Services should also be administratively accessible. For example, a specific residence requirement might limit accessibility for homeless, travelling, or otherwise mobile women. Similarly, the normal route of access to antenatal care by way of general practitioner referral will obviously not be possible for women who are not registered with one. Women with behavioural problems such as drug use may have difficulty in finding a general practitioner who will accept them as patients and they may be allocated to general practitioners' lists on a short-term rotating basis. They may not know with whom they are registered at any given time, or may not manage to arrange referral before their allocation is changed to another doctor. Greater flexibility is therefore essential and for such women access should be possible by any route, including self-referral.

Multidisciplinary care

Multidisciplinary care has many benefits for women with special needs (Hepburn 1991). Such women may have many problems with different degrees of urgency. As a result, housing, financial problems, or the needs of other children may take priority over attendance for antenatal care. Provision of help with all problems within a multidisciplinary service will facilitate

199

attendance for antenatal care which coincidentally will provide an opportunity to deal with problems which might otherwise be neglected. These may relate to the woman herself, as in the screening of prostitutes for sexually transmitted diseases, or her family, as in the case of a partner's problem drug or alcohol use. While within a multidisciplinary team some redefinition of individual roles may be necessary, this approach allows service providers to recognize their limitations and collaborate with other services rather than attempt to provide aspects of care for which they lack the necessary skills. In a multidisciplinary clinic, obstetric need will not be the only criterion for attendance and all participants will not make equal contributions to all consultations. Hence while the total number of attendances may be less than the cumulative total for all services, it may be greater than the total required by any individual service. But the brief yet frequent contacts which this provides can help in the assessment of women's problems and overall stability.

Staff attitudes

Negative staff attitudes to women with special needs and especially behavioural problems are common. Whether real or perceived, attitudinal problems can discourage not only disclosure but also attendance and so prevent effective service delivery. They may result from disapproval of a woman's behaviour or lifestyle *per se*, or the perceived effects of this on the baby as in the case of maternal drug use. Staff may doubt a woman's ability to care for a child because of her lifestyle or other problems such as learning or physical disabilities. Prejudice may be caused by the worker's past experience or may be due to ignorance or fear, while perceived conflict between the rights of mother and baby may cause difficulties. Staff involved in a supportive relationship with a pregnant woman may find it difficult to contribute to a negative decision about child custody, or to acknowledge this contribution to the woman, and this may prejudice their relationship with her.

Non-attendance

Non-attendance for maternity care is often attributed to parental inadequacy but is more commonly due to inappropriate services. As discussed, services may be effectively inaccessible because of design or delivery. Women with special needs may also have other more urgent demands on their time. Dealing with all these problems may require additional input from standard services; or sometimes the need for dedicated specialist services when providing comprehensive care within a multidisciplinary clinic will provide the most effective solution with the benefits discussed above. Community clinics in the WRHS are staffed by an obstetrician and a midwife, but also by a health visitor, a member of social services staff, and a drugs worker. All women see all members of the team with the exception of the drugs worker who is only seen if the woman or her partner has a drug problem or if the woman requests a consultation. Availability of help with all problems within one clinic will encourage attendance and improve contact with all relevant services. In the WRHS the average booking gestation is now comparable to the overall hospital rate (Hepburn 1997).

Women reluctant to attend clinics for whatever reason may be encouraged by initial contact elsewhere, including in their own homes (Olds *et al.* 1988). A home visit may be seen either as simply a means of making initial contact or as an opportunity to deliver care, but should not be seen as a substitute for clinic attendance. Efforts should always be made to encourage women to attend services to demonstrate stability of lifestyle and to assume some responsibility for their own care.

Care providers

Continuity of care is important, and the need for one individual to be identified as the principal care-giver or at least care coordinator is especially important when many individuals or services are involved. Socio-economic deprivation is associated with increased perinatal mortality and morbidity. While women with deprivation-linked special needs are therefore unsuitable for total midwifery management, much of their care can be delivered by midwives. For women with problems which have long-term social implications, the contributions of the general practitioner and the primary care team are also critically important as is input from the social services. Although the planning of her care will jointly involve the woman, midwife, obstetrician, general practitioner, social worker, and other professionals as necessary, the midwife is often the most appropriate individual to coordinate care and provide the first point of contact. Current trends in maternity care are towards a one-to-one relationship with a named midwife. However, in the care of women with some categories of special needs, particularly where these are associated with difficulties in relating to other people, an exclusive relationship may reinforce communication problems and encourage dependency. Therefore, in the care of such women it is essential to identify a named midwife that the woman can contact about any aspect of her care and with whom she can develop a close relationship, but this midwife should avoid being perceived as the sole care provider. Such a midwife, if she has a large case-load, may be unable to guarantee she will be available at all stages of the woman's care and the best compromise will depend on the individual woman's needs. For example, experience in the WRHS has shown that for women with social problems, continuity of care antenatally and postnatally is vital. While they also want to see someone familiar when in labour, intermittent contact with their named midwife or another team member is sufficient and they do not consider it necessary for that individual to deliver their baby. However, for the woman with a history of sexual abuse, delivery by her named midwife may be the overriding priority.

Communications

Case records

The 'shared care' card is the traditional route for communications between health care professionals providing maternity care. Current trends are towards giving women their complete case record, and *Changing Childbirth* (Department of Health 1993) states that women should be given the option of carrying their own case notes. While for the vast majority of women this is an excellent and practical objective, there are potential pitfalls for some women with special needs and especially lifestyle problems. Theoretically, it should resolve the problem of women not attending the same clinic on every occasion, particularly if they arrive at a different clinic without warning. However, women who do not stay in one place, whether because of homelessness or chaotic lifestyle – the very women most likely to attend at a variety of clinics – are often those who have difficulty keeping possession of a shared-care card let alone bringing it to all consultations. This is not necessarily indicative of irresponsibility. While women under the influence of drugs may lose the card they are also frequently robbed, especially when working as prostitutes. Women who are homeless may have to find temporary accommodation with family or friends on a day-to-day basis. Some may find their house boarded up as a result of inability to pay the rent or following absence interpreted by housing authorities as abandonment, while some may have to leave suddenly due to a violent partner. Consequently, despite their best efforts women may lose or at least mislay their card. An informal review in the WRHS revealed not only a significant rate of loss but also anxiety caused by this loss, and many women expressed the view that being given responsibility for their entire case record would prove very stressful.

A second problem arises from the information recorded. Many women with special needs have partners or families unaware of their problems. While sometimes it would be helpful if they were aware, many women either do not want them to know, feel unable to tell them, or require time to do so. They are also often unable to prevent them from seeing the card, so in such situations the information recorded must be an even more abridged version of the full record. Such contentious information is often useful to carers but not invariably vital to management. Some of it could therefore be omitted from the full case record but, inevitably, some would have to remain and it could be very stressful for women to have possession of their record containing information they do not want others to know. Again, informal review suggests many such women would prefer not to carry their case records but if the offer were made in the presence of their partner, refusal might prove difficult. While women should always have the option of involvement of their partners in their antenatal care, it is important to remember it may be inappropriate to make this offer in the partner's presence. Secondly, even if the offer is accepted it should be remembered that seemingly innocuous questions such as the offer of carrying the full case record may carry wider implications. Sometimes the woman herself may not have thought of such implications so, as noted earlier, no matter how supportive her partner or family may appear it is important that some time is spent with the woman on her own.

Interdisciplinary communications

Women with special needs will often benefit from multidisciplinary care whether or not it is delivered from a single site. The need for integrated multidisciplinary care for women with medically based special needs is well recognized, but the relevance of social problems to obstetric management is less fully appreciated. Communication between the agencies concerned often only occurs when or if specific problems arise. However, in the care of women whose problems may affect child care or even jeopardize child custody, it is vital that medical and social management should be jointly planned, and regular meetings of all concerned are essential.

Confidentiality

In many cases of special needs, women may want the information to remain known to only an individual or group of individuals and steps should be taken to ensure this confidentiality. Where the information is essential to others, women can usually be persuaded to agree to this provided they retain a sense of control over disclosure. It is therefore important that time is taken to obtain their permission. Consideration should be given to methods of documentation to limit disclosure to those with an agreed and acknowledged need to know.

Service content

Medical care

The content of care should not be rigidly defined but should depend on individual needs and wishes. For example, routine weighing at every clinic visit, although largely abandoned in standard maternity care, is valuable in the regular assessment of drug users as an indicator of stability of an individual's drug use. It is also something which many women want to know, but those from deprived backgrounds often do not own scales. Cervical cytology (if due) is often deferred until after delivery. However, women who do not attend for antenatal care often fail to attend for postnatal care, while those who are very mobile may have moved on. Not only do such women risk missing postnatal screening but they are often the very women most likely to have been missed by regular screening programmes, while some will also be at greater risk of abnormal cytology. Contact in the antenatal period may provide an invaluable opportunity both to take a cervical smear and also to screen for genital infections where indicated. Pelvic examination may seem particularly inappropriate for some types of special needs, such as a history of sexual abuse. However, such women, especially if exposed to early sexual contact with many partners, may be those for whom screening is particularly relevant. Even if not appropriate at the booking clinic, screening may be possible later in the antenatal period when a supportive relationship has developed between the woman and her carer. In making recommendations to women, all the arguments for and against any intervention should be carefully considered.

Dietary advice

It is important to ensure information given is appropriate to the woman, and this is particularly true of dietary advice. Many women from deprived backgrounds have inadequate and inappropriate diets. This is partly due to financial difficulties exacerbated by women's tendency to give priority to their children and partners. However, the standard dietary advice is often also unappealing because of differences in culture or eating habits and can be impractical for women without adequate cooking facilities or the ability to use them. Therefore, while addressing their financial problems will be helpful, it will not necessarily improve their diet.

Preparation for parenthood

Women prepare for childbirth and parenthood in different ways. Some want to know as much as possible about what will happen to them, why it will happen, and what options they have. For them, knowledge and involvement in decision-making produce a reassuring sense of control. Some women, however, and especially those from deprived backgrounds, find the information anything but reassuring and claim they prefer not to have prior knowledge of the process of childbirth. In the Glasgow WRHS this, together with embarrassment at receiving information in the company of other women, was given as a major reason for non-attendance at antenatal classes. Women attending the service are now provided, either in small groups or on a one-to-one basis, with the information they consider important (mostly relating to diagnosis of labour, availability and effectiveness of epidural anaesthesia, and necessary length of postnatal stay). Such arrangements, while still underused, were at least judged favourably by the women. However, while formal evaluation of women's views confirmed the popularity of this approach, it also confirmed inadequate understanding of intrapartum events. Interestingly, while concerned by their lack of knowledge, the women failed to recognize the information they lacked as that which they had rejected antenatally or indeed to see any connection between their lack of knowledge and rejection of antenatal education (Hepburn and Elliott 1997). This demonstrates clearly that what women want and what they need may not be identical. It is therefore important to look for ways of bridging the gap and finding a compromise solution acceptable to all.

Postnatal contraception

Special needs which affect compliance may influence contraceptive method, timing, and delivery. In such circumstances contraceptive choice should be discussed early and repeatedly during pregnancy. Commencement prior to postnatal discharge may be indicated and maternity services should contribute to discussions about provision of postnatal contraception (Hepburn 1995*b*).

Women's choices

Planning care

Changing Childbirth (Department of Health 1993) correctly emphasized the importance of involving women in decisions about their care and allowing them to choose how, where, and by whom they should be managed. However, the existence of sometimes inevitable restrictions should be recognized. For example, home birth may not be an option for women with inadequate or unstable housing. It will also not be feasible for those who will require intensive support or supervision to acquire or confirm satisfactory parenting skills. Some women will require input from social services if they are to retain child custody but may be reluctant to accept such involvement. While women should always be encouraged to exercise choice, choice is not always an option. In such situations they should be helped by reassurance and persuasion to accept unavoidable restrictions, to view such interventions as supportive rather than punitive and authoritarian, and to work with services to secure the best possible outcome.

Care in labour and postnatally

Ensuring appropriate support and advocacy for the woman is also important when helping her make plans for her labour. As already discussed, it should be remembered that the woman's partner may not be male or may not be the father of her child – whether knowingly or unknowingly – while the pregnancy may be the result of an abusive relationship with her partner or someone else. It should not be assumed that a woman has only one sexual partner. The possibility of doubt about paternity should be borne in mind even if this is not totally acknowledged by the woman and/or her partner as, for example, when a woman has been involved in prostitution. Where uncertainty is acknowledged it is important that staff should avoid actions which might cause rather than resolve problems. Thus requests for paternity testing should be treated with caution, remembering that testing will not necessarily prove who is the father and may only prove that the woman's partner is not the father. It should also be remembered that women not in a stable relationship, as well as some who are, may want someone other than a regular partner to be with them during labour. Some women will be aware they will not, or are unlikely to get, custody of the baby while some may have decided voluntarily to give the baby for adoption. Such situations may affect all aspects of a woman's care and should be discussed with her. She should be asked whether or to what extent she would want to receive antenatal care (including preparation for parenthood) or postnatal care in the company of other women and what contact, if any, she would like to have with the baby.

Specific special needs

The following is not intended as a comprehensive list of circumstances incurring special needs nor as a comprehensive list of special needs associated with these problems. It merely lists some examples of special needs to illustrate how these may influence both the care which women need and the way they receive it. Women's need for modified care and their ability to access services should always be individually assessed. It should also be remembered that some of the issues discussed here, such as Hepatitis B and HIV infection, are relevant to all women and not only those with special needs.

Problem drug and alcohol use

Women with problem drug or alcohol use may not be registered with a general practitioner, may present late for antenatal care, and may have difficulty keeping appointments. Many will have consequent health problems. Problem drug use but not alcohol use is associated with socio-economic deprivation, but the need to finance a habit may cause or exacerbate poverty and may result in criminal activities and/or legal problems. Women with problem drug or alcohol use may have precarious accommodation, be mobile, or even homeless. They may have a partner with problem drug or alcohol use, be at risk of violence from their partner, have to finance a partner's use and, if involved in prostitution, be at risk of sexually transmitted infections and/or violence from their clients. The paternity of their baby may be uncertain with or without their partner's knowledge. They will need input from social services, including drug or alcohol services, but may not want this if their partner and/or family are unaware of their problems or because they fear loss of custody of their child(ren). This may further compromise attendance for care. Confidentiality will be an important issue.

When a woman is identified as having a drug or alcohol problem it is important to identify all associated medical and social problems. Like all pregnant women she should receive information about and the offer of testing for Hepatitis B and/or HIV infection, and in this case infection with Hepatitis C will also be particularly relevant. With her permission, involve other relevant services and ensure she is registered with a supportive general practitioner. Establish effective communication with other services since this will also help maintain contact with the woman. Planning meetings should be held involving all concerned, including the woman, her partner, her family, and other supportive individuals or agencies to identify needs, establish goals, and monitor progress (LGDF and SCODA 1997). Potential problems in labour should be discussed, including neonatal complications, and the woman prepared for such events. Again, with her permission, ensure those who will provide care in labour or who will care for the baby are aware of all relevant facts. The possibility of a prolonged postnatal stay in hospital should be raised and plans made for provision of support after discharge. Remember the possibility of psychological problems, including postnatal depression after birth and especially after she returns home.

Poverty

Poverty may make attendance for antenatal care difficult and may prevent the woman from making adequate preparations for the new baby. It may jeopardize housing or accommodation and may lead to criminal activities and consequent legal problems. Women's financial circumstances should always be explored and referral to relevant services arranged if necessary. It is important to also be aware of the possible impact on existing children. Remember severe poverty may make a woman's accommodation unsuitable not just for home birth but also for subsequent care of a new baby. Again, ensure there is involvement of all relevant services, that effective communication is established with them, and that planning meetings take place to arrange ongoing support, including psychological support. Check these are all in place before the woman is discharged home postnatally.

Homelessness

Always check not only a woman's address but also whether she lives there and any other addresses where she may spend time. Establish details of her accommodation, including security of residence, and if she is homeless or mobile obtain details of others with permanent addresses who can be contacted if she moves. Ensure she is in contact with relevant agencies, is registered with a general practitioner, and knows how and where to obtain help if she is suddenly obliged to move. While it may be helpful for her to have possession of at least an abbreviated form of her medical records in case she has to attend elsewhere, giving her sole responsibility for her records may cause problems for her. Similar restrictions will apply regarding choice of place for delivery and a longer postnatal stay in hospital may be necessary. Again, remember the need for psychological support and the risk of mental health problems.

Travelling women

As in the case of homeless women, travelling women may experience problems due to mobility. They may have difficulty attending at one site for all their antenatal care and may move to another area before the baby is born. They may not be registered with a general practitioner or may have to change if they move. Some but not all travelling women also suffer from poverty or from limitations in suitability of their accommodation either for delivery or care of a young baby. Check details of their accommodation and if it is inadequate ensure they are in contact with the relevant services. Ask how long they intend to remain in the area and if they know where or when they will move. Provide adequate medical details to be presented at another centre if necessary, contact services elsewhere if possible, and make sure they know how to make contact themselves.

Institutionalized women

Women may live in various types of institutions either because of problems with housing or because they need support as a result of other special needs such as learning difficulties. They may be temporarily living in an institution because of problem drug or alcohol use or because they are serving a custodial sentence. Establish the terms under which they are living in the institution, whether they will be there permanently or at least for the foreseeable future or, if temporarily, when and where they will be moving. Identify other causal or incidental factors incurring special needs and ensure these are also addressed. Check involvement with primary care services. Consider where delivery will take place and whether the woman's choices in labour will be restricted. Check whether the institution has facilities for babies and, if not, whether the woman will have to leave after delivery or, if this is not an option, whether the baby will have to be received into care. Again, remember the possibility of mental health problems arising or becoming worse after delivery.

Prostitution

Find out whether the woman is engaged in commercial sex because of poverty *per se* or because of a need to finance a drug habit. Ensure she receives help with any causal factors. Remember the possibility of sexually transmitted infections. Screen for genital infections antenatally and, as for all women, provide information with the offer of screening for HIV and Hepatitis B infections. Be aware that paternity may be uncertain. Her partner may not be aware of either her involvement in prostitution or any underlying problems such as drug use, but conversely he may not only be aware of it but may be actively encouraging or even controlling her activities and/or using the money she earns to finance his own lifestyle. Confidentiality will be an important issue both antenatally and during labour.

HIV infection

Women may know they are infected with HIV before conception or may discover this following antenatal screening. Whatever the circumstances, the woman known to be HIV positive needs information about implications for her own and her baby's health, and specifically about the risk of vertical transmission and possible interventions aimed at reducing this risk. Her own and her baby's management should be discussed and agreed with her. Most women with HIV infection will want this information to be made available only to those who need to know, and these will be determined by her choice of management. Remembering that all pregnant women may be infected with HIV, knowledge of status is never justified on grounds of infection control and confidentiality should be observed throughout pregnancy, delivery, and the puerperium according to the woman's wishes. All those involved in the woman's care should participate in joint planning throughout and, as with any potential paediatric problem, this will include those who will care for the baby. The many potential medical and social problems make multi-disciplinary care particularly essential for women with HIV infection, but it should also be appreciated that such women may not perceive HIV infection as their most immediate problem.

Violence/abuse

This is an underdetected problem which occurs throughout the social spectrum and all pregnant women should be routinely asked whether they have suffered violence and/or abuse. Remember the current pregnancy may be the result of abuse and the abuser may or may not be her partner. Women who report abuse should be asked about supportive people in their lives and given information about agencies which could help. They may want help to leave an abusive relationship immediately or to develop contingency plans in case they need to leave at a later date. If they leave they may experience many of the other problems discussed, including mobility and/or homelessness, financial hardship, and social isolation. Screening for sexually transmitted infections may be relevant. Check who she wants to have with her during labour and with her permission ensure the person in charge of her care in labour is aware of the circumstances. Post-partum she may be returning to circumstances of continuing abuse.

Young age

As with all women, check the circumstances of the pregnancy and whether it was intended and/or wanted. If the woman is under 16 years old, the age of her partner should be asked, remembering that he has committed an offence. Consider whether screening for sexually transmitted infections is relevant, remembering that her young age may make her more vulnerable to infections such as chlamydia. If family or others will be essential for child care, their views should also be sought. Contact should be made with other appropriate agencies, particularly social services, although their degree of involvement will depend on individual circumstances. She may need considerable support during pregnancy, and especially during labour, and possibly individualized child-care tuition. Accommodation and finance may be important issues as well as the question of ongoing education.

Learning difficulties

Again it is important to establish the circumstances of the pregnancy, the relationship with the baby's father, and whether he also has learning difficulties. With significant disability, involvement of social services and other agencies will be necessary. Consider whether the mother will be able to care for the baby independently or with the help of her partner, whether other family members will be partially or wholly responsible for child care, whether supported accommodation will be an option, and whether statutory measures of care will be necessary. Adequate and appropriate preparation for labour will be essential, with involvement of those who will care for her and provide support. If it is hoped the mother will care for the baby herself, she will need help to develop the necessary child-care skills as well as intensive support during her postnatal stay in hospital and after her return to the community. Screening for sexually transmitted infections may be indicated. Whether or not the woman has an ongoing relationship with the baby's father and whether or not she retains custody of the baby, contraception will be an important issue.

Mental health problems

The nature and pattern of the illness should be established. If the woman is continuously sufficiently unwell to prejudice child care, the problems and appropriate management will be similar to those for women with learning difficulties. If the woman is only periodically unwell, plans are necessary to deal with these episodes, remembering that when she is unwell she may be unaware of this and not only fail to seek help but resist any intervention, so that maintaining contact and providing effective supervision may be difficult or impossible.

Sexual orientation

Lesbian women in stable relationships may seek advice or help preconceptionally but, if not, should be identified by an adequate booking history. The circumstances of conception should be established and, if not already requested, the offer of screening for sexually transmitted infections may be appropriate. As with all pregnant women, her partner may participate to varying degrees during pregnancy, labour, and postnatally. In some cases the father of the baby may also be involved and, as for all women, staff should discuss the individual woman's circumstances to plan her management according to her wishes.

Staff training

It is unrealistic and unnecessary to expect all staff to possess the expertise to manage all problems incurring special needs. It is, however, essential that all who come in contact with women presenting for maternity care are aware of, and can identify, such problems so that women can be offered appropriate help. How this is provided will vary from centre to centre, according to local circumstances.

Staff education and training should also deal with communication difficulties, including attitudinal problems which staff may experience. Caring for some groups of women with some types of special needs can be extremely stressful and demanding, and the need for support for staff should also be recognized. In such circumstances, participation in a multidisciplinary team can provide one useful source of support.

Conclusions

Health care providers therefore need to be aware of factors which carry specific service requirements, have the skills to identify them, and understand their implications for care provision. They also need to be aware that women often have multiple problems. The special needs discussed here are only examples to heighten awareness while the management issues discussed are only examples of problems which may be associated with them. Many will be associated with other problems or will coexist; management should not be rigidly defined but in every case should be determined by individual assessment.

References

Bassuk, E. L. and Weinreb, L. (1993). Homeless pregnant women: two generations at risk. *American Journal of Orthopsychiatry*, 63(3), 348–57.

Benzeval, M., Judge, K., and Whitehead, M. (1995). *Tackling inequalities in health: an agenda for action.* King's Fund, London.

Borgford-Parnell, D., Hope, K. R., and Deisher, R. W. (1994). A homeless teen pregnancy project: an intensive team case management model. *American Journal of Public Health*, 84(6), 1029–30.

Bradley, P. J. and Martin, J. M. (1994). The impact of home visits on enrolment patterns in pregnancy-related services among low-income women. *Public Health Nursing*, 11(6), 392–8.

Cardale, P. (1992). Springing the poverty trap. *Nursing Times*, 88(29), 66–7.

Cook, V. (1995). An inner-urban funded maternity care programme: maternity information and advice centre. *Midwives*, 108, 142–5.

Cowl, J. (1995). Diverse needs, diverse choice – developing ethnically sensitive maternity services. *Changing Childbirth Update*, 3, 6–10.

Department of Health (1993). Changing childbirth. Report of the Expert Maternity Group. HMSO, London.

Dickinson, C. P., Jackson, D. J., Swartz, W. H. (1994). Making the alternative the mainstream: maintaining a family-centred focus in a large free-standing birth centre for low-income women. *Journal of Nurse-Midwifery*, 39(2), 112–18.

Dineen, K., Rossi, M., Lia-Hoagberg, B., and Keller, L. O. (1992). Antepartum home-care services for high-risk women. *Journal of Obstetric, Gynaecologic, and Neonatal Nursing*, 21(2), 121–5.

Hepburn, M. (1991). Social problems. In: *Antenatal care: clinical obstetrics and gynaecology, international practice and research* (ed. M. H. Hall). Vol. 4. Bailliere Tindall, London.

Hepburn, M. (1995a). The Glasgow Women's Reproductive Health Service. *Changing Childbirth Update*, 3, 11.

Hepburn, M. (1995b). Factors influencing contraceptive choice. In: *Handbook of family planning and reproductive health care* (eds. N. Loudon, A. Glasier, and A. Gebbie). Churchill Livingstone. London, pp. 19–36.

Hepburn, M. (1997). Horses for courses: developing services for women with special needs. *British Journal of Midwifery*, 5(8), 482–4.

Hepburn, M. and Elliott, L. (1997). A community obstetric service for women with special needs – consumer views. *British Journal of Midwifery*, 5(8), 485–6.

Levy, S. R., Perhats, C., Nash-Johnson, M., and Welter, J. F. (1992). Reducing the risks in pregnant teens who are very young and those with mild mental retardation. *Mental Retardation*, **30**(4), 195–203.

Local Government Drugs Forum (LGDF) and the Standing Conference on Drug Abuse (SCODA) (1997). *Drug-using parents: policy guidelines for inter-agency working*. Local Government Association publication, London.

Marcenko, M. O. and Spence, M. (1994). Home visitation services for at-risk pregnant and post-partum women: a randomized trial. *American Journal of Orthopsychiatry*, **64**(3), 468–78.

Mayer, J. P., Blakely, C. H., and Johnson, C. D. (1990). Formative evaluation of a community-based maternity services program for the uninsured. *Family and Community Health*, 13(3), 18–26.

Miller, W. H., Bloom, J. D., Resnick, M. P. (1992). Prenatal care for pregnant chronic mentally ill patients. *Hospital and Community Psychiatry*, 43(9), 942–3.

O'Connell, M. L. (1993). Childbirth education classes in homeless shelters. *AWHONN's Clinical Issues in Perinatal and Women's Health Nursing*, 4(1), 102–12.

Olds, D., Henderson, C., Tatelbaum, R., and Chamberlin, R. (1998). Improving the life course development of socially disadvantaged mothers : a randomized trial of nurse home visitation. *American Journal of Public Health*, **78**, 1436–45.

Ovrebo, B., Ryan, M., Jackson, K., and Hutchinson, K. (1994). The homeless prenatal program: a model for empowering homeless pregnant women. *Health Education Quarterly*, 21(2), 187–98.

Reilly, R. A. (1993). Homelessness: a midwifery perspective. *Midwives' Chronicle and Nursing Notes*, **106**(1271), 486–90.

Rodriguez, R., McFarlane, J., Mahon, J., and Fehir, J. (1993). De madres a madres: a community partnership to increase access to prenatal care. *Bulletin of the Pan American Health Organization*, 27(4), 403–8.

Thomas, V. and Dines, A. (1994). The health care needs of ethnic minority groups: are nurses and individuals playing their part? *Journal of Advanced Nursing*, **20**, 802–8.

Townsend, P. and Davidson, N. (1982). *Inequalities in health: the Black Report*. Penguin, Harmondsworth.

Vernon, D. (1994). The health of traveller gypsies. *British Journal of Nursing*, 3(18), 969–72.

Woodard, G. R. B. and Edouard, L. (1992). Reaching out: a community initiative for disadvantaged pregnant women. *Canadian Journal of Public Health*, 83(3), 188–90.

Yordan, E. E. and Yordan, R. A. (1993). The maternity home for adolescents: a concept from the past fulfilling a contemporary need. *Connecticut Medicine*, 57(2), 65–8.

CHAPTER THIRTEEN

The use of technology in
maternity care

James P. Neilson

Introduction

This chapter will concentrate on the use of machines to complement or replace the clinical care of women during pregnancy or childbirth by doctors and midwives. The use of equipment is not necessarily bad if it clearly produces tangible benefits compared with standard clinical care alone, but it is the responsibility of proponents of new techniques and/or equipment to demonstrate such benefits before these are accepted into practice. It has been realized belatedly that the rigorous processes of evaluation that are necessary before a new drug can be given to patients have not been applied to new machines or techniques. In consequence, many uses of technology are of questionable value and others may be downright harmful.

The burden of responsibility to prove the effectiveness of new technologies should rest with their proponents because:

- the technologies may be expensive and deflect scarce resources from activities of greater value such as the salaries of midwives and other staff
- they may be potentially dangerous either by immediate effects (e.g. damage to the fetus from invasive prenatal diagnostic procedures), delayed effects (e.g. prenatal X-rays), or through the generation of misleading information, encouraging, for example, inappropriate termination of pregnancy or planned delivery
- they may constitute a barrier between a woman and her care-provider (a midwife may be distracted from care of a woman in labour by an electronic fetal monitor that is malfunctioning or even one that is functioning correctly)
- they may appear intimidating
- they may restrict activities and postures that the woman might otherwise choose
- they may exclude certain care-givers, particularly those working in the

213

community, and encourage the 'medicalization' of pregnancy and child-birth.

The use of technology is now very widespread in maternity care in the industrialized world (Wheble *et al.* 1989). A recent survey in the UK has shown that 77% of maternity units offer women a routine early booking ultrasound scan to establish gestational age, and 82% of units offer a routine detailed scan in mid-pregnancy to screen for structural fetal abnormalities (Whittle, personal communication).

It is important for community-based clinicians to understand the techniques to be able to deliver appropriate advice where necessary, even if they do not actually use the equipment themselves. Certain technologies can be used in the community – cardiotocography can be performed in the homes of women and, if necessary, the signals can be transmitted electronically to a base unit (Dawson *et al.* 1988) or a printout can be faxed; portable ultrasound scanners can also be used in the community; indeed, one new technology (home uterine activity monitoring) was designed primarily for community use. The technological barriers to the use of these techniques in the community can be overcome and are of little interest. What is much more important is whether the information derived from these tests is of sufficient value in any setting as to justify seeking to overcome these barriers.

This chapter will rely heavily on the systematic reviews of randomized controlled trials of technological interventions during pregnancy. The randomized controlled trial is widely seen as providing the gold standard method of assessing the effectiveness of new treatments or tests or other procedures by minimizing bias (Chalmers 1989). In the perinatal field, large numbers of women or babies are usually needed to address important research questions about outcomes that may be rare. Such questions may be tackled by mounting large studies or by pooling data from a number of different trials of similar structure and purpose (meta-analysis) (Peto 1987). Meta-analysis is a component of a systematic (or scientific) review and these are increasingly being produced to inform clinical practice and health planning. An international research network, the Cochrane Collaboration, aims to produce up-to-date, high-quality systematic reviews of all aspects of health care (Chalmers *et al.* 1992); there are already many such reviews from the pregnancy and childbirth field published electronically in the Cochrane Library (and previously in the Cochrane Pregnancy and Childbirth Database).

In this chapter, reference will be made where possible to an up-to-date Cochrane review and the individual trials from which the systematic review is derived will not be cited unless there is a specific issue of note that arises from a single trial. If there is only a single trial of substance in a specific area of interest, that will be cited rather than the Cochrane review.

Antenatal technology

The use of technology during antenatal care has almost exclusively been applied to fetal assessment – of either structural abnormality, growth or size, or well-being.

Ultrasound

Ultrasound, as a diagnostic procedure, developed from the studies of Ian Donald, Regius Professor of Midwifery (Obstetrics and Gynaecology) at the University of Glasgow. Starting during the 1950s, the story is an interesting one (Willocks 1993) and illustrates not only vision and innovation but also the lack of formal evaluation of new health technologies. The initial imaging was very crude but technological advances have produced increasingly clear images of the fetus and other intrauterine structures and have ensured that ultrasound equipment is increasingly easy to use. These phenomena have produced difficulties. Thus:

- quantum leaps in imaging resolution may make evaluations of effectiveness redundant before they are completed

- similarly, such advances may demonstrate features not previously seen and whose significance may be completely unknown; a good example is the choroid plexus cyst. These cysts have no functional significance and almost universally disappear during the course of pregnancy. They have, however, been linked to chromosomal abnormality in the fetus (especially Edward's syndrome or trisomy 18 – usually a lethal abnormality), but there remains a lack of consensus about whether this occurs with sufficient frequency to justify offering amniocentesis or other invasive investigations to women whose fetuses are shown to have these. The news that their baby has a 'brain abnormality' is, of course, very alarming

- the ease of use is a double-edged sword. On the one hand, the equipment may be used by less extensively trained operators, thus being employed on delivery units, by midwives, and sometimes in the community; on the other hand, they may be used by individuals without appropriate training and skill. Ultrasound is dependent on the skill of the operator, and highly misleading information may follow inexpert use.

Specific examinations

There are many specific clinical situations in which the use of ultrasound is seen as desirable. These include bleeding in early pregnancy (to confirm pregnancy viability) and late pregnancy (to exclude placenta praevia), suspected multiple pregnancy, investigation of clinically identified oligo- or polyhydramnios, and investigation of the clinically small fetus. The use of ultrasound in these specific circumstances has not been subjected to rigorous assessment by randomized trial, and probably never will. Controversy has surrounded, instead, the other type of ultrasound use, i.e. as a screening technique in all pregnancies.

Screening examinations

Screening examinations may be performed in early, mid, or late pregnancy. The rationale for routine ultrasound in early/mid-pregnancy is:

- better assessment of gestational age
- earlier detection of multiple pregnancies
- detection of unsuspected fetal abnormalities (or, conversely, reassurance of apparent structural normality).

There is evidence from randomized controlled trials (Neilson 1997*a*) that routine ultrasound is associated with:
- fewer inductions of labour for 'post-term' pregnancies, presumably because of better dating
- earlier diagnosis of multiple pregnancies (although this has not been converted into an improvement in the high perinatal mortality rate associated with multiple pregnancies)
- no change in substantive clinical outcomes *unless* detection of fetal malformation is seen as an important priority and a screening process is implemented to permit accurate prenatal diagnosis in a community in which most women will opt for termination of pregnancy if there is a major fetal malformation. These conditions were met in a Finnish study (Saari-Kemppainen *et al.* 1990) and, in consequence, there was a lower perinatal mortality rate among the screened women. This of course represents in most cases the conversion of a perinatal death to a termination of pregnancy rather than beneficially altering the fundamental outcome of the pregnancy, and the absolute value of this could be debated. These conditions were not met by the large American RADIUS trial (Ewigman *et al.* 1993) whose findings have provoked considerable debate – the detection of fetal abnormalities was considerably less than that achieved in both the Finnish trial and also in some observational studies performed in district hospitals (e.g. Chitty *et al.* 1991; Shirley *et al.* 1992). In the RADIUS trial, only 17% of fetuses with major anomalies were detected. Thus, the RADIUS figures may represent an accurate picture of ultrasound screening in primary care settings but not of secondary or tertiary care. Clearly, it would be difficult to justify anomaly screening in primary care on the basis of these figures.

There are, likewise, legitimate grounds for debate about whether routine ultrasound is desirable in any setting. Some would see the data concerning reduced induction of labour for post-term pregnancy (as, in part, a surrogate index of better gestational age assessment) and earlier diagnosis of multiple pregnancies as sufficient gains to justify routine screening; others would not. In countries with especially restricted health resources, as in the developing world, it would be very difficult indeed to justify routine ultrasound during pregnancy (Munjanja 1993; Geerts *et al.* 1996).

What is clear is that if an ultrasound examination is being performed, the woman should have clear access to images on the screen and information about the scan (Neilson 1995*a*).

Nuchal translucency screening

Where anomaly screening by ultrasound has been adopted, examinations are usually performed between 18 and 22 weeks. The later gestational weeks have been favoured by some because of the greater likelihood of detection of structural heart defects in the fetus (often very rarely identified). Recently, it has been suggested that nuchal translucency screening (identifying and, if appropriate, measuring a fluid-filled space at the baby's neck) may provide a useful screening method for the identification of Down's syndrome at an earlier stage than alternative screening techniques (Nicolaides *et al.* 1996). This technique is now being studied in the UK in a major research project (SURUSS).

Prenatal diagnosis

Amniocentesis

Sampling amniotic fluid for, mainly, chromosome studies is a well-established technique. It is usually performed at around 16 weeks and carries an additional risk of miscarriage in the range of 1% (Neilson *et al.* 1995). With technical advances in laboratory cytogenetics, it has proven possible to consider sampling earlier in pregnancy ('early amniocentesis') and with high-resolution modern ultrasound imaging for guidance, sampling can be performed in experienced hands without undue difficulty at around 10–12 weeks. However, available trial evidence points towards a higher pregnancy loss rate than after chorion villus sampling (Alfirevic *et al* 1997*a*). Thus, except under highly specific circumstances, this procedure does not at present seem justified without further controlled trials. A large ongoing study in Canada will hopefully provide more precise estimates of risks and benefits in the not too distant future.

Chorion villus sampling

Chorion villus sampling (CVS) was first developed in the 1970s as a blind procedure in China to sex fetuses as a response to the one child policy in that country. It was introduced to the West through workers in the Soviet Union. The technique has the advantage of earlier and more rapid diagnosis than conventional amniocentesis, but processing is more time-consuming and expensive in the laboratory. The popularity of the test has, undoubtedly, decreased in recent years partly because of anxieties about associated limb defects in babies (if performed before 11 weeks) (Jackson and Wapner 1993) and other safety issues. Thus, meta-analysis (Alfirevic *et al.* 1997*b*) of the three randomized controlled trials suggests an increase of around 30% in the number of preterm deliveries and of small-for-dates babies born to women allocated to CVS. More importantly, these women had a 33% increased risk in the odds of pregnancy loss.

Fetal blood sampling

Also called cordocentesis or percutaneous umbilical blood sampling (PUBS), this is a still more specialized technique in which fetal blood is obtained for testing, for example in chromosomal studies or haemoglobin estimation (in Rhesus sensitized women), or viral studies. The risk from the procedure will vary according the underlying problem that provoked testing in the first place.

Biochemical screening

Biochemical screening by maternal serum alpha-fetoprotein (MSAFP) assay has been in use for some years in certain parts of the world, with a high incidence of neural tube defects (spina bifida, anencephaly, etc.). It was discovered that in pregnancies in which the fetus has Down's syndrome, the MSAFP result tends to be lower. This observation evolved into a biochemical screening test in which MSAFP is combined with human chorionic gonadotropin (hCG) estimation, sometimes with oestradiol included. Further refinements have included free beta-hCG estimation and study of pregnancy-associated placental protein A (PAPPA) and inhibin as adjunctive tests. A great deal of research effort is, at present, attempting to drive the screening time into the first trimester of pregnancy to facilitate earlier, and safer, termination of pregnancy in the event of a positive diagnosis.

Earlier screening would pose clinical difficulties in addition to logistical demands. Thus, if a woman were to be 'screen positive' on biochemical testing at 11 weeks, there would be a need for a diagnostic procedure to clarify the baby's karyotype. Her options would be to wait until around 16 weeks which would impose what would seem an intolerable strain, or to have an immediate invasive procedure – chorion villus sampling or early amniocentesis – which seem to have a higher loss rate associated with them. An additional potential disadvantage is that some chromosomally abnormal pregnancies that would otherwise have aborted spontaneously between 11 and 16 weeks will be diagnosed through screening and subsequent diagnostic testing with the end result that a unnecessary burden of guilt is transferred to the woman through her need to consider termination of pregnancy. Manifestly, there is an absolute need to test formally, by randomized trial, any first-trimester screening strategies before they are introduced into clinical practice.

Fetal well-being

Routine late pregnancy ultrasound

The main rationale for routine late pregnancy ultrasound screening examinations is the detection of the clinically unsuspected small-for-gestational-age fetus. The deficiencies of clinical detection of small-for-gestational-age fetuses are well documented, and intrauterine growth retardation represents the major avoidable cause of perinatal mortality (Neilson 1994). Attempts to prevent intrauterine growth retardation by prophylactic low-dose aspirin has proven, as with pre-eclampsia, largely disappointing (Collins 1995).

Limited information is available from the randomized controlled trials of routine fetal measurements in the third trimester and meta-analysis does not at present encourage this screening procedure (Neilson 1995b). Not all of the trials, however, employed effective measurement techniques, and the sensitivity of detection of small-for-gestational-age fetuses was very variable.

One third trimester screening examination that has shown more promise than routine fetal measurement is the examination of 'placental texture' by ultrasound. Morphological changes of the placenta can be detected by ultrasound as pregnancy advances and it was hoped by early investigators that the detection of 'advanced' grades would allow confirmation of fetal lung maturity in the absence of invasive testing. This was not shown to be sufficiently reliable to be implemented but it was observed that mature appearances were sometimes seen before term in pregnancies complicated by pre-eclampsia, intrauterine growth retardation, and maternal smoking. A single trial (Proud and Grant 1987) has assessed the impact of routine placental ultrasonography on pregnancy outcome, and has reported fewer stillbirths in the screened group. This observation supports the reporting of placental texture appearances during ultrasound examinations during the third trimester. Whether universal screening is merited requires confirmation by additional and much larger trials; it seems unlikely that these will now be done.

Antepartum cardiotocography

Cardiotocography is a very widely used method of assessing fetal well-being that is suitable for use in both the community and the hospital or clinic. Four randomized controlled trials have been performed and these show an *increased* perinatal mortality associated with the use of antepartum cardiotocography in 'high-risk' pregnancies (Neilson 1995c). These trials may not be clearly applicable to modern maternity care – they were performed at a time when concepts of obstetric risk and clinical care were considerably different. However, they do clearly raise questions about the effectiveness of antepartum cardiotocography as a monitoring tool. It is possible, for example, that false reassurance may be derived from a normal trace in a situation of genuine fetal compromise. It may well be that the place of cardiotocography is where there are reasons for anxiety about the acute state of fetal well-being (such as after an antepartum haemorrhage, or when a woman presents with decreased movement) rather than as an intermittent monitoring test in a high-risk pregnancy. The newer computerized equipments that assess fetal heart rate variability as an indicator of fetal 'reserve' have not yet been assessed in randomized trials.

Biophysical profile

The biophysical profile was developed as a type of intrauterine Apgar score and the original profile was based on five parameters: fetal movement, breathing, and tone; amniotic fluid volume; cardiotocography (Manning *et al.* 1980). Minor modifications have been suggested by some authors. Very limited information is available from randomized controlled trials despite large published observational series that are difficult to interpret because the results were made available to clinical staff during the period of assessment. Data from the two small randomized controlled trials that are available do not encourage the use of biophysical testing during antenatal care (Alfirevic and Neilson 1997).

Doppler ultrasound

In contrast, Doppler ultrasound has been tested much more rigorously and extensively. The first report of the use of Doppler ultrasound to assess the pattern of blood flow in the umbilical artery appeared in 1979 (Fitzgerald and Drumm 1979). The feto-placental circulation should be a low-resistance vascular system with forward flow of blood throughout the cardiac cycle but, in uteroplacental insufficiency, resistance may increase with cessation of blood flow (and even reversal of flow) during diastole. Similar findings may be detected in the uteroplacental circulation on the maternal side of the placenta although this a more complex circulation in its anatomy and physiology, and in its ease of study. With the development of colour-flow imaging, small fetal vessels can also be identified and studied and patterns of flow have been seen that are compatible with the 'brain-sparing' effect seen in hypoxaemic fetuses studied in animal models. More recently, there has been interest in the study of fetal veins (inferior vena cava, ductus venosus, umbilical vein) to complement better established study of fetal arteries (e.g. cerebral vessels, aorta, renal arteries). The study of internal fetal vessels has not been subjected to randomized controlled trial.

Eleven randomized controlled trials have been completed to assess the use of Doppler ultrasound in high-risk pregnancies (usually pregnancies complicated by hypertension or suspicion that the fetus is small for gestational age). Meta-analysis (Neilson and Alfirevic 1997) shows that the use of Doppler ultrasound was associated with a 29% reduction in overall perinatal mortality, with confidence intervals that are compatible with a reduction of as much as 50% or with no effect. There was no obvious effect on indices of neonatal morbidity but women in the Doppler group were less likely to be admitted to hospital antenatally and less likely to have labour induced.

Many would see these findings as providing strong evidence that access to Doppler ultrasound examination of the umbilical artery is important in high-risk pregnancies.

Intrapartum technology

Care of the mother

The rapid, and largely unevaluated, introduction of technology into the labour wards of the 1970s provoked a backlash among many users of the maternity services that has led, ultimately, to improvements in the quality of care. Questioning of the value of established techniques also encouraged research studies that have helped to clarify what measures are effective and what are not.

Thus the routine use of many of the ritual procedures of the past can be discarded on the basis of research evidence, including perineal shaving (Renfrew 1995) and the use of enemas (Hay-Smith 1995). On a more positive note, there is good evidence from research studies that psychological support of women during labour (by professionals or lay women) is beneficial not only in improving women's feelings about labour and delivery, but also by decreasing medical interventions and adverse clinical outcomes (Hodnett 1997a). This may seem self-evident to some but there are many parts of the world in which women do not receive such support during labour in institutional settings. Indeed, in many under-resourced settings, these data should provide support for the use of scarce finances in employing people rather than buying technology. Psychological support is important in affluent countries as well and economic quandaries also apply with conflicting demands; in the words of the relevant Cochrane reviewer: 'Hospitals which are considering renovations of their labour wards (into 'birth centres') should be made aware that there is much stronger evidence to support the need for changes in care-givers' behaviour than there is to support the need for structural changes to labour wards' (Hodnett 1997b).

Many of the effects of common interventions during labour represent a trade-off between advantage and disadvantage, and application should be tailored to individual circumstances and women's preferences. Thus:

- amniotomy (artificial rupture of the membranes) reduces the duration of labour (if this is seen as a benefit, as it often is) and the number of babies with depressed five-minute Apgar scores, but does not decrease the number of Caesarean sections (indeed the trend, though not statistically significant, is towards more Caesarean sections) (Fraser et al. 1997)

- the use of epidural analgesia provides, in general, better pain relief than alternative methods but more frequent operative deliveries (Howell 1995)

- active management of the third stage of labour by the use of oxytocic drugs will decrease maternal blood loss and the need for blood transfusion, although at the cost of more frequent nausea and vomiting (Prendiville et al. 1997).

For other interventions, the issues are more clear cut, for example, the advantages of a restrictive policy of performing episiotomy (Carroli et al. 1997).

Fetal assessment

Labour poses a potentially damaging stress to the fetus mainly because of the effects of uterine contractions in interrupting uteroplacental blood flow. In consequence, considerable efforts have gone into the development of technological methods of assessing fetal well-being during labour.

Trials that have compared continuous electronic fetal heart rate monitoring during labour with intermittent auscultation have been reviewed recently (Thacker *et al.* 1997). Continuous electronic fetal heart rate monitoring was associated with a statistically significant reduction in the risk of the baby having a one-minute Apgar score of less than 4, and of neonatal seizures. No significant differences were observed in one-minute Apgar scores of less than 7, rate of admission to neonatal intensive care units, and perinatal death. An increase was seen, with the use of continuous electronic fetal heart rate monitoring, in the rate of Caesarean section and total operative delivery rate.

Trials of intermittent electronic monitoring (e.g. Herbst and Ingemarsson 1994) were not included in this systematic review.

New techniques of fetal assessment are being tested – fetal ECG waveform analysis shows promise ((Westgate *et al.* 1993); fetal pulse oximetry may soon overcome the technical difficulties that have bedevilled progress to be ready for trials of effectiveness.

Technology could potentially help not only with detection of problems during labour, but also with their resolution without the need for operative delivery. Amnioinfusion, for example, is associated with a reduction in Caesarean sections, low Apgar and cord pH scores, and a clinical diagnosis of 'birth asphyxia' when used for umbilical cord compression during labour (Hofmeyr 1997).

Conclusion

Although the introduction of technology into maternity care has occurred in the past with unbridled enthusiasm and without the benefit of proper evaluation, this trend seems to be abating and there is certainly wider understanding of the processes through which the evaluation of new technologies should be channelled before any thought of introduction into practice. It will be interesting to observe screening for fetal chromosomal abnormalities by nuchal translucency scanning to see if the scientific and clinical community and health planners demand proper health technology evaluation of it, or are content to see its premature establishment through a process of insidious and patchy introduction (Neilson 1997*b*). Pregnant women are entitled to better than this. In the eloquent words of someone who has made an enormous contribution to the development of evidence-based maternity care, Murray Enkin:

'In most fields of medical care, persons come to a doctor because they are ill and seek a cure or relief. In obstetrics, pregnant women come to us healthy but with an iatrogenic belief that obstetrical care will further improve the excellent outcomes that nature has already provided for them. The professionally engendered nature of our care increases our responsibility. The presence of the baby, who has no choice in the matter, doubles it' (Enkin 1996).

References

Alfirevic, Z. and Neilson, J. P. (1997). Biophysical profile for fetal assessment in high-risk pregnancies. In: Pregnancy and Childbirth Module of the Cochrane Database of Systematic Reviews [updated 1 Sept. 1997] (ed. J. P. Neilson, C. A. Crowther, E. D. Hodnett, and G. J. Hofmeyr.). Available in the Cochrane Library. The Cochrane Collaboration. Issue 4. Update Software, Oxford. Updated quarterly.

Alfirevic, Z., Gosden, C. M., and Neilson, J. P. (1997a). Early amniocentesis versus chorion villus sampling. In: Pregnancy and Childbirth Module of the Cochrane Database of Systematic Reviews [updated 1 Sept. 1997] (ed. J. P. Neilson, C. A. Crowther, E. D. Hodnett, and G. J. Hofmeyr.). Available in the Cochrane Library. The Cochrane Collaboration. Issue 4. Update Software, Oxford. Updated quarterly.

Alfirevic, Z., Gosden, C. M., and Neilson, J. P. (1997b). Chorion villus sampling versus amniocentesis. In: Pregnancy and Childbirth Module of the Cochrane Database of Systematic Reviews [updated 1 Sept. 1997] (ed. J. P. Neilson , C. A. Crowther, E. D. Hodnett, and G. J. Hofmeyr). Available in the Cochrane Library. The Cochrane Collaboration. Issue 4. Update Software, Oxford. Updated quarterly.

Carroli, G. Belizan, J., and Stamp, G. (1997). Episiotomy policies in vaginal births. In: Pregnancy and Childbirth Module of the Cochrane Database of Systematic Reviews [updated 1 Sept. 1997] (ed. J. P. Neilson, C. A. Crowther, E. D. Hodnett, and G. J. Hofmeyr). Available in the Cochrane Library. The Cochrane Collaboration. Issue 4. Update Software, Oxford. Updated quarterly.

Chalmers, I. (1989). Evaluating the effects of care during pregnancy and childbirth. In: Effective care in pregnancy and childbirth. (ed. I. Chalmers, M. Enkin, and M. J. N. C. Keirse), pp. 3–38. Oxford University Press, Oxford.

Chalmers, I., Dickersin, K., and Chalmers, T. (1992). Getting to grips with Archie Cochrane's agenda. *British Medical Journa*, 305, 786–7.

Chitty, L. S., Hunt, G. H., Moore, J., and Lobb, M. O. (1991). Effectiveness of routine ultrasonography in detecting fetal structural abnormalities in a low-risk population. *British Medical Journal*, **303**, 1165–9.

Collins, R. (1995). Antiplatelet agents for IUGR and pre-eclampsia. In: Pregnancy and Childbirth Module (ed. M. J. N. C. Keirse, M. J. Renfrew, J. P. Neilson, and C. A. Crowther). Cochrane Database of Systematic Reviews. Published through Cochrance Updates on Disk, Oxford. Update Software, Disk issue 2.

Dawes, G. S., Lobb, M., Moulden, M., Redman, C. W. G., and Wheeler, T. (1992). Antenatal cardiotocogram quality and interpretation using computers. *British Journal of Obstetrics and Gynaecology*, **99**, 791–7.

Dawson, A. J., Middlemiss, C., Jones, E. M., and Gough, N. A. J. (1988). Fetal heart rate monitoring by telephone. I. Development of an integrated system in Cardiff. *British Journal of Obstetrics and Gynaecology,* **95,** 1018–23.

Enkin, M. W. (1996). The need for evidence-based obstetrics. *Evidence-based Medicine,* **1,** 132–3.

Ewigman, B. G., Crane, J. P., Frigoletto, F. D., LeFevre, M. L., Bain, R. P., McNellis, D., *et al.* (1993). Effect of prenatal ultrasound screening on perinatal outcome. *New England Journal of Medicine,* **329,** 821–7.

Fitzgerald, D. E. and Drumm, J. E. (1979). Non-invasive measurement of the human circulation using ultrasound. *British Medical Journal,* **2,** 1450–1.

Fraser, W. D., Krauss, I., Brisson-Carrol, G., Thornton, J., and Breart, G. (1997). Amniotomy to shorten spontaneous labour. In: Pregnancy and Childbirth Module of the Cochrane Database of Systematic Reviews [updated 1 Sept. 1997] (ed. J. P. Neilson, C. A. Crowther, E. D. Hodnett, and G. J. Hofmeyr). Available in the Cochrane Library. The Cochrane Collaboration. Issue 4. Update Software, Oxford. Updated quarterly.

Geerts, L. T. G. M., Brand, E. J., and Theron, G. B. (1996). Routine ultrasound examinations in South Africa: cost and effect on perinatal outcome – a prospective randomized controlled trial. *British Journal of Obstetrics and Gynaecology,* **103,** 501–7.

Hay-Smith, J. (1995). Routine enema on admission in labour. In: Pregnancy and Childbirth Module (ed. M. J. N. C. Keirse, M. J. Renfrew, J. P. Neilson, and C. A. Crowther). Cochrane Database of Systematic Reviews. Published through Cocharane Updates on Disk, Oxford. Update software, Disk issue 2.

Herbst, A. and Ingemarsson, I. (1994). Intermittent versus continuous electronic fetal monitoring in labour: a randomized study. . *British Journal of Obstetrics and Gynaecology,* **101,** 663–8.

Hodnett, E. D. (1997*a*). Support from care-givers during childbirth. In: Pregnancy and Childbirth Module of the Cochrane Database of Systematic Reviews. [updated 1 Sept. 1997] (ed. J. P. Neilson, C. A. Crowther, E. D. Hodnett, and G. J. Hofmeyr). Available in the Cochrane Library. The Cochrane Collaboration. Issue 4. Update Software, Oxford. Updated quarterly.

Hodnett, E. D. (1997*b*). Alternate versus conventional delivery settings. In: Pregnancy and Childbirth Module of the Cochrane Database of Systematic Reviews [updated 1 Sept. 1997] (ed. J. P. Neilson, C. A. Crowther, E. D. Hodnett, and G. J. Hofmeyr). Available in the Cochrane Library. The Cochrane Collaboration. Issue 2. Update Software, Oxford. Updated quarterly.

Hofmeyr. G. J. (1997). Amnioinfusion for intrapartum umbilical cord compression (potential, or diagnosed by electronic fetal heart rate monitoring). In: Pregnancy and Childbirth Module of the Cochrane Database of Systematic Reviews [updated 1 Sept. 1997] (ed. J. P. Neilson, C. A. Crowther, E. D. Hodnett, and G. J. Hofmeyr). Available in the Cochrane Library. The Cochrane Collaboration. Issue 1. Update Software, Oxford. Updated quarterly.

Howell, C. J. (1995). Epidural vs non-epidural analgesia in labour. In: Pregnancy and Childbirth Module (ed. M. J. N. C. Keirse, M. J. Renfrew, J. P. Neilson, and C. A. Crowther). Cochrane Database of Systematic Reviews. Published through Cocharane Updates on Disk. Update Software, Oxford. Disk issue 2.

Jackson, L. and Wapner, R. J. (1993). Chorionic villus sampling. In: *Essentials of prenatal diagnosis* (ed. J. L. Simpson and S. Elias), pp.45–62. Churchill Livingstone, New York.

Manning, F. A., Platt, L. D., and Sipos, L. (1980). Antepartum fetal evaluation: development of a fetal biophysical profile score. *American Journal of Obstetrics and Gynecology*, 136, 787–95.

Munjanja, S. P. (1993).Ultrasound in the developing world: appropriate technology?. In: *Obstetric ultrasound 1* (ed. J. P. Neilson and S. Chambers), pp.189–202. Oxford University Press, Oxford.

Neilson, J.P. (1994). Perinatal loss and appropriate fetal surveillance. In: *A critical appraisal of fetal surveillance* (ed. H. P. van Geijn and F. J. A. Copray), pp.16–24. Excerpta Medica, Amsterdam.

Neilson, J. P. (1995*a*). High vs low feedback to mothers at fetal ultrasonography. In: Pregnancy and Childbirth Module (ed. M. J. N. C. Keirse, M. J. Renfrew, J. P. Neilson, and C. A. Crowther). Cochrane Database of Systematic Reviews. Published through Cocharane Updates on Disk. Update Software, Oxford. Disk issue 2.

Neilson, J. P. (1995*b*). Routine fetal anthropometry in late pregnancy. In: Pregnancy and Childbirth Module (ed. M. J. N. C. Keirse, M. J. Renfrew, J. P. Neilson, and C. A. Crowther). Cochrane Database of Systematic Reviews. Published through Cochrance Updates on Disk. Update Software, Oxford. Disk issue 2.

Neilson, J. P. (1995*c*). Antepartum cardiotocography. In: Pregnancy and Childbirth Module (ed. M. J. N. C. Keirse, M. J. Renfrew, J. P. Neilson, and C. A. Crowther). Cochrane Database of Systematic Reviews. Published through Cocharane Updates on Disk. Update Software, Oxford. Disk issue 2.

Neilson, J. P. (1997*a*). Routine ultrasound in early pregnancy. In: Pregnancy and Childbirth Module of the Cochrane Database of Systematic Reviews [updated 1 Sept. 1997] (ed. J. P. Neilson, C. A. Crowther, E. D. Hodnett, and G. J. Hofmeyr). Available in the Cochrane Library. The Cochrane Collaboration. Issue 4. Update Software, Oxford. Updated quarterly.

Neilson, J. P. (1997*b*). Assessment of fetal nuchal translucency test for Down's syndrome. *Lancet*, **350**, 754–5.

Neilson, J. P., Alfirevic, Z., and Gosden, C. (1995). Genetic amniocentesis at 16 weeks' gestation. In: Pregnancy and Childbirth Module (ed. M. J. N. C. Keirse, M. J. Renfrew, J. P. Neilson, and C. A. Crowther). Cochrane Database of Systematic Reviews. Published through Cocharane Updates on Disk. Update Software, Oxford. Disk issue 2.

Neilson, J. P. and Alfirevic, Z. (1997). Doppler ultrasound in high-risk pregnancies. In: Pregnancy and Childbirth Module of the Cochrane Database of Systematic Reviews [updated 1 Sept. 1997] (ed. J. P. Neilson, C. A. Crowther, E. D. Hodnett, and G. J. Hofmeyr). Available in the Cochrane Library. The Cochrane Collaboration. Issue 4. Update Software, Oxford. Updated quarterly.

Nicolaides, K. H., Sebire, N. J., Snijders, R. J. M., and Johnson, S. (1996). Down's syndrome screening in the UK. *Lancet*, **347**, 906–7.

Peto, R. (1987). Why do we need systematic overviews of randomized trials? *Statistics in Medicine*, 6, 233–40.

Prendiville, W. J., Elbourne, D., and McDonald, S. (1997). Active versus expectant management of the third stage of labour. In: Pregnancy and Childbirth Module of the Cochrane Database of Systematic Reviews [updated 1 Sept. 1997] (ed. J. P. Neilson, C. A. Crowther, E. D. Hodnett, and G. J. Hofmeyr). Available in the Cochrane Library. The Cochrane Collaboration. Issue 4. Update Software, Oxford. Updated quarterly.

Proud, J. and Grant, A. (1987). Third trimester placental grading by ultrasonography as a test of fetal well-being. *British Medical Journal*, **294**, 1641–7.

Renfrew, M. J. (1995). Routine perineal shaving on admission in labour. In: Pregnancy and Childbirth Module (ed. M. J. N. C. Keirse, M. J. Renfrew, J. P. Neilson, and C. A. Crowther). Cochrane Database of Systematic Reviews. Published through Cocharane Updates on Disk. Update Software, Oxford. Disk issue 2.

Saari-Kemppainen, A., Karjalainen, O., Ylostalo, P., and Heinonen, O. P. (1990). Ultrasound screning and perinatal mortality: controlled trial of systematic one-stage screening in pregnancy. *Lancet*, 336, 387–91.

Shirley, I. M., Bottomly, F., and Robinson, V. P. (1992). Routine radiographer screening for fetal abnormalities in an unselected low-risk population. *British Journal of Radiology*, **65**, 564–7.

Thacker, S. B., Stroup, D. F., and Peterson, H. B. (1997). Continuous electronic fetal heart rate monitoring during labour. In: Pregnancy and Childbirth Module of the Cochrane Database of Systematic Reviews [updated 1 Sept. 1997] (ed. J. P. Neilson, C. A. Crowther, E. D. Hodnett, and G. J. Hofmeyr). Available in the Cochrane Library. The Cochrane Collaboration. Issue 4. Update Software, Oxford. Updated quarterly.

Westgate, J., Harris, M., Curnow, J. S. H., and Greene, K. R. (1993). Plymouth randomized trial of cardiotocogram only vs ST waveform plus cardiotocogram for intrapartum monitoring in 2400 cases. *American Journal of Obstetrics and Gynecology*, **169**, 1151–60.

Wheble, A. M., Gilmer, M. D. G., Spencer, J. A. D., and Sykes, G. S. (1989). Changes in fetal monitoring practice in the UK: 1977–1984. *British Journal of Obstetrics and Gynaecology*, **96**, 1140–7.

Willocks, J. (1993). Ian Donald and the birth of obstetric ultrasound. In: *Obstetric ultrasound* (ed. J. P. Neilson and S. Chambers), pp.1–18. Oxford University Press, Oxford.

CHAPTER FOURTEEN

Born too soon or too small or both

Sheila MacPhail, Stephen Walkinshaw, and
Stuart Walton

Born too soon

One in every 200 births occurs at less than 28 weeks' gestation, and three in 200 at less than 32 weeks' gestation. Over 11 000 babies are therefore born before 32 weeks in the UK, with 3750 of these before 28 weeks. Almost a half of all deaths occurring in liveborn infants in the first month of life in England, Wales, and Northern Ireland are the consequence of premature birth and, in 1994, over 1500 babies died because they were born too soon. Survival is highly dependent on actual gestation, but at least one third of infants born at 24 weeks' gestation would be expected to survive (Rennie 1996). By a gestation of 28 weeks, expectations are of 95% survival (Hagan *et al.* 1996). Survival prospects change rapidly over time, and many published figures examine cohorts of infants from the 1980s. Liverpool data have shown a consistent improvement in survival throughout the 1980s . Northern regional data demonstrate substantial differences in survival at all gestations above 24 weeks between 1983–1986 and 1991–1994 (Tin *et al.* 1997). Even these data may be an underestimate of survival as antenatal steroids were not widely utilized in that region during that time period. Developments in coordinated perinatal care, active use of steroids, and artificial surfactant are likely to produce even better results.

By definition, 3% or 5% of all infants are born less than the third or fifth centiles for gestation. Between 23 000 and 38 000 infants are therefore born classified as small for gestation. Around two thirds of stillbirths have no specific cause, and approximately one quarter of these, from regional series, are a consequence of growth restriction. There is a widespread belief that many more so-called unexplained stillbirths are a consequence of growth failure – the 'growth-restricted appropriate for gestation' fetus. Mortality may be related to the degree of smallness . Swedish and American studies have demonstrated a two to fourfold increase in risk of perinatal death in growth-restricted infants (Wennergren *et al.* 1988; Piper *et al.* 1996). In 1994 in the UK, nearly 600 fetuses died before birth because they grew poorly.

Although the deaths from being born too soon are of serious concern, they actually hide a much larger problem – that of long-term handicap and underachievement.

Many survivors of neonatal intensive care are handicapped in some way. Around 7–8% will have cerebral palsy. A small percentage will be visually handicapped, and a slightly higher proportion will have hearing problems. Long-term intellectual impairment will occur in around 5–10% of survivors, and is heavily gestation dependent. Many will have respiratory problems over the first year, although it appears that long-term lung function is near normal. Only 23% of women having a baby at 24 weeks and 29% of those having a baby at 26 weeks will go home with a child free from some form of moderate to severe handicap (Rennie 1996). By 30–32 weeks this has increased to almost 95%. Intriguingly, although changes in mortality have been documented over time, the proportion of severe handicap does not appear to have followed the same trend (Tin *et al.* 1997). Issues are compounded by the fact that many preterm infants are growth restricted, with almost 20% of infants admitted to Liverpool Women's Hospital Regional Neonatal Intensive Care Unit prior to 32 weeks, being less than the fifth centile for gestation.

Defining the morbidity due to impaired fetal growth is more difficult. Numerous studies have tried to evaluate the relationship between growth and long-term intellectual outcome. The data remain conflicting. Some studies demonstrate differences in school performance and development (Ounsted *et al.* 1984; Rantakillo 1985), while others do not find differences in long-term outcome. Recent information on term growth-restricted infants from black American low-income groups have demonstrated a reduction in IQ scores and an increase in mental retardation even after correction for home environment (Goldenberg *et al.* 1996). All data are confounded by the poor definitions of growth restriction used in most studies.

Even more recently, matters have been complicated further by an understanding that the indication for preterm birth may itself influence outcome. Thus, for a given gestation, infants born under different circumstances may have markedly different expectations for both survival and handicap. Preterm rupture of the membranes and antepartum haemorrhage, in particular, may impart poorer outcome. All of these factors make it difficult to give individual parents hard data on the chances for their child.

Other information has highlighted that the consequences of being born small may last into middle age and impart serious risk of disease and early death (Barker and Clark 1997; Chapter 15).

The magnitude of the task in reducing the consequences of being born too soon which faces those caring for women during their pregnancies is formidable. The remainder of this section will concentrate on how we can identify women at risk and how we might prevent or minimize the harm of these complications.

Predicting from past history

In order to determine strategies for the prevention of preterm birth, two important factors must be possible. Either we must be able to identify women at risk of this complication from clinical findings, or there must be a universal screening test of sufficient accuracy.

Preterm birth is heterogeneous, consisting of births after spontaneous preterm labour, births after complex preterm labour such as those precipitated by placental abruption, and elective preterm births for major pregnancy complications such as growth restriction. There are likely to be differences in outcomes depending on why the preterm birth took place, and there is preliminary evidence that this is true of cerebral palsy following preterm delivery.

Classically, poverty and disadvantage are the main determinants of preterm birth. However, it is likely that the relative importance of individual factors may vary depending on the precise mechanism of preterm birth. Important distinctions particularly are becoming evident between spontaneous preterm birth after labour and as a consequence of preterm premature rupture of the membranes (preterm PROM). This is particularly true of smoking and second-trimester bleeding, which are more powerful risk factors for preterm PROM (Hargar *et al.* 1990). Table 14.1 lists, with relative risks where available, the demographic variables of women at risk of spontaneous preterm birth.

Teasing apart the various factors can be difficult given the interdependence of many. It would be difficult to base a strategy for prevention on identification of these factors, but they might serve as a first step in identifying those who might benefit from other types of screening. Women

Table 14.1 *Factors associated with spontaneous preterm birth*

Factors	Odds ratio (where available)
Social class	1.7–2.3
Unemployed	2.0–2.6
Primiparity	
Ethnicity	2.2
Age under 20 years	
Marital status	1.7
Cigarette smoking	1.1–1.65
Opiate abuse	3.0
Cocaine abuse	2.4
Heavy/stressful work	
Psychological stress	
Assisted conception (singletons)	3.0
Congenital uterine abnormality	3.1

should be made aware of these risk factors, preferably before pregnancy. Especially for primigravida there should be more detailed discussion about signs and symptoms of labour prior to 28 weeks. There is evidence from US studies that early presentation may improve outcome . It would be common sense to deduce that early contact with health professionals, even if not preventing delivery, would allow time for effective interventions to improve neonatal survival. For most women, discussion about labour does not occur until parent education classes begin in the third trimester: this is patently too late. Given the importance of preterm birth, a radical rethink of this approach is long overdue.

Assisted conception may impart increased risk in singleton pregnancies, independent of age and parity. This risk is across gestations and appears to be about threefold (Lumley 1993). This has been attributed to stress, infection (a cause of infertility), cervical problems (as these women have often undergone numerous gynaecological procedures), or problems with implantation.

The role of stressful lifestyle and events remains one of the controversial areas in the genesis of preterm labour. Past reproductive performance plays the most crucial role in predicting a further preterm birth (Lumley 1993) (Table 14.2). As important is the striking relationship between the gestation of the first preterm birth and the likelihood of delivering at that gestation subsequently. Thus, women who deliver before 27 weeks are 20 times more likely to do the same again, and thus have an 8% chance of delivering before 27 weeks and a 12% chance of delivering between 28 and 35 weeks (Hoffman and Bakketeig 1984).

Predicting from current pregnancy complications

Many events which develop during pregnancy increase the risk of spontaneous preterm birth (Lumley 1993). The most obvious of these is multiple pregnancy. These make up one in six of births before 28 weeks and one in five of those between 28 and 31 weeks.

Table 14.3 lists those factors linked with spontaneous preterm labour and delivery.

Table 14.2 *Relative risk of subsequent preterm birth*

Three previous first-trimester losses	1.1
One previous first-trimester loss	1.7
Two previous first-trimester losses	2.9
Three previous first-trimester losses	5.9
One previous preterm birth	2.2
Two previous preterm births	3.7
Three previous preterm births	4.9

Source: Lumley (1993).

Table 14.3 *Factors arising during pregnancy predisposing to preterm birth*

Factors	Odds ratio (where available)
Urinary tract infection	
Asymptomatic bacteriuria	
Appendicitis	2.8
Hyperemesis	4.1
Retained IUCD	
Anaemia (< 7.0 g/dl)	4.2
Abruptio placentae	8.0
First or second-trimester bleeding	2.1
Polyhydramnios	2.6

Source: Lumley (1993).

Role of infection

It is now widely accepted that the major aetiological factor in spontaneous preterm labour is local infection (Walkinshaw 1995). Evidence of association has accrued from studies of the placenta (Hillier *et al.* 1988), from amniotic fluid (Romero *et al.* 1988), and from numerous studies of vaginal and cervical microbiology (McDonald *et al.* 1991; Kurki *et al.* 1992). The range of bacterial organisms implicated is vast and there may be regional variations. There are differences between the organisms implicated in labour with intact membranes and in preterm PROM (McDonald *et al.* 1991). There may be gestation-dependent differences in the rates of infection, with increased rates of bacterial isolation in the extremely preterm cases.

The mechanism by which these organisms initiate preterm labour or rupture of the membranes is complex, with enzymatic digestion and direct and indirect stimulation of cytokine and prostaglandin pathways being the key elements.

At a practical level, prospective studies have begun to quantify the risk of preterm delivery in low-risk populations and work is in progress on the practicalities of how women could be screened (Hay *et al.* 1994). The commonest findings are of bacterial vaginosis, bacteriodes, and of a mixed group of gram-negative pathogens. Bacterial vaginosis is a common condition. It is also relatively simple to diagnose, both clinically and in the laboratory. Until more information is available, it would seem prudent to advise and screen women with a past history of this condition.

Prediction of preterm labour

Understanding the aetiology of a condition is not the same as the capacity to screen or predict the development of the condition. A number of strategies have been developed to try to select out a group at high risk.

Risk scoring

Given the numerous demographic variables, it would seem reasonable to attempt to combine these in a clinical risk score. However, in practice these have proven very disappointing (McLean *et al.* 1993). They have failed to identify most women (sensitivity 40%), and have falsely labelled many women with normal pregnancies as at risk (false positive rate of 80%). As such they may expose large numbers of women and fetuses to potentially hazardous interventions.

Cervical assessment

Two approaches need to be considered. First, do changes in the cervix predict delivery in women already identified as high risk? Advances in ultrasound equipment allow accurate determination of cervical length by transabdominal and particularly transvaginal ultrasound. Single measurements between 20 and 24 weeks is the most pragmatic approach, and there is increasing evidence that a length less than 25 mm at this time increases the risk of subsequent preterm delivery by a factor of four (Berghella *et al.* 1997). A similar approach may be useful in multiple pregnancy, although the cervical length measure with most sensitivity may be 35 mm.

More difficult to determine is whether universal screening would be effective. In work from France, where there have been attempts to educate the public about preterm labour and birth, a short cervix doubled the risk in normal primigravidae (Papiernik 1993). Others have shown very little value in this approach, although most studies are of relatively small number. Recent large studies have suggested that routine cervical length screening, especially using transvaginal scanning, may usefully identify women at risk (Iams *et al.* 1996).

Home uterine activity monitoring

It is now possible to monitor uterine activity at remote locations using sophisticated telemonitoring. This approach has been used to monitor high-risk pregnancies. Women attach the monitor for a fixed period each day, the results being fed down a telephone link. Increase in uterine activity using this technique can be demonstrated in the 24 to 48 hours prior to delivery . Sensitivities of up to 80% have been shown for preterm delivery (Main *et al.* 1988). Although predictive, the lack of an effective tocolytic reduces the value of the information.

Microbiological screening

With the known link with genital infection, screening for the relevant organisms in all women is an attractive approach. Such testing would need to be quite sophisticated since the range of organisms is wide. Large studies seem capable of quantifying risk (McDonald *et al.* 1991). Screening for bacterial vaginosis alone would be feasible, and as there is effective treatment this is an attractive possibility. It remains to be demonstrated whether treatment of low-risk women will reduce the preterm birth rate. It is also unclear how women would feel about such a relatively invasive approach and the resource implications are considerable.

In women at very high risk, for example by previous obstetric history, there is likely to be microbiological and histological information from the previous pregnancy. In these circumstances, screening may be indicated and be helpful.

Biochemical screening (fetal fibronectin)

Until recently, the search for a biochemical marker of preterm labour has been fruitless. The discovery of fetal fibronectin has radically altered our views on this approach.

Fetal fibronectin is a specific protein of this family which is found only in the extracellular matrix of the decidua basalis. It should not be present in cervical secretions unless there is some disruption of this layer. This occurs in late pregnancy in a proportion of women (Blanch *et al.* 1996). There is now little argument about its predictive value in high-risk women, although less than the original studies of Lockwood and colleagues (Lockwood *et al.* 1991). The advantage of this test is that it may predate delivery by several weeks, allowing time for intervention. It is a simple bedside testing kit, not unlike a pregnancy testing kit, and could be carried out in any location.

As further data have accumulated, many hospital departments now incorporate testing at 24–28 weeks as part of the investigation of women at risk of very preterm delivery (Leeson *et al.* 1996). Its other role may be in the delivery suite where it may prove a good discriminator in women admitted with uterine activity, perhaps allowing clinicians to withhold tocolysis.

As a screening test in low-risk women it has a lower predictive value, but its simplicity and the possibility of screening in the community make it the current front runner. There are close links between fetal fibronectin testing and bacterial vaginosis, suggesting possible therapeutic options such as prophylactic antibiotics.

Prevention of preterm birth

Although the development of screening tools may be progressing, such advances need to be accompanied by methods by which we could actually prevent premature labour or rupture of the membranes. There is less hope in this area.

Education programmes

One hypothesis is that if women, both low and high risk, were more aware of the problems of prematurity and the symptoms of preterm labour, then preterm birth could be reduced. This might occur via avoidance of risk factors such as smoking, stress, or heavy work, or via earlier presentation resulting in more effective use of tocolysis to prevent birth. Observational population studies have shown a reduction in preterm birth over time (Papiernik *et al.* 1985). However, randomized trials of such interventions have not shown any benefit from this approach (Collaborative Group on Preterm Birth Prevention 1993).

It remains to be studied if early identification followed by delay in delivery of 48–72 hours with use of steroids, or other treatments aimed at improving outcome, would reduce morbidity and mortality from preterm birth.

Home uterine monitoring

Following the excellent predictive value of this type of home monitoring, a number of trials have been performed. There does seem to be an effect, with perhaps a reduction by one third in preterm births being observed. Recent large trials have confirmed this effect (Colton *et al.* 1995). Such a technique has not yet found favour in the UK.

Cervical cerclage

In a small group of very high-risk women, namely those having three or more previous preterm deliveries, cervical cerclage does have value in prevention (MRC/RCOG Working Party on Cervical Cerclage 1993).

Pharmacological intervention

Beta-mimetic and other uterine suppressive drugs used orally in the prevention of preterm labour have not yet demonstrated benefit. Antibiotics for asymptomatic bacteriuria is of proven benefit, reducing the odds of preterm birth by one third.

The value of antibiotic use where there is preterm PROM is still debated. There does seem evidence that it delays delivery, but as yet no evidence that it prevents morbidity or mortality. It is too early to tell if the use of antibiotics against genital infection earlier in pregnancy will prevent preterm birth, although early studies are promising. There are several ongoing studies and at present this seems the most likely approach to have real impact.

One other simple measure also has potential merit. In many parts of the world, magnesium is used as an acute tocolytic drug. There are several trials examining whether oral supplementation with magnesium reduces the incidence of preterm birth (Sibai *et al.* 1989). Although not based on very large numbers, a reduction in preterm labour has been shown. This simple and risk-free approach demands larger definitive studies.

Prevention of poor outcome

As prediction and prevention seem some way off, there has been more concentration on prenatal therapies which might improve neonatal outcome (Table 14.4).

Short-term delay of delivery

For any of such therapies to be effective some short-term delay must be achieved. This is the current aim of tocolytic therapy. There is no ideal drug. All have side-effects on either the mother , the fetus, or both. Both ritodrine hydrochloride and indomethacin, the drugs commonly in use in the UK,

Table 14.4 *Interventions which may improve outcome*

Intervention	Result
Tocolysis	Short-term delay in delivery
Antibiotics	Short-term gain in preterm PROM
Antenatal steroids	Reduction in death and serious morbidity
Antenatal TRH	No proven benefit
Antenatal phenobarbitone	Possible benefit in extreme preterm

appear to buy a short period of time, usually 48 hours (Zuckerman *et al.* 1984; King *et al.* 1988). The use of ritodrine is limited by its maternal side-effects, whereas indomethacin is limited by its possible fetal side-effects . Other drugs, such as calcium channel blockers or newer oxytocin antagonists, have yet to demonstrate advantages over conventional treatment. Nitric oxide donors, such as the trinitrates, are at an experimental stage. *In vitro* work is not encouraging, and clinical trials are still ongoing.

Antibiotics, especially for preterm PROM, may also buy time (Crowley 1993*a*), but their precise value is still in question and the subject of the large ORACLE trial.

Antenatal corticosteroids

There is now no argument that widespread use of corticosteroids in the days before preterm birth imparts tremendous advantage to the infant. There are reductions in death, hyaline membrane disease, ventricular haemorrhage, and necrotizing enterocolitis (Crowley *et al.* 1990). There appear no disadvantages either to the mother or to the infant on long-term follow-up. Doses equivalent to 24 mg of beta-methasone need to be given in a 24-hour period. Maximum advantage is obtained if birth occurs 24 hours to one week after completion of treatment. Steroid-use rates of 80% of all preterm deliveries are achievable in well-organized and motivated units. The advantage is maintained where delivery follows preterm PROM (Crowley 1993*b*).

Thyroid-releasing hormone (TRH)

Thyroid hormone is involved in lung maturation, and has been found experimentally to be synergistic with corticosteroids. As thyroid hormone itself does not cross the placenta, clinical trials have utilized TRH, which does. Results have been conflicting, with some trials conferring benefit and others showing no benefit. Overview of the results currently does not favour treatment and the recent MRC trial was abandoned following the most recent overview.

Antenatal phenobarbitone

Phenobarbitone reduces the peaks of blood pressure in very preterm infants which are thought to contribute to periventricular bleeding and subsequent cerebral damage. Because of the timing of action, attempts have been made to prepare newborn infants by maternal administration of phenobarbitone to prevent intracranial bleeding. Early studies were very encouraging, but recent large studies have shown little benefit (Thorpe *et al.* 1994; Shankaran *et al.* 1996). The issue still needs to be resolved, especially in the extremely preterm at highest risk.

The birth

Where birth is inevitable, it is important that it takes place in circumstances geared to achieve the best outcome. Experienced midwifery support is essential to reassure and guide through a highly stressful event.

Good analgesia should be available if required but opiates should be avoided if possible as they may complicate the neonatal resuscitation.

Electronic fetal monitoring is not essential, there being no evidence in this group as in the general population that it is of value. If it is to be utilized then there must be clinical staff with experience of interpreting the preterm cardiotocograph, as there are many pitfalls for the inexperienced or unwary.

Where labour is spontaneous, there are no data to support the use of Caesarean section in either the preterm cephalic or breech presentation. Where the indication for preterm birth is more complex, there is often justifiable recourse to abdominal delivery.

The parents

Throughout the process of considering preterm birth, parents must be given all available information. They must have ample opportunity to ask questions and a chance to meet staff.

Information must be honest, even if distressing. Unrealistic expectations should not be fostered. Between obstetrician, paediatrician, midwife, and parents there should be a clear view about the fetus, its expectations, and the indications for intervention. This should include, if required, instructions on when not to intervene.

Follow-up, both within the hospital service and in the community, is vital. Parents need an opportunity to go through issues with senior staff both at the time and at a later date. They need to be able to question and to plan for the future. They will need reassurances that it 'was not their fault'.

Summary

Birth of infants 'too soon' remains one of the great health challenges. There is a gradually improving understanding of the aetiology of spontaneous preterm labour. Over the last few years the emphasis has therefore shifted from therapy to contain premature labour to strategies to prevent preterm birth. Although these remain crude, they begin to hold out promise of actually reducing the numbers of infants at risk. This has been coupled with better use of known effective therapies in both obstetric and neonatal care which reduce the risk of death and major handicap.

Most of the strategies will need to be community based, and some will be complex . A wide range of health care professionals will need to coordinate their roles if these approaches are to come to fruition.

Born too small

The size we are at birth clearly influences not only our immediate chances of survival but may also modify our life expectancy (Barker 1992; Barker and Fall 1993; Barker et al. 1993; Barker 1995). It is only relatively recently that newborn infants have been weighed, and some early reports of birthweight were often wildly inaccurate such that William Smellie in 1752 was reported to consider a normal newborn to weigh between 10 and 16 lbs. The adult consequences of being born too small are addressed in Chapter 15 and are a testament to the accurate records which have been maintained over a generation. It is our purpose to focus on the detection, diagnosis, and management of the small baby in the peri-partum period.

It is disappointing that, despite careful antenatal care with attention directed specifically to the identification of fetal growth problems, we continue to fail to identify the majority of small-for-gestational-age infants. Clinical suspicion of small-for-gestational-age fetuses identifies only around 10% of such cases. Babies with a birthweight less than 2.5 kg are responsible for 30% of total perinatal loss and, although most are preterm, about 20% are considered to be small for dates.

How small is too small?

The term 'small for gestational age' (SGA) is generally given to babies born with a birthweight less than the 10th centile, but growth failure can not be defined by a population-based weight centile as fetal weight is dependent upon constitutional as well as pathological factors. However, fetal size and fetal growth are often confused in clinical practice. It is not unusual to see birthweight for gestation charts described as fetal growth charts and a weight for gestation below some arbitrary centile described as intrauterine growth retardation (IUGR). It is important to realize that the terms SGA and IUGR are not synonymous. Growth can not be estimated without two or more measurements of size and it is not clinically useful to compare size in late pregnancy with measurements obtained at the routine anomaly scan. It is important to limit the term IUGR to those fetuses with evidence of growth restriction but to remember that most infants with IUGR will be small for gestational age. The infant who falls from the 90th to the 30th centile in a short period of time may be at greater risk than a small baby who is growing steadily along the fifth centile. The importance of the distinction between smallness and growth restriction continues into the postnatal period as there is conclusive evidence that perinatal morbidity is increased in the group who are small with additional evidence of growth restriction (Patterson and Pouliot 1987; Vilar et al. 1990; Fay et al. 1991).

Determinants of birth weight

The weight at birth reflects the intrinsic weight potential of the individual and the extent to which it has been achieved. This in turn is determined by a combination of fetal and parental factors, although maternal characteristics are predominant and are reflected in animal hybrid models where foals from Shetland mares are lighter than foals from Shire mares (Walton and Hammond 1938). Determinants of human fetal growth include both physiological and environmental factors. Some factors, such as gestational age, fetal sex, fetal abnormality, multiple pregnancy, maternal height and weight, weight gain during pregnancy, bleeding in pregnancy, hypertension, diabetes, ethnic group, and parity, may highlight an at-risk pregnancy but not be directly amenable to professional modification. Some environmental factors, such as smoking, may be altered by appropriate professional advice.

Accurate assessment of gestational age is vital to interpretation of weight at delivery. Determining the date of delivery by early ultrasound scan is clearly better than menstrual dates when these are uncertain or unknown, and there is evidence that measurements obtained before 25 weeks' gestation may even be better than accurate menstrual dates (Geirsson 1991). While it is known that ethnic group may be associated with birthweight there is evidence that second-generation Asian women who are born in the UK may give birth to babies who are significantly heavier than first-generation women who were themselves born in the Indian subcontinent (Dhawan 1995).

Screening tests for the SGA infant

Abdominal palpation is the oldest method of estimating fetal size but appears to be of little diagnostic benefit. Twenty per cent of such assessments just before birth are not within 450 g of the actual birthweight, and the errors are greatest at the extremes of the range which is just where the greatest precision is required. Direct measurement of the maternal abdomen should provide more reproducible information and attempts have been made to measure either symphysis fundal height (SFH) or maternal abdominal girth at the level of the umbilicus. Several studies have looked at symphysis fundal height but have shown sensitivities varying from 27–86% in detecting birthweight less then the 10th centile (Bailey and Grant 1995). As a single measurement at 32–34 weeks, SFH can have a sensitivity of 69–85% and a specificity of approaching 96%. If SFH is taken serially by the same observer, an indication of growth rather than size can be objectively obtained. However, it may be that more appropriate use of SFH measurement will be encouraged with the development of customized growth charts (see later) and the identification of the fetus which is not reaching its growth potential. Fetal activity may be reduced in the compromised fetus and it was hoped that maternal perception of fetal movement might help identify the fetus at risk of dying *in utero*. However, prospective randomized studies have shown no evidence that routine fetal movement counting reduces the incidence of fetal death in late pregnancy.

Antenatal risk factors have not proved helpful for the identification of the SGA infant (Galbraith *et al.* 1979; Wennergren *et al.* 1982) and it would appear that ultrasound involving either morphometric measurements or Doppler assessment of blood velocity is the most sensitive method. There was considerable interest in the potential ability of Doppler ultrasound to characterize the uteroplacental circulation at an early point in gestation and identify women at risk of hypertension or growth restriction. However, although initial work was encouraging (Bewley *et al.* 1991; Campbell *et al.* 1991), the positive predictive value was low (25%) and in subsequent screening studies the sensitivities were improved but the false positive rate was unacceptably high (Bower *et al.* 1993). This has implications for the provision of resources in the subsequent monitoring of such women and highlights the lack of any effective intervention in modifying the outcome. Randomization of a general population of women into antenatal care schedules with or without routine Doppler assessment failed to show any improvement in neonatal outcome in the Doppler group (Davies *et al.* 1992; Newnham *et al.* 1993). Thus screening of general populations with Doppler has not been demonstrated to be of value.

Customized growth charts

In order to address the problems of poor identification of the at-risk fetus, considerable attention has been directed to the development of customized fetal growth charts in the hope that more of the at-risk population would be identified (Leeson and Aziz 1997). These charts are designed to have gestational age on the x-axis and can have both ultrasound estimated fetal weight and symphysis fundal height on opposing y-axes. This allows clinical screening for growth retardation with measurement of symphysis fundal height by all involved in antenatal care. The values, ideally obtained by a single observer throughout an individual pregnancy, can be plotted on a customized chart carried in the woman's records. Deviation from the expected growth would result in direct referral for ultrasound assessment of fetal size. Large multicentre prospective studies are required to determine if this approach will identify an appropriate high-risk group without an excessive number of false positives and make an important contribution to the identification of fetal malnutrition.

Diagnosis of smallness

A recent review of all published English-language data over a 15-year period (Chang *et al.* 1994) suggested that measurement of fetal abdominal circumference and estimated fetal weight were better at predicting an SGA fetus than other morphometric or Doppler measurements. However, the clinically important distinction is between the fetus who is small but well and the fetus who is small and retarded in growth. In a study of 156 women with SGA fetuses, Chang and colleagues showed that fetal growth failure was better identified with serial assessment of abdominal circumference and estimated weight than with umbilical artery pulsatility index (PI) or the aortic to middle cerebral PI ratio (Chang *et al.* 1993).

There seems little doubt that the combination of serial measurements of SFH and ultrasonically derived abdominal circumference values in those fetuses found to be falling behind their normal growth patterns will result in consistent identification of those babies requiring more intensive monitoring, with sensitivity rates of 93% and a positive predictive value of 85% (Leeson and Aziz 1997).

Doppler

Doppler studies of umbilical artery flow revealed that when absent or reversed end-diastolic flow velocity is demonstrated, this represents a major defect in uteroplacental perfusion and is associated with intrauterine growth restriction, fetal hypoxia, and acidaemia. Detection can therefore lead to action, thus reducing perinatal mortality and morbidity (Alfirevic and Neilson 1995). Using this test as a screening test, however, has little value when applied to a low-risk population other than to increase the number of attendances, subsequent ultrasound examinations, and inevitably the anxiety of the screened mothers (Goffinet *et al.* 1997). There seems little doubt therefore that the benefit of umbilical artery Doppler is in those 'high-risk' pregnancies where the possibility of growth restriction exists. Nevertheless, there is some hope that Doppler flow measurements in early pregnancy may lead to the identification of women at high risk from developing hypoxaemia. Recent studies at St. George's Hospital have , by using a multivariate analysis, shown that differences in uterine and umbilical artery Doppler blood flow indices at 12–16 weeks can be used in selecting those which will develop pre-eclampsia and IUGR (Harrington *et al.* 1997). It must not be forgotten that in a significant proportion (around 25%) of those pregnancies where there are abnormal Doppler patterns, there is a risk of aneuploidy (Kingdom *et al.* 1997).

Antenatal management of the small baby

Once a small baby has been identified antenatally, the challenge for the clinical team is the organization of subsequent monitoring and determining the optimal time of delivery. Most centres would adopt some form of monitoring strategy but the threshold for intervention is highly variable and dependent on many factors, including prior experience, monitoring expertise, and the neonatal facilities available locally. This uncertainty about management was highlighted by the pilot phase of the GRIT study (Growth Restriction Intervention Study) where a group of 'experts' were asked what sort of test results would lead them to recommend immediate delivery or further conservative management. There was a clear area of clinical uncertainty which is the rationale behind the GRIT study.

In developing a strategy for antenatal detection and supervision of this high-risk group, the community team must be included in a collaborative approach with the technical, obstetric, and neonatal services. Common protocols must be agreed, including check-lists of predisposing and compounding factors coupled with adherence to plans of antenatal monitoring. Early gestational assessment by ultrasound will establish accurate dating and serial symphysis fundal height measurements by the same observer (easier to arrange in the community clinic than at hospital) will identify those women who will require extra ultrasonic and Doppler surveillance. The use of customized fetal growth assessment may assist in the identification and monitoring of high-risk women, although whether growth-retarded fetuses as defined by customized charts are at actual risk when compared with those identified on population charts still needs testing by randomized controlled trials.

Once detected , the management of these women can still involve community-based care-givers and, indeed, there may be a case for continuing care in the community provided a strict protocol is adhered to. The institution of weekly Doppler measurements will supplement the intensive clinical attendance and, when compared with antenatal cardiotocography, can provide an earlier warning of impending asphyxia. In addition, it reduces the number of additional hospital antenatal visits, in-patient days of stay, and out-patient episodes without affecting outcome (Haley *et al.* 1997). Intrapartum management remains under the hospital team but the importance of maintaining continuity is important, particularly if serious morbidity and, indeed, mortality results. The community carers are pivotal in the overall antenatal and postnatal and preconceptional care of the individual women.

References

Alfirevic, Z. and Neilson, J. P. (1995). Doppler ultrasonography in high-risk pregnancies: systematic review with meta-analysis. *American Journal of Obstetrics and Gynecology*, 172, 1379–87.

Bailey, S. M. and Grant, J. M. (1995). Clinical detection of the small fetus: requiem for the symphysis-fundal height. In: *The yearbook of the Royal College of Obstetricians and Gynaecologists* (ed. J. Studd), pp.231–8. RCOG Press, London.

Barker, D. J. (1992). Fetal growth and adult disease. *British Journal of Obstetrics and Gynaecology*, **99**, 275–6.

Barker, D. J. (1995). Fetal origins of coronary heart disease [review]. *British Medical Journal*, **311**, 171–4.

Barker, D. J. and Fall, C. H. (1993). Fetal and infant origins of cardiovascular disease [review]. *Archives of Disease in Childhood*, **68**, 797–9.

Barker, D. J., Gluckman, P. D., Godfrey, K. M., Harding, J. E., Owens, J. A., and Robinson, J. S. (1993). Fetal nutrition and cardiovascular disease in adult life [see comments] [review]. *Lancet*, **341**, 938–41.

Barker, D. J. P. and Clark, P. M. (1997). Fetal undernutrition and disease in later life. *Reviews in Reproduction*, **2**, 105–12.

Berghella, V., Tolosa, J., Kuhlman, K., Weiner, S., Bolognese, R., and Wapner, R. (1997). Cervical sonography compared with manual examination as a predictor of preterm delivery. *American Journal of Obstetrics and Gynecology*, **176**, S7.

Bewley, S., Cooper, D., and Campbell, S. (1991). Doppler investigation of uteroplacental blood flow resistance in the second trimester: a screening study for pre-eclampsia and intrauterine growth retardation [see comments]. *British Journal of Obstetrics and Gynaecology*, **98**, 871–9.

Blanch, G., Olah, K. S. J., and Walkinshaw, S. A. (1996). The presence of fetal fibronectin in the cervicovaginal secretions of women at term: its role in the assessment of women before labour induction and in the investigation of the physiological mechanisms of labour. *American Journal of Obstetrics and Gynecology*, **174**, 262–6.

Bower, S., Schuchter, K., and Campbell, S. (1993). Doppler ultrasound screening as part of routine antenatal scanning: prediction of pre-eclampsia and intrauterine growth retardation. *British Journal of Obstetrics and Gynaecology*, **100**, 989–94.

Campbell, S., Vyas, S., and Nicolaides, K. H. (1991). Doppler investigation of the fetal circulation. *Journal of Perinatal Medicine*, **19**, 21–6.

Chang, T. C., Robson, S. C., Spencer, J. A., and Gallivan, S. (1993). Identification of fetal growth retardation: comparison of Doppler waveform indices and serial ultrasound measurements of abdominal circumference and fetal weight. *Obstetrics and Gynecology*, **82**, 230–6.

Chang, T. C., Robson, S. C., Spencer, J. A., and Gallivan, S. (1994). Prediction of perinatal morbidity at term in small fetuses: comparison of fetal growth and Doppler ultrasound. *British Journal of Obstetrics and Gynaecology*, 101, 422–7.

Collaborative Group on Preterm Birth Prevention (1993). Multicenter randomized controlled trial of a preterm birth prevention program. *American Journal of Obstetrics and Gynecology*, **169**, 352–66.

Colton, T., Kayne, H. L., Zhang, Y., and Heeren, T. (1995). A meta-analysis of home uterine activity monitoring *American Journal of Obstetrics and Gynecology*, **172**, 1499–505.

Crowley, P. (1993a) Antibiotics for prelabour preterm rupture of the membranes. In: Pregnancy and Childbirth Module of the Cochrane Database of Systematic Reviews (ed. M. Enkin, M. Keirse, M. Renfrew, and J. Neilson). Update Software, Oxford . Review 04391, issue 2.

Crowley, P. (1993b) Corticosteroids after prelabour preterm rupture of the membranes. In: Pregnancy and Childbirth Module of the Cochrane Database of Systematic Reviews (ed. M. Enkin, M. Keirse, M. Renfrew, and J. Neilson). Update Software, Oxford .Review 04395, issue 2.

Crowley, P., Chalmers, I., and Keirse, M. J. N. C. (1990). The effects of corticosteroid administration before preterm delivery: review of evidence from controlled trials. *British Journal of Obstetrics and Gynaecology*, 97, 11–25.

Davies, J. A., Gallivan, S., and Spencer, J. A. (1992). Randomized controlled trial of Doppler ultrasound screening of placental perfusion during pregnancy. *Lancet*, **340**, 1299–303.

Dhawan, S. (1995). Birthweight of infants of first-generation Asian women in Britain compared with second-generation Asian women [clinical research editorial]. *British Medical Journal,* 311, 86–8.

Fay, R. A., Dey, P. L., Saadie, C. M., Buhl, J. A, and Gebski, V. J. (1991). Ponderal index: a better definition of the 'at-risk' group with intrauterine problems than birthweight for gestational age in term infants. *Australian and New Zealand Journal of Obstetrics and Gynaecology,* 31, 17–19.

Galbraith, R. S., Karchmar, E. J., Piercy, W. N., and Low, J. A. (1979). The clinical prediction of intrauterine growth retardation. *American Journal of Obstetrics and Gynecology,* 133, 281–6.

Geirsson, R. T. (1991). Ultrasound instead of last menstrual period as the basis for gestational age assessment. *Ultrasound in Obstetrics and Gynecology,* 1, 212–19.

Goffinet, F., Paris-Llado, J., Nisand, I., and Breart,G. (1997. Umbilical artery Doppler velocimetry in unselected and low-risk pregnancies: a review of randomized controlled trials. *British Journal of Obstetrics and Gynaecology,* 104, 425–30.

Goldenberg, R. L., DuBard, M. B., Cliver, S. P., *et al.* (1996). Pregnancy outcome and intelligence at age 5 years. *American Journal of Obstetrics and Gynecology,* 175, 1511–15.

Hagan, R., Benninger, H., Chiffings, D., Evans, S., and French, N. (1996). Very preterm birth: a regional study. Part 2: The very preterm infant. British Journal of Obstetrics and Gynaecology, 103, 239–45.

Haley, J., Tuffnell, D. J., and Johnson, N. (1997). *British Journal of Obstetrics and Gynaecology,* 104, 431–5.

Hargar, J. H., Hsing, A., Tuomala, R. E., *et al.* (1990). Risk factors for preterm premature rupture of the fetal membranes : a multicenter case–control study. *American Journal of Obstetrics and Gynecology,* 163, 130–7.

Harrington,K., Carpenter,R. G., Goldfrad,C., and Campbell, S. (1997). Transvaginal Doppler ultrasound of the uteroplacental circulation in the early prediction of pre-eclampsia and intrauterine growth retardation. *British Journal of Obstetrics and Gynaecology,* 104, 682–8.

Hay, P. E., Lamont, R. F., Taylor-Robinson, D., Morgan, D. J., Ison, C., and Pearson, J. (1994). Abnormal bacterial colonization of the genital tract and subsequent preterm delivery and late miscarriage. *British Medical Journal,* 308, 295–8.

Hillier, S. L., Martius, J., Krohn, M., Kiveat, N., Holmes, K. K., and Eschenbach, D. A. (1988). A case–control study of chorioamniotic infection and histologic chorioamnionitis in prematurity. *New England Journal of Medicine,* 319, 972–8.

Hoffman, H. J. and Bakketeig, L. S. (1984). Risk factors associated with the occurrence of preterm birth. *Clinical Obstetrics and Gynaecology,* 27, 539–52.

Iams, J. D., Goldenberg, R. L., Meis, P. J., *et al.* (1996). The length of the cervix and the risk of spontaneous preterm delivery. *New England Journal of Medicine,* 334, 567–72.

King, J. F., Grant, J. M., Keirse, M. J. N. C., and Chalmers, I. (1988). Beta-mimetics in preterm labour: an overview of randomized controlled trials. *British Journal of Obstetrics and Gynaecology,* 95, 211–22.

Kingdom, J. C. P., Rodek,C. H.,and Kaufmann,P. (1997). Umbilical artery Doppler – more harm than good? *British Journal of Obstetrics and Gynaecology,* 104, 393–5.

Kurki, T., Sivonen, A., Renkonen, O., Savia, E., and Ylikorkala, O. (1992). Bacterial vaginosis in early pregnancy and pregnancy outcome. *Obstetrics and Gynecology*, **80**, 173–7.

Leeson, S. and Aziz, N. (1997). Customized fetal growth assessment. *British Journal of Obstetrics and Gynaecology*, **104**, 648–51.

Leeson, S. C., Maresh, M. J., Martindale, E. A., *et al.* (1996). Detection of fetal fibronectin as a predictor of preterm delivery in high-risk asymptomatic pregnancies. *British Journal of Obstetrics and Gynaecology*, **103**, 48–53.

Lockwood, C. J., Senyei, A. E., Dische, M. R., *et al.* (1991). Fetal fibronectin in cervical and vaginal secretions as a predictor of preterm delivery. *New England Journal of Medicine*, **325**, 669–74.

Lumley, J. (1993). The epidemiology of prematurity. *Balliere's Clinical Obstetrics and Gynaecology*, **7**, 477–98.

McDonald, H. M., O'Loughlin, J. A., Jolley, P., Vigneswaran, R., and McDonald, P. J. (1991). Vaginal infection and preterm labour. *British Journal of Obstetrics and Gynaecology*, **98**, 427–35.

McLean, M., Walters, W. A., and Smith, R. (1993). Prediction and early diagnosis of preterm labour : a critical review. *Obstetrics and Gynecological Survey*, **48**, 209–25.

Main, D. M., Katz, M., Chiu, G., *et al.* (1988). Intermittent weekly contraction monitoring to predict preterm labour in low-risk women : a blinded study. *Obstetrics and Gynecology*, **72**, 757–61.

MRC/RCOG Working Party on Cervical Cerclage (1993). Final report of the MRC/RCOG multicentre randomized trial of cervical cerclage. *British Journal of Obstetrics and Gynaecology*, **100**, 516–23.

Newnham, J. P., Evans, S. F., Michael, C. A., Stanley, F. J., and Landau, L. I. (1993). Effects of frequent ultrasound during pregnancy: a randomized controlled trial. *Lancet*, **342**, 887–91.

Ounsted, M. K., Moar, V. A., and Scott, A. (1984). Children of deviant birthweight at the age of seven years: health, handicap, size, and developmental status. *Early Human Development*, **9**, 323–40.

Papiernik, E. (1993). Prevention of preterm labour and delivery. *Balliere's Clinical Obstetrics and Gynaecology*, **7**, 499–522.

Papiernik, E., Bouyer, J., Dreyfus, J., *et al.* (1985). Prevention of preterm birth : a perinatal study in Haguenau, France. *Paediatrics*, **76**, 154–8.

Patterson, R. M. and Pouliot, R. N. (1987). Neonatal morphometrics and perinatal outcome: who is growth retarded? *American Journal of Obstetrics and Gynecology*, **157**, 691–3.

Piper, J. M., Xenakis, E. M., McFarland, M., Elliot, B. D., Berkus, M. D., and Langer, O. (1996). Do growth-retarded preterm infants have different rates of perinatal morbidity and mortality than appropriately grown preterm infants? *Obstetrics and Gynecology*, **87**, 169–75.

Rantakallio, P. (1985). A 14-year follow-up of children with normal and abnormal birthweight for their gestational age. *Acta Paed.Scand.*, **74**, 62–9.

Rennie, J. M. (1996). Perinatal management at the lower margin of viability. *Archives of Diseases in Childhood*, **74**, F214 – F218.

Romero, R., Emamian, M., and Quintero, R. (1988). The value and limitations of the gram stain in the diagnosis of intraamniotic infection. *American Journal of Obstetrics and Gynecology*, **159**, 114–19.

Shankaran, S., Woldt, E., Nelson, J., Bedard, M., and Delaney-Black, V. (1996). Antenatal phenobarbital therapy and neonatal outcome. II: neurodevelopmental outcome at 36 months. *Paediatrics*, 97, 649–52.

Sibai, B. M., Villar, M. A., and Bray, E. (1989). Magnesium supplementation during pregnancy: a double blind randomized controlled trial. *American Journal of Obstetrics and Gynecology*, **161**, 115–19.

Thorpe, J. A., Parriott, J., Ferette-Smith, D., Meyer, B., Cohen, G., and Joynson, J. (1994). Antepartum vitamin K and phenobarbital for preventing intraventricular haemorrhage in the premature newborn: a randomized, double blind, placebo-controlled trial. *Obstetrics and Gynecology*, 83, 70–6.

Tin, W., Wariyar, U., and Hey, E. (1997). Changing prognosis for babies of less than 28 weeks' gestation in the north of England between 1983 and 1994. *British Medical Journal*, **314**, 107–11.

Vilar, J., de Onis, M., Kestler, E., Bolanos, F., Cerezo, R., and Bernedes, H. (1990). The differential neonatal morbidity of the intrauterine growth retardation syndrome. *American Journal of Obstetrics and Gynecology*, **163**, 151–7.

Walkinshaw, S. A. (1995). Preterm labour and delivery of the preterm infant. In: *Turnbull's obstetrics* (ed. G. Chamberlain). Churchill Livingstone, Edinburgh.

Walton, A. and Hammond, J. (1938). The maternal effects on growth and conformation in Shire horse–Shetland pony crosses. *Proceedings of the Royal Society*, 125, 311–25.

Wennergren, M., Karlsson, K., and Olsson, T. (1982). A scoring system for antenatal identification of fetal growth retardation. *British Journal of Obstetrics and Gynaecology*, **89**, 520–4.

Wennergren, M., Wennergren, G., and Vilbergsson, G. (1988). Obstetric characteristics and neonatal performance in a four-year small-for-gestational-age population. Obstetrics and Gynecology, 72, 615–20.

Zuckerman, H., Shalev, E., Gilad, G., and Katzuni, E. (1984). Further study of the inhibition of premature labour by indomethacin. Part 2. Double blind study. *Journal of Perinatal Medicine*, **12**, 25–9.

CHAPTER FIFTEEN

Fetal origins of adult disease

Louise Parker

Life expectancy

Life expectancy has increased dramatically over the last century as a consequence of improved social conditions, better nutrition, and advances in medicine. A baby born in 1900 had a life expectancy of under 50 years whereas a child born in 2000 will be expected to live for over 80 years (Central Statistics Office: Social Trends 1996). This dramatic change is due in part to the fact that infectious diseases are now both preventable and curable and are no longer a major cause of death. In 1921, 15% (70 497) of deaths in England and Wales were from infection (Registrar-General's Statistical Review of England and Wales 1921). By 1971 this figure had dropped to 3300, and the rate continues to fall (Registrar General's Statistical Review of England and Wales 1921, 1971, 1992). Deaths from infection now make up fewer than 0.5% of all deaths in England and Wales.

Premature mortality

Premature adult mortality (deaths < 65 years) has fallen by half since 1950 and is now 190 per 100 000 for women and 280 per 100 000 for men (Central Statistics Office: Social Trends 1996). The major causes of premature adult death are the non-communicable diseases, especially circulatory disease, including cardio- and cerebrovascular, and respiratory disease. For men under the age of 65, the greatest single cause of death is heart disease, although this has fallen by one half in the last two decades to 74 per 100 000 in 1994. In women under 65 years, heart disease is similarly a major cause of death (though at a rate around one third of that in men). Deaths from stroke in men and women also make a major contribution to premature mortality.

The non-communicable diseases

Non-insulin-dependent diabetes (NIDD) and glucose intolerance have increased in recent decades to become a major public health problem in several parts of the world (Fain 1993). The prevalence of NIDD varies substantially between countries with estimates for the UK being around 4% of adults (Lee *et al.* 1993), whilst in some groups it is much higher, for example in Pima Indians in the USA, prevalence is over 50% (Mitchell and Stern 1992). Together, morbid obesity (body mass index $\geqslant 40\%$) and NIDD are two of the most common serious diseases of today. Glucose intolerance, obesity, and especially NIDD are major risk factors for the circulatory diseases, including ischaemic heart disease (IHD) and stroke (Fuller *et al.* 1980; Modan *et al.* 1985).

The circulatory and respiratory diseases and NIDD bring with them a substantial burden of both mortality and morbidity, and whilst they are often treatable they are not curable. The solution must therefore lie in prevention and the first step towards this is the identification of the causes of these diseases. Established risk factors are related to adult lifestyle, in particular diet, smoking, alcohol intake, obesity, and exercise (Kannell and Larson 1993). A general trend to a healthier diet can be observed at a national level, but the changes are small and occur slowly, showing how resistant adults are to changes in behaviour (Gregory *et al.* 1990).

'Lifestyle factors' are not by themselves an adequate explanation, for example for a non-smoking man of average build with a 'healthy' diet who takes regular exercise, ischaemic heart disease is still the major single cause of death; and there are wide and persistent geographical variations in health which are not explained by differences in lifestyle (Gardner *et al.* 1984; Rose 1985). Mortality from all causes is higher in areas of high social deprivation and there are particularly strong gradients in death from circulatory and respiratory disease even when differences in levels of smoking (a major risk factor for both diseases) are taken into account (Townsend *et al.* 1988). Ischaemic heart disease was a disease of affluence but is now, like the other non-communicable diseases, more prevalent in the less advantaged.

Any explanation of the causes of these diseases must account for these complex geographic and demographic trends.

Introduction to the Barker hypothesis

The 'Barker' hypothesis postulates that the non-communicable diseases responsible for premature mortality and morbidity in adults have their origin in fetal and early infant life. Thus an individual's predisposition to develop these diseases when challenged by lifestyle and dietary factors is set – 'programmed' – by the time of birth or shortly afterwards.

Barker's proposal is that fetal undernutrition during pregnancy results in selected and specific perturbations in fetal growth and metabolism which can be recognized at birth by the anthropometric characteristics of the infant, including its weight, ponderal index (birthweight /[length]^3) and 'thinness'. These characteristics are related to the risk of developing high blood pressure, cardiovascular disease, diabetes or stroke as adults. Suboptimal fetal development can then be compounded by poor growth during the first year of life with further consequences for the risk of other chronic diseases – such as of the respiratory system. Thus growth and development *in utero* and during the first year of life are vital in determining the risk of adult disease (Barker 1992, 1994).

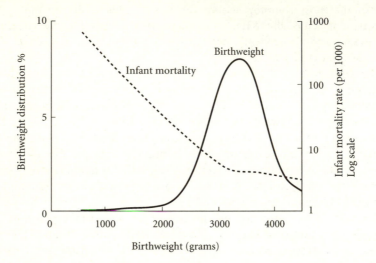

Figure 15.1 *Birthweight and infant mortality in England and Wales (Alberman 1991).*

The evidence for consequences of fetal undernutrition

Birthweight is an important predictor of morbidity and mortality in infants (Alberman 1991). The lowest infant mortality is associated with a birthweight about 1000 grams heavier than the mode (Figure 15.1). An implication of this is that the *majority* of babies experience suboptimal conditions *in utero* and thus fail to realize their full growth potential.

Birthweight, growth during childhood and adult height

That the consequences of lower birthweight reach beyond infancy has been demonstrated in a number of studies. One of the first, The Thousand Families Study, was an investigation of over 900 children born in the city of Newcastle in 1947, which clearly showed that birthweight predicts height throughout life (Figure 15.2) (Spence *et al.* 1954; Miller *et al.* 1960: Miller *et al.* 1974).

The Thousand Families Study data also demonstrate the tendency of physiological parameters to 'track' during life. The lighter babies remain shorter throughout their lives and the heavier babies remain taller and the absolute values of the measurements tend to diverge so that the differences between the top and bottom ranges becomes greater as time passes.

Birthweight and blood pressure

Wadsworth *et al.* (1985) reported an inverse association between birthweight and diastolic blood pressure at age 36 years in 5362 men and women recruited

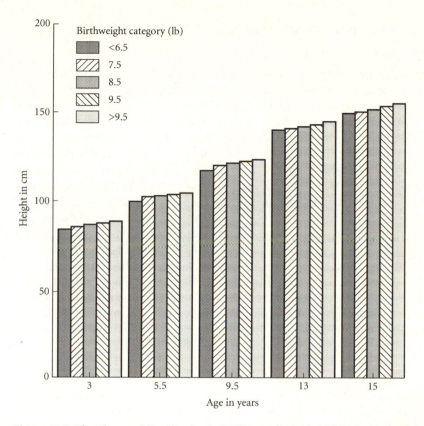

Figure 15.2 *The Thousand Families Study (Miller et al. 1974).* Height by birthweight.

into the National Birth Cohort Study of 1946; that is, the children with the lowest birthweights grew up to be the adults with the highest blood pressures.

This observation has since been repeated by many researchers who have almost universally reported an inverse or more complex relationship between birthweight and blood pressure which is present from childhood (Law *et al.* 1991; Whincup *et al.* 1992; Launer *et al.* 1993). The exceptions have been studies in adolescents though a possible explanation of this is that of the large perturbations in growth velocity at this age (Barker and Law 1994; Davis 1994; Matthes 1994).

Thus birthweight is related to both stature and blood pressure in adult life – characteristics which are known to be risk factors for circulatory disease – implying that birthweight is an important marker of many important aspects of fetal development (Waaler 1984; Barker *et al.* 1990; Kannel and Larson 1993; Frankel *et al.* 1996).

Birth characteristics and adult disease

Geographical studies

Barker's first observations were from 'ecological studies' in which he examined the relationship between past infant mortality and current adult deaths. Barker and Osmond (1986) found that there was significant correlation between mortality rates in adults aged 35–74 years occurring within a local authority district between 1968–1978 and infant mortality in the same place during 1921–1925. One of the difficulties in interpreting the results of this type of study is that areas with the highest levels of social deprivation in the 1920s largely continue to suffer the same relative disadvantage today. Indeed, in an earlier study in Norway, Forsdahl (1977) made a similar observation but interpreted the association between past infant mortality and current adult mortality as reflecting the legacy of lifetime deprivation. In a second study in three towns in Lancashire (Burnley, Nelson, and Colne), Barker and Osmond (1987a) found that the current mortality rates from coronary heart disease reflected the levels of infant mortality in the early years of the century, despite the fact that the towns are now of similar socio-economic status. They concluded that experiences in prenatal and early postnatal life predispose to IHD rather than the risk arising from the experience of continued deprivation throughout life.

In a separate study, Barker and Osmond (1987b) showed similar correlation between deaths from stroke, in particular in adults during 1968–1978, and maternal mortality some 60 years previously and concluded that the health and physique of mothers are important determinants of the adult risk of stroke in their offspring: not only is good nutrition during pregnancy vital to provide the optimal milieu for fetal growth and development but maternal health before pregnancy also plays an essential role.

Evidence on mortality from retrospective cohort studies

Barker et al. (1989) were fortunate in locating a unique set of health visitor records for 17 464 boys born in Hertfordshire from 1911 to 1930. Attempts were made to follow them up through the National Health Service Central Register (NHSCR) which was established during the Second World War to assist with issuing food ration coupons and began as a set of ledgers with a one-line entry for each individual alive in Great Britain at that time. On death, the entry in the NHSCR is 'flagged' with a code which allows the death certificate to be located.

Women who were married by the 1940s were registered under their married name only and so would be difficult to identify from their name at birth. Hence men born before the 1930s are more likely to be successfully traced than women.

NHSCR successfully traced 5654 of the Hertfordshire men and provided the death certificates of the 1186 who had died between 1951 and 1987. The results showed a clear trend for increasing mortality from IHD and chronic obstructive lung disease with decreasing birthweight and decreasing weight at one year in men (Table 15.1).

These results were confirmed in a similar study of mortality rates in 1586 men born in the Jessop Hospital in Sheffield from 1907 to 1923 (Barker *et al.* 1993*b*). For this cohort length was available and it was possible to calculate ponderal index, which is a measure of proportionate growth. Barker found that mortality rate from cardiovascular disease, especially in those aged under 65, was much lower in those who were fat at birth, as shown by a high ponderal index (standardized mortality rate 69), than in those who were thin (standardized mortality rate 118). The conclusions from these studies were that reduced growth in fetal and infant life are associated with increased risk of cardiovascular disease in later life.

Evidence of disease risk factors from follow-up studies

Barker and his colleagues furthered their investigations by examining the relationship between birth characteristics and physiological measurements of disease risk. They studied two groups of men: 825 from the Hertfordshire cohort described above and 142 men born in Preston during 1935–1943 who again had records of birth measurements. A third group of 227 men and women, aged 50–53 years old and for whom detailed birth records were available at the Jessop Hospital in Sheffield, was also identified.

Table 15.1 *Standardized mortality rates according to weight at one year and birthweight*

Weight (lb)	Cause of death		
	Ischaemic heart disease	Chronic obstructive lung disease	All causes
At one year			
⩽ 18	111	129	89
19–20	81	86	89
21–22	98	41	85
23–24	71	61	68
25–26	68	52	73
⩾ 27	42	29	58
At birth			
⩽ 5.5	104	93	101
6–6.5	77	59	69
7–7.5	90	75	83
8–8.5	85	50	80
9–9.5	62	69	70
⩾ 10	81	33	77
Total (n=5654)	82 (n=434)	61 (n=43)	79 (n=1186)

Heart disease

Circulating plasma fibrinogen, factor VII, and cholesterol concentrations are all known to be risk factors for ischaemic heart disease (Kannel and Larsen 1993). In 597 Hertfordshire men, increasing birthweight and increasing weight at one year were both associated with lower levels of fibrinogen and factor VII, and hence a lower risk of IHD (Barker *et al.* 1992*b*). Blood pressure showed a similar trend. In the younger men of the Preston cohort there was no such trend with birthweight for either factor VII or fibrinogen, but simultaneous analysis of birthweight and placental weight showed that fibrinogen levels tended to fall with increasing birthweight (p=0.06) and rise with increasing placental weight (p=0.03).

Serum cholesterol levels were measured in the 227 men and women born in Jessop Hospital, Sheffield (Barker *et al.* 1993*a*). They found that in men who had been thin babies, cholesterol and associated lipids were higher than those who had been fatter at birth. The trend was not as marked for women. Abdominal circumferences at birth reflect the size of the liver and so Barker concluded that thin babies with poor liver development have impaired fat metabolism in adult life.

Lung disease

Barker *et al.* (1991) measured lung function in 825 men from the Hertfordshire cohort. The results showed that, when adjusted for adult height, there was a trend for forced expiratory volume in one second to increase with birthweight. There was no trend with weight at one year, suggesting that impaired growth in infancy does not affect this aspect of lung function.

Hypertension

Barker confirmed the association between birthweight and blood pressure throughout childhood and adult life in several studies. He further demonstrated, in the Preston cohort, that for any birthweight, thin babies had higher adult blood pressure than fat babies (Barker *et al.* 1992*a*). He also showed that for any birthweight, adult blood pressure is higher in those with higher placental weights – a high placenta:birthweight ratio indicating a pregnancy during which the placenta has hypertrophied to compensate for impoverished nutritional supply.

Diabetes and glucose intolerance

Barker and his colleagues successfully performed glucose tolerance tests on 370 men from the 1920s Hertfordshire birth cohort (Hales *et al.* 1991). Of these, 93 were found to have glucose intolerance or previously undiagnosed diabetes. The results showed increasing risk of glucose intolerance and diabetes with decreasing birthweight and decreasing weight at one year, consistent with impaired glucose metabolism associated with suboptimal growth *in utero* and in infancy.

Obesity: abdominal fatness

Obesity is associated with increased risk of cardiovascular disease and diabetes. In addition, the distribution of body fat is in itself a marker of disease risk and accumulation of fat on the abdomen (as measured by the waist:hip ratio) in particular, is associated with high risk of diabetes and heart disease which is reflected in associated high rates of glucose intolerance and plasma fibrinogen and factor VII concentrations.

Waist:hip ratio was measured in 845 of the Hertfordshire men and 252 men from the Preston cohort. Barker found that the waist:hip ratio was inversely correlated with birthweight (after adjustment for body mass index) and that for any birthweight, waist:hip ratio increased with increasing placental weight. Thus the babies who showed by having a lighter birthweight and a heavier placenta that their *in utero* environment had been least optimal, were most likely to store fat abdominally as adults and consequently be at higher risk of the diseases associated with this tendency.

The mechanism of fetal programming

The Dutch hunger winter

The Dutch hunger winter of 1944–45 provided a natural experiment in the effect of severe malnutrition during pregnancy (Stein *et al.* 1975). Following a general rail strike in Holland, the German army retaliated by stopping food transportation into Holland in October 1944. By June 1945, when the war ended, mean daily calorie intake was below 1000 KCals per person. Babies who were exposed to the famine during the second half of gestation were thin at birth and, on average, were 350 grams lighter. They have remained thin as adults, possibly due to a reduction in the total number of fat cells. The birthweight of the babies who were exposed to the famine conditions only during the first half of pregnancy were largely unaffected but as adults they have had a tendency to obesity, possibly due to inappropriate setting of hypothalamic control of appetite. Recent studies have also shown decreased glucose tolerance in adulthood in these babies, especially those exposed during late gestation (Ravelli *et al.* 1998). The next generation of babies, the grandchildren of the women who were pregnant during the hunger winter, were of lower birthweight (Lumley 1992).

These data demonstrate clearly how complex the relationship is between dietary intake, fetal nutrition, and fetal development since even under these extreme circumstances the birthweight of the infants was little affected, though their metabolism was apparently altered irrevocably. Of great importance is the study of the grandchildren, demonstrating how the mother's own fetal growth and development affects her subsequent ability to nurture her infants.

Growth in pregnancy

Barker (1994) postulates that suboptimal nutrition of the fetus during each of the three trimesters of pregnancy results in differential programming of the fetus, which can be observed firstly by differences in the anthropometric indices of the newborn and secondly by adult disease and disease risk factors.

First trimester

During implantation, the embryo is particularly sensitive to low glucose levels to which it responds by growth retardation, which will then 'track' at a low level for the remainder of the pregnancy, infancy, and childhood. The baby will be light and proportionately small and will be a small child who will grow into a short adult. Adult blood pressure will be raised and risk from haemorrhagic stroke will be increased. Clearly, the nutritional requirement of the developing baby during the first few weeks of pregnancy is very low and only in cases of severe malnutrition will maternal stores be inadequate at this early stage of pregnancy.

Second trimester

The placenta and fetus both grow rapidly during the second trimester. During this phase maternal undernutrition results in placental hypertrophy, but only when malnourishment is severe will fetal weight be reduced. The placental weight:fetal weight ratio will be high and the baby will be light and thin at birth, though weight may catch up during infancy to result in a normal weight at one year. The baby born after undernourishment in this phase of pregnancy will, as an adult, tend to have high blood pressure, insulin resistance, and glucose intolerance.

Third trimester

In the third trimester, fetal growth is most rapid and slows immediately if the delivery of nutrients is restricted. The physiological response of the fetus will be to spare brain growth at the expense of trunk. The baby will be normal weight but short, and weight at one year will be reduced as the slower growth trajectory is maintained.

The adult will have higher blood pressure, cholesterol, and fibrinogen, and will be at risk from coronary heart disease and thrombocytic stroke.

Programming disease

Heart disease

Lipid metabolism, especially cholesterol and triglyceride metabolism, are of central importance in heart disease. Thin babies have smaller livers than fat babies and Barker suggests that lipid metabolism is permanently affected as a consequence of poor liver development resulting from undernutrition in the final trimester of pregnancy. The liver also plays an important role in regulating fibrinogen and factor VII, both of which are also risk factors for heart disease and which are also raised in those of lower birthweight and who were thin at birth (Barker *et al.* 1992*b*)

Lung disease

The associations between birthweight and mortality from obstructive lung disease and lung function is interpreted by Barker as evidence that suboptimal conditions during a critical period of rapid lung growth in mid to late pregnancy results in restricted growth of the airways, which is irreversible. Respiratory tract infections in early childhood have also been shown to have long-term effects on lung function but Barker proposes that this effect is of minor significance compared with the dominant effect of impaired lung growth *in utero*.

Hypertension

Folkow suggested that hypertension is the consequence of two processes: an initiating event followed by a chronic process which continues to amplify the elevation of blood pressure (Folkow 1987). This is supported by observations that blood pressures 'track' during life (Andersen and Haraldsottir 1993). Since birthweight but not weight gain in infancy is predictive of blood pressure, the initiating event most probably occurs before birth and is probably a permanent change in the structure of the blood vessel walls, resulting perhaps from hormonal exposures *in utero* (Marty *et al.* 1995). It may also be related to a reduced number of nephrons in the poorly grown kidney (MacKenzie and Brenner 1995). The amplification process may involve progressive changes in the structure and elasticity of the vessel walls (Law *et al.* 1993).

Evidence from Whincup *et al.* (1996), however, suggests that deprivation during childhood may also be important determinants of adult blood pressure.

Diabetes and glucose intolerance

Glucose intolerance and NIDD are more prevalent in adults who were lighter babies, especially in those that were thin. 'Syndrome X' (insulin resistance syndrome), which is characterized by impaired glucose tolerance, hypertension, and hyperlipidaemia, is five times more common in those who had a birthweight < 5.5 lb than in those with a birthweight > 9 lb. Fetal insulin and insulin-like growth factors (IGFs) have a central role in the regulation of fetal growth, and the pancreas grows rapidly during the second trimester of pregnancy and is largely complete within a few months of birth. Hales and Barker (1992) have proposed the 'thrifty phenotype' hypothesis to explain the fetal origins of syndrome X: poor nutrition in fetal and early life limits the development and function of the beta cells of the islets of Langerhans and also induces persistent changes in the production of, and response to, IGFs, especially in muscle, which makes them insulin resistant. Together the insulin resistance and limited number of beta cells, which declines further as a consequence of the normal ageing process, predispose to NIDD. NIDD is thus the outcome of under-nourishment during early life; the inheritance for a nutritionally thrifty fetus is diabetes in the face of a challenge from overnutrition and a sedentary lifestyle which as an adult he or she cannot meet.

Undernutrition in pregnancy

Fetal undernutrition remains ill-defined by Barker and his colleagues but is clearly not determined in any straightforward way by the diet of the mother during her pregnancy. Nutritional status is the net result of the interaction between genetic and environmental influences and nutritional intake. In addition for the fetus, nutrition reflects the complex interplay between the mother, placenta, and fetus.

The efficacy of the maternal–placenta–fetal unit in delivering oxygen and nutrients is a vitally important determinant of fetal growth and development.

Supported by the evidence from the Dutch hunger winter, Hytten and Leitch concluded that within wide limits 'the fetus of a reasonably healthy woman is remarkably unaffected by dietary inadequacy during pregnancy and is difficult to damage by overall restriction of food' (Hytten and Leitch 1971).

Many of the metabolic adjustments of pregnancy occur very early in pregnancy and anticipate the needs of the developing infant. The adjustments are profound, as Hytten reflects: 'The entire maternal metabolism is working from a different base; the mother is almost another species.'

In the normal pregnancy, the overall nutritional balances are positive, i.e. anabolic for both mother and fetus, but understanding of the metabolic adjustments during pregnancy is still far from complete (Hytten et al. 1980).

Lipid metabolism changes radically from the very onset of pregnancy. Circulating triglycerides at term are almost three times that of pre-pregnancy and glycerol, cholesterol, phospholipid, and NEFA levels rise by up to 50%.

Glucose homeostasis changes so that by the end of pregnancy fasting glucose levels are 20% lower and the peak insulin response to an oral glucose tolerance test increases by almost 50%.

Thus, the nutrient delivery to the fetus from the maternal circulation which originates from both dietary intake and maternal stores is achieved by complex metabolic control which no doubt reflects the programming of the mother's homeostatic mechanisms in her fetal and early infant life as well as the influences of her genetic constitution.

The role of the placenta

One per cent of human life is spent *in utero*. During this time, 42 of the 47 cycles of cell division which are estimated to occur between conception and adulthood occur and the fetus achieves around 5% of adult weight. During this time, the placenta acquires and transfers all the substances required for fetal growth and, like the fetus, it continues to grow throughout pregnancy and has substantial functional reserve (Fox 1978). The placenta is not merely a conduit for the transfer of nutrients and oxygen from mother to fetus. It acts alone and together with the fetus and mother, as part of the maternal–feto–placental unit, to fulfill an enormous range of endocrine functions, and in so doing it produces huge quantities of a greater range of hormones than any other endocrine organ. The placenta undoubtedly plays a major role in ensuring adequate nutrition and metabolic control of the fetus.

What can be done?

If the major causes of premature mortality do indeed have their roots in the nutrition of fetal and infant life, then they can be prevented.

However, action to ensure optimal fetal nutrition and thereby to safeguard the long-term health of children must begin long before pregnancy. The nutritional status of the fetus reflects the efficacy with which the mother has been prepared for pregnancy throughout her life, starting with the nutritional provision she herself received as a fetus and continuing with her diet and lifestyle during childhood and the adequacy of her nutritional stores at the onset of pregnancy. Finally, her diet and lifestyle during pregnancy plays an important role in the nourishment of her baby.

The conclusion is clear: the health and welfare of the woman throughout her life is important in ensuring optimal growth and development of her children and her grandchildren.

Preparing for pregnancy

There is nothing to be done about a woman's own fetal life or childhood, but her nutritional status and general health as she enters pregnancy is vitally important. Women in a poor nutritional state at the beginning of pregnancy will produce light babies despite large weight gains; and the opposite is also true – obese women will produce large babies even though they may gain little weight during pregnancy, demonstrating the importance of mobilization of maternal stores in the nutritional provision of the fetus (Naeye 1990).

Many young women yield to the constant media assault on body image by restricting their diet to an extent that they become very thin. If prolonged, this will certainly put their own health at risk, but it could have even more damaging consequences for their as yet unconceived offspring and even for their grandchildren. Embarking upon pregnancy with diminished nutrient stores will result in a fetus suffering from nutritional disadvantage at key stages of pregnancy with major consequences for his or her health throughout life.

Women can, and should, prepare in advance for pregnancy and dietary advice should be a key component of preconception care. It is well established that preconceptional folic acid supplementation reduces the risk of neural tube defects, though the benefit of other dietary supplementation of fetal growth and development is more obscure (MRC Vitamin Study Group 1991). However, women can ensure that they eat a healthy diet, rich in iron and protein and adequate in calories, so that they do not enter pregnancy whilst in the middle of a weight-reducing diet or when anaemic since this is known to have profound effects on the development of the placenta (Hytten and Leitch 1971).

Nutritional status, as discussed previously, is not merely a reflection of dietary intake. It is well established that lifestyle has substantial effects on metabolic regulation – reflected in blood pressure and circulating lipid levels. It is probably important that a woman considering pregnancy maintains not only a 'healthy' diet but also a healthy lifestyle with adequate exercise, modest alcohol intake, and not too much stress since it would appear that her own metabolic regulation is the starting point for that of her baby.

The evidence suggests that whilst a good diet during pregnancy may mitigate against, it will not compensate for, a poor pre-pregnancy nutritional status.

Diet during pregnancy

Nutrition during pregnancy is undoubtedly important. The health of the children and grandchildren born to women after the Dutch hunger winter is testament to this. However, the results of studies of nutritional supplementation during pregnancy demonstrate the complexity of the relationship between maternal diet in pregnancy and fetal growth. In a study of women in Southampton, Godfrey and colleagues (1996) have shown that a high carbohydrate intake during the early months of pregnancy or a low meat and dairy protein diet results in reduced fetal and placental weights at birth. In other studies, protein supplementation has resulted in lighter babies and there is little correlation between maternal weight gain, fetal weight, and calorific intake during pregnancy.

Some specific groups of women are at increased dietary risk during pregnancy; for example, vegetarians and especially vegans may wish to consider taking additional vitamins and minerals during pregnancy, though as with all women they should be wary of taking too large a dose of vitamin A as high intake may be associated with increased fetal anomalies (DHSS 1990). Adolescents who are still growing themselves and women with eating disorders may well require special dietary advice to ensure that as well as the vitamin and mineral content of their diet, the protein and fat content is adequate. These groups make up only a small proportion of the women contemplating pregnancy, but early nutritional advice and support could have major benefits for the babies both in the short and long term.

Infant feeding

Barker has shown that risk of heart disease is related not only to low birthweight but also to low weight of the infant at one year. This implies that the risk for heart disease in a baby of lower birthweight may be lowered by optimizing weight gain during the first year of life. Infant feeding is therefore vitally important.

All the evidence suggests that breastfeeding for the first four to six months of life is the preferred option (DHSS 1980). Breastfed babies not only have a nutritional advantage over formula-fed infants, they also are at reduced risk of infective illnesses for two reasons: firstly, because of the passive immunity they get from maternal antibodies present in breast milk; and secondly, because the opportunity for bacterial contamination of breast milk is small (Howie *et al.* 1990; Wilson *et al.* 1998).

Breastfed babies are less likely to develop allergic conditions such as asthma and eczema, and are conferred some intellectual advantage either as a consequence of the intimacy involved in breastfeeding or as a result of specific growth factors which promote neural development and are of particular importance for the premature infant (Lucas *et al.* 1992; Pollock 1994).

National trends: what is happening now?

Birthweight

The trends in birthweight indicate the nation's future health. Data from Scotland show that birthweight is increasing; in particular, the proportion of all babies weighing over 3.5 kg at birth increased from 33.5% to 40.2% in the 20-year period 1975–1994 (Power 1994). Birthweight in England and Wales is similarly increasing (Alberman 1991). This is despite an increase in the overall proportion of first births (which tend to be lighter) from 37% in 1958 to 43% in 1985 as family size is falling.

Overall, the demographic trends towards increasing maternal height and birthweight are favourable and, if they continue, will be reflected in a healthier adult population for this generation and those to come.

Breastfeeding

Whilst up to 60% of babies are breastfed initially, only one quarter are still being breastfed by the time they are four months of age, and those born into the lower social classes are least likely to be breastfed (Botting 1995). Babies born to women of lower social classes are generally of lower birthweight (even after adjusting for smoking) and are more likely to be premature and have health problems. Despite the fact that neonatal mortality has fallen dramatically over recent decades, babies born to women of social class 5 are still twice as likely to die in the neonatal period than those of social class 1 and babies born to single mothers are at an even higher risk. Because so few women in lower social classes breastfeed their babies, the babies who have most to gain from breast milk are the least likely to be given it. There is clearly a vital need to encourage women to breastfeed their babies – and to persevere for months rather than weeks. Education of the mothers about the benefits of breastfeeding by their health care team during pregnancy, and continued practical support afterwards, are obviously essential to meet this objective (Chapter 24).

Cigarette smoking

Overall, smoking in the UK is declining. However, of concern is the fact that in one sector of the population, which includes young women of childbearing age, rates are increasing (OPCS 1991). Smoking during pregnancy is known to affect the development of the fetus. Birthweight is reduced by up to 175 g by smoking – almost as much as the reduction in weight of the children born after the famine of the Dutch hunger winter (Rush and Cassano 1970). The immediate consequences of reduced birthweight in terms of infant mortality and morbidity are obvious. It is probable that the adult diseases associated with lower birthweight will be more prevalent in exposed infants. Passive smoking also has detrimental effects on children's health and has been implicated in several conditions of childhood, including sudden infant death (Blair *et al.* 1996).

Add to this the fact that children of smokers are themselves more likely to smoke and that smoking accounts for around one third of all premature mortality, there can be absolutely no doubt that encouraging and supporting women in cessation of smoking during or preferably before pregnancy will have a profound effect not only on their health but also on the health of their children for the rest of their lives (Goddard 1990; Peto *et al.* 1994).

Social inequalities

A major implication of the Barker hypothesis is that exposing young women to poverty and social disadvantage has consequences not only for their own long-term health but also for the long-term health of their children and grandchildren. In some of the Western countries, for example in the UK and the USA, there is increasing divide between the wealthy and the poor and the effect of this is seen in the current health of the populations (Phillimore *et al.* 1994; Ben-Shlomo *et al.* 1996; Kaplan *et al.* 1996). This increasing social disadvantage will have consequences for the health of the nation for generations to come and this should be given consideration in social and health planning (Davey-Smith 1996).

We have seen that women from more disadvantaged backgrounds are more likely to smoke, less likely to breastfeed, and may well have difficulty in maintaining a 'healthy' diet and lifestyle. The primary health care team has an important role to play in the provision of information and support to these women before, during, and after their pregnancies.

Future research: the unanswered questions

It is likely that Barker's hypothesis of the fetal and infant origins of adult disease at least partly explains the aetiological mechanisms of the adult disease as discussed in this chapter. Impaired fetal growth and development is probably one of the first steps on the pathway to diseases of complex aetiology. However, it is probably equally true that our genetic heritage and the accumulated experiences – good and bad – over the course of a lifetime also play an important role in the occurrence of disease (Scrimshaw 1997). That lifestyle is important in the causation of disease is clearly shown in the Whitehall studies (in which a large cohort of civil servants was followed in detail): there is continuous improvement in adult health with increasing adult social status, at whatever resolution economic status and health can be measured (Marmot *et al.* 1991). The interaction of impaired *in utero* growth and development with adult lifestyle factors is reflected in the results of several studies, including that of Leon *et al.* (1996) who concluded that failure to realize the full growth potential *in utero* (as indicated by being light at birth but tall as an adult) is associated with raised adult blood pressure, but that a substantial increase in adult BP only occurs in those who become obese. Many researchers also consider that genetic predisposition may play a substantial role in the aetiology of these diseases, and gene–environment interaction must be an important factor influencing the substantial differences in the prevalence of non-communicable diseases between different populations (Turner *et al.* 1993; Humphries 1995).

An alternative hypothesis suggests that the pattern of emergence of cardiovascular disease is consistent with that of a disease in which there is early exposure to the causative agents and it has been suggested recently that cardiovascular disease may be related to inflammatory response following infection, in particular that resulting from *Helicobacter pylori* or *Chlamydia pneumoniae* to which there may be differences in genetic susceptibility (Patel *et al.* 1995). However, the hypothesis of an infective aetiology is difficult to reconcile with some of the risk factors for cardiovascular disease, for example short stature, and Danesh and Peto (1998) have carried out a meta analysis of 18 published studies reporting cardiovascular risk factors in relation to *Helicobacter Pylori* infection and conclude that the evidence does not support a causal association.

Within a group of individuals the observed pattern of disease reflects a balance of the influences of genetics, fetal growth, and lifetime experience which may be unique to that population. Another group of individuals will have a different disease pattern influenced by a different balance of these factors. This could go some way to explaining the different observations from studies of different populations.

Distinguishing the relative contributions to adult disease of fetal growth, genetic predisposition, and life experience is the challenge for future research. Low birthweight and social disadvantage at birth are correlated both with each other and with social disadvantage throughout childhood and many studies have not been able to address the possible confounding effects of a lifetime of social deprivation and hence to distinguish whether the importance of birth characteristics are that they act as a surrogate measure of 'what is yet to come' or reflect what has already past (Ben-Shlomo and Davey Smith 1991; Elford *et al.* 1991; Bartley *et al.* 1994).

Future research will need to address the different pathways to disease in individuals to better understand the relative contribution and interplay between the potential disease risk factors of genetics, lifetime experiences, and fetal and childhood growth and development. Of particular relevance in the ability to explore these issues are two important cohort studies which began 50 years ago. These cohorts are unique in the extent and duration for which they have been studied and are amongst the best sources of data for testing the Barker hypothesis in the world.

A thousand families in Newcastle upon Tyne

In 1946, Sir James Spence began the Thousand Families Study in an attempt to understand the causes of the high rate of infective illness prevalent in infants in Newcastle upon Tyne. All 1142 babies born in the city of Newcastle in May and June of 1947 were recruited and 967 took part fully in the first-year study in which an extensive data-collection exercise was performed by a team of paediatricians and health visitors. Antenatal and delivery records were collected to provide the team with the earliest data on the infants. Subsequently, the families were visited regularly by the study team. Not only was the health, development, and nutrition of the children documented in great detail, but also the wealth and social circumstance of the families were recorded and the city council performed a detailed housing survey. Newcastle had a substantial proportion of disadvantaged families in 1947; for example, 30% of the families lived in overcrowded conditions and 15% in houses which were classified as unfit for habitation. Illnesses were investigated and recorded and by the end of the first year 1393 episodes of acute infection, including 800 respiratory tract infections, had been documented.

The conclusions of the first-year study were of the strong relationship between social circumstances and infant health and the importance of good mothering skills in all aspects of nurture and child health and development. The details of the first-year study are recounted in the book *A thousand families in Newcastle upon Tyne* (Spence *et al.* 1954).

The study of the cohort was extended to include investigation of the health and development of the cohort until 1962 when they attained school-leaving age. Two further volumes completed the trilogy of the original Thousand Families Study (Miller *et al.* 1960, 1974).

The Thousand Families Study is a uniquely detailed chronicle of the childhood of a complete birth cohort who were 50 years old in 1997. The study was not, of course, set up to explore the Barker hypothesis and so the subtleties of anthropometry at birth that may be important clues to fetal development, e.g. ponderal index, abdominal circumference, placental weight, and head circumference, are not available. However, in addition to birthweight and weights during childhood, there are very detailed records of health, growth and development, social circumstances, and nutrition over the first 15 years of life. The Thousand Families cohort therefore provides a framework within which the question of birthweight marking 'the past' or 'the future' can be addressed. The Wellcome Trust funded a three-year project, beginning in 1996, for the author and her colleagues at the Departments of Child Health and Medicine at Newcastle University to evaluate the current health and lifestyle of the original Thousand Families cohort to investigate the extent to which risk factors for adult diseases are related both to childhood and adult health and lifestyle and to what extent their disease risk was programmed *in utero*.

The National Survey of Health and Development

In 1946, a birth cohort study was set up by James Douglas who was concerned about the apparent decline in fertility and wanted to know what was putting people off having children (Wadsworth 1991). The original 1946 birth cohort study involved over 13 500 babies, 91% of all those born in Great Britain from 3 to 9 March 1946. One important observation to come out of the early study was that only 20% of the mothers received any form of pain relief during labour; indeed reports from this study led to a private member's bill in the House of Commons in the 1950s which brought a change in the regulations on the administration of analgesia, making it more readily available to women giving birth at home, as the majority of the women in the study had done. The original concerns of the study were ameliorated somewhat by the postwar baby boom, but nevertheless the study continued on a representative sample of 5362 children born in England, Scotland, and Wales. Every two years over the next two decades the development of the cohort was followed up by health visitors, teachers, and school doctors and nurses. A wide range of measurements were made, including height, weight, and blood pressure. Infant mortality fell by over 50% in the six years following 1946, from 55 to 26 per 1000, but the 1946 birth cohort study clearly showed that children from poorer backgrounds were still vulnerable as they grew up – the legacy of early deprivation continued to be observed. Much of the study is described in a book *The imprint of time* (Wadsworth 1991), and it was in this cohort that the association between birthweight and adult blood pressure was first observed.

The cohort has been followed up at regular intervals throughout life and, together with the Thousand Families cohort, it provides a unique series for testing Barker's hypothesis and exploring the relative contribution of adult disease experiences throughout life. Professor Michael Wadsworth of the MRC Unit, University College, London has recently embarked upon the latest follow-up study of this cohort which will provide a valuable contribution to the understanding of adult disease and early life experience.

References

Alberman, E. (1991). Are our babies becoming bigger? *Journal of the Royal Society of Medicine*, **84**, 257–60.

Andersen, L. B. and Haraldsdottir, J. (1993). Tracking of cardiovascular disease risk factors, including maximal oxygen uptake and physical activity from late teenage to adulthood. An 8-year follow-up study. *Journal of Internal Medicine*, **234**(3), 309–15.

Barker, D. J. P. (1992). *Fetal and infant origins of adult disease.* BMJ Publications, London.

Barker, D. J. P. (1994). *Mothers, babies, and disease in later life.* BMJ Publications, London.

Barker, D. J. P. and Osmond, C. (1986). Infant mortality, childhood nutrition, and ischaemic heart disease in England and Wales. *Lancet*, **I**, 1077–81.

Barker, D. J. P. and Osmond, C. (1987a). Inequalities in health in Britain: specific explanations in three Lancashire towns. *British Medical Journal*, **294**, 749–52.

Barker, D. J. P. and Osmond, C. (1987b). Death rates from stroke in England and Wales predicted from past maternal mortality. *British Medical Journal*, **295**, 83–6.

Barker, D. J. P., Winter, P. D., Osmond, C., Margetts, B., and Simmons, S. J. (1989). Weight in infancy and death from ischaemic heart disease. *Lancet*, **II**, 577–80.

Barker, D. J. P., Osmond, C., and Golding, J. (1990). Height and mortality in the counties of England and Wales. *Annals of Human Biology*, **17**(1), 1–6.

Barker, D. J. P., Godfrey, K. M., Fall, C., Osmond, C., Winter, P. D., and Shaheen, S. O. (1991). Relation of birthweight and childhood respiratory infection to adult lung function and death from chronic obstructive airways disease. *British Medical Journal*, **303**, 671–5.

Barker, D. J. P., Godfrey, K. M., Osmond, C., and Bull, A. (1992a). The relation of fetal length, ponderal index, and head circumference to blood pressure and the risk of hypertension in adult life. *Paediatric and Perinatal Epidemiology*, **6**(1), 35–44.

Barker, D. J. P., Meade, T. W., Fall, C. H., Lee, A., Osmond, C., Phipps, K., *et al.* (1992b). Relation of fetal and infant growth to plasma fibrinogen and factor VII concentrations in adult life. *British Medical Journal*, **304**, 148–52.

Barker, D. J. P., Martyn, C. N., Osmond, C., Hales, C. N., and Fall, C. H. D. (1993a). Growth *in utero* and serum cholesterol concentrations in adult life. *British Medical Journal*, **307**, 1524–7.

Barker, D. J. P., Osmond, C., and Wield, G. A. (1993b). The relation of small head circumference and thinness at birth to death from cardiovascular disease in adult life. *British Medical Journal*, **306**, 422–6.

Barker, D. J. P. and Law, L. M. (1994). Birthweight and blood pressure in adolescence: studies may be misleading. *British Medical Journal*, **308**(6944), 1634.

Bartley, M., Power, C., Blane, D., Davey Smith, G., and Shipley, M. (1994). Birthweight and later socioeconomic disadvantage: evidence from the 1958 British cohort study. *British Medical Journal*, **309**, 1475–9.

Ben-Shlomo, Y. and Davey Smith, G. (1991). Deprivation in infancy or in adult life: which is more important for mortality risk? *Lancet*, **337**, 530–4.

Ben-Shlomo, Y., White, I. R., and Marmot, M. (1996) Does the variation in the socio-economic characteristics of an area affect mortality? *British Medical Journal*, **312**, 1013–14.

Blair, P. S., Fleming, P. J., Bensley, D., Smith, I., Bacon, C., Taylor, E. E., *et al.* (1996). Smoking and the sudden infant death syndrome: results of 1993–95 case–control study for confidential inquiry into stillbirths and deaths in infancy. *British Medical Journal*, **313**, 195–8.

Botting, B. (ed.) (1995). *The health of our children*. Decennial supplement, OPCS. HMSO, London.

Central Statistics Office (1996). *Social trends*. HMSO, London.

Danesh, J. and Peto, R. (1998). Risk factors for coronary heart disease and infection with Heliocobacter pylori: meta analysis of 18 studies. *British Medical Journal*, **316**, 1130–2.

Davey-Smith, G. D. (1996). Income inequality and mortality: why are they related? [editorial].*British Medical Journal*, 312, 987–8.

Davis, J. A. (1994). Birthweight and blood pressure in adolescence: findings could be influenced by the stage of puberty. *British Medical Journal*, 308(6944), 1634.

DHSS (1980).*Present-day practice in infant feeding*. Report on Health and Social Subjects No. 20. HMSO, London.

DHSS (1990). Vitamin A and pregnancy. PL/CMO (90) II PL/CNO (90).

Elford, J., Whincup, P., and Shaper, A. G. (1991). Early life experience and adult cardiovascular disease: longitudinal and case–control studies. *International Journal of Epidemiology*, 20(4), 833–44.

Fain, J. A. (1993). National trends in diabetes: an epidemiologic perspective. *Nursing Clinics of North America*, 28(1), 1–7.

Folkow, B. (1987). Cardiovascular structural adaptation: its role in the initiation and maintenance of primary hypertension. *Clinical Science*, 55, S3–S22.

Forsdahl, A. (1977). Are poor living conditions in childhood and adolescence an important risk factor for arteriosclerotic heart disease? *British Journal of Preventive Social Medicine*, 31, 91–5.

Fox, H. (1978). *Pathology of the placenta*. W. B. Saunders, Philadelphia.

Frankel, S., Elwood, P., Sweetnam, P., Yarnell, J., and Davey Smith, G. (1996). Birthweight, adult risk factors and incident coronary heart disease: the Caerphilly Study. *Public Health*, 110, 139–43.

Fuller, J. H., Shiplet, M. J., Rose, G., Jarrett, R. J., and Keen, H. (1980). Coronary heart disease risk and impaired glucose tolerance. *Lancet*, I, 1376–6.

Gardner, M. J., Winter, P. D., and Barker, D. J. P. (1984). *Atlas of mortality from selected diseases in England and Wales 1968–1978*. Wiley, Chichester.

Goddard, E. (1990). *Why children start smoking*. OPCS, HMSO, London.

Godfrey, K., Robinson, S., Barker, D. J. P., Osmond, C., and Cox,V. (1996). Maternal nutrition in early and late pregnancy in relation to placental and fetal growth. *British Medical Journal*, 312, 410–14.

Gregory, J., *et al.* (1990). *The dietary and nutritional survey of British adults*. HMSO, London.

Hales, C. N., Barker, D. J. P., Clark, P. M., Cox, L. J., Fall, C., Osmond, C., *et al.* (1991). Fetal and infant growth and impaired glucose tolerance at age 64 . *British Medical Journal*, 303, 1019–22.

Hales, C. N. and Barker, D. J. P. (1992). Type 2 (non-insulin-dependent) diabetes mellitus: the thrifty phenotype hypothesis. *Diabetologia*, 35, 595–601.

Howie, P. W., Stewart-Forsyth, J., Ogston, S. A., Clark, A., and Florey, C. D. (1990). Protective effect of breastfeeding against infection. *British Medical Journal*, 300, 11–16.

Humphries, S. E. (1995). Genetic regulation of fibrinogen. *European Heart Journal*, 16(Suppl. A), 16–19.

Hytten, F. E. (1980). In: *Clinical physiology in obstetrics* (ed. F. E. Hytten and G. Chamberlain). Blackwell Scientific Publications, Oxford.

Hytten, F. E. and Leitch, I. (1971). *The physiology of human pregnancy* (2nd edn). Blackwell Scientific Publications, Oxford.

Kannel, W. B. and Larson, M. (1993). Long-term epidemiologic predictions of coronary disease: the Framingham experience. Cardiology, **82**(2–3), 137–52.

Kaplan, G. A., Pamuk, E. R., Lynch, J. W., Cohen, R. D., and Balfour, J. L. (1996). Inequality in income and mortality in the United States: analysis of mortality and potential pathways. *British Medical Journal*, **312**, 999–1003.

Launer, L., Hoffman, A., and Grobbee, D. E. (1993). Relation between birthweight and blood pressure: longitudinal study of infants and children. *British Medical Journal*, **307**, 1451–4.

Law, C. M., Barker, D. J. P., Bull, A. R., Osmond, C. (1991). Maternal and fetal influences on blood pressure. *Archives of Disease in Childhood*, **6**, 1291–5.

Law, C. M., de Swiet, M., Osmond, C., Fayers, P. M., and Barker, D. J. P. (1993). Initiation of hypertension *in utero* and its amplification throughout life. *British Medical Journal*, **306**, 24–7.

Lee, A. J., Lowe, G. D., Woodward, M., and Tunstall-Pedoe. H. (1993). Fibrinogen in relation to personal history of prevalent hypertension, diabetes, stroke, intermittent claudication, coronary heart disease, and family history: the Scottish Heart Health Study. *British Heart Journal*, **69**(4), 338–42.

Leon, D. A., Koupilova, I., Lithell, H. O., Berglund, L., Mohsen, R., Vagero, D., *et al.* (1996). Failure to realize growth potential *in utero* and adult obesity in relation to blood pressure in 50-year-old Swedish men. *British Medical Journal*, **312**, 401–6.

Lucas, A., Morley, R., Cole, T. J., Lister, G., and Leeson-Payne, C. (1992). Breast milk and subsequent intelligence quotient in children born preterm. *Lancet*, **339**, 261–4.

Lumley, L. H. (1992). Decreased birthweights in infants after maternal *in utero* exposure to the Dutch famine of 1944–1945. *Pediatric Epidemiology*, **6**, 240–53.

MacKenzie, H. S. and Brenner, B. M. (1995). Fewer nephrons at birth: a missing link in the etiology of essential hypertension? *American Journal Kidney Disease*, **26**(1), 91–8.

Marmot, M. G., Davey-Smith, G. D., Stansfield, S., Patel, C., North, F., Head, J., *et al.* (1991). Health inequalities among British civil servants: The Whitehall II study. *Lancet*, **337**, 1387–93.

Marty, C. N., Barker, D. J. P., Jespersen, S., Greenwald, S., Osmond, C., and Berry, C. (1995). Growth *in utero*, adult blood pressure and arterial compliance. *British Heart Journal*, **73**(2), 116–21.

Matthes, J. W., Lewis, P. A., Davies, D. P., and Bethel, J. A. (1994). Relation between birthweight at term and systolic blood pressure in adolescence. *British Medical Journal*, **308**(6936), 1074–7.

Medical Research Council Vitamin Study Group (1991). Prevention of neural tube defects: Results of the MRC Vitamin Study. *Lancet*, **238**, 131–7.

Miller, F. J. W., Court, S. D. M., Walton, W. S., and Knox, E. G. (1960). *Growing up in Newcastle upon Tyne*. Oxford University Press, Oxford.

Miller, F. J. W., Court, S. D. M., Knox, E. G., and Brandon, S. (1974). *The school years in Newcastle upon Tyne*. Oxford University Press, Oxford.

Mitchell, B. D. and Stern, M. P. (1992). Recent developments in the epidemiology of diabetes in the Americas. *World Health Statistics Quarterly Report*, 45(4), 347–9.

Modan, M., Halikin, H., Almog, S., *et al.* (1985). Hyperinsulinaemia: a link between hypertension, obesity, and glucose intolerance. *Journal of Clinical Investigation*, 75, 809–17.

Naeye, R. L. (1990). Maternal bodyweight and pregnancy outcome. *American Journal of Clinical Nutrition*, 52, 273–9.

Office of Population Censuses and Surveys (1991). *General household survey: cigarette smoking. 1972–1990.* OPCS monitor SS 91/3.

Patel, P., Mendall, M., Carrington, D., Strachan, D., Leatham, E., and Molineaux, N. (1995). Association of *Helicobacter pylori* and *Chlamydia pneumoniae* infections with coronary heart disease and cardiovascular risk factors. *British Medical Journal*, 311, 711–14.

Peto, R., Lopez, A. D., Boreham, J., Thun, M., and Heath Jr., C. (1994). *Mortality from smoking in developed countries 1950–2000. Indirect estimates from national statistics.* Oxford University Press, Oxford.

Phillimore, P., Beattie, A., and Townsend, P. (1994). Widening inequality of health in northern England, 1981–1991. *British Medical Journal*, 308, 1125–8.

Pollock, J. I. (1994). Long-term associations with infant feeding in a clinically advantaged population of babies. *Development and Child Neurology*, 36(5), 429–40.

Power, C. (1994). National trends in birthweight: implications for future adult disease. *British Medical Journal*, 308, 1270–1.

Ravelli, A. C. J., van der Meulen, J. H. P., Michels, R. P. J. *et al.* (1998). Glucose tolerance in adults after prenatal exposure to famine. *Lancet*, 351, 173–7.

Registrar General's statistical review of England and Wales 1921. HMSO, London.

Registrar General's statistical review of England and Wales 1971. HMSO, London.

Registrar General's statistical review of England and Wales 1992. HMSO, London

Rose, G. (1985). Sick individuals and sick populations. *International Journal of Epidemiology*, 14, 32.

Rush, D. and Cassano, P. (1970). Relationship of cigarette smoking and social class to birthweight and perinatal mortality among all births in Britain. *Journal of Epidemiology and Community Health*, 90, 1040–5.

Scrimshaw, N. S. (1997). The relationship between fetal malnutrition and chronic disease in later life [editorial]. *British Medical Journal*, 315, 825–6.

Spence, J., Walton, W. S., Miller, F. J. W., and Court, S. D. M. (1954). *A thousand families in Newcastle upon Tyne.* Oxford University Press, Oxford.

Stein, Z., Susser, M., Saenger, G., and Marolla, F. (1975). *Famine and human development: in the Dutch hunger winter of 1944–45.* Oxford University Press, New York.

Townsend, P., Phillimore, P., and Beattie, A. (1988). *Health and deprivation: inequalities and the North.* Croom Helm Ltd, Beckenham, Kent.

Turner, R. C., Levy, J. C., and Clark, A. (1993). Complex genetics of type 2 diabetes: thrifty genes and previously neutral polymorphisms. *Quarterly Journal of Medicine*, 86(7), 413.

Waaler, H. T. (1984). Height, weight, and mortality. The Norwegian experience. *Acta Medica Scandinavia*, 79(Suppl.), 1–56.

Wadsworth, M., Cripps, H., Midwinter, R, and Colley, J. (1985). Blood pressure in a national birth cohort at the age of 36 years related to social and familial factors, smoking, and body mass. *British Medical Journal*, 291, 1534–8.

Wadsworth, M. E. J. (1991). The imprint of time: childhood, history, and adult life. Clarendon, Oxford.

Whincup, P. H., Cook, D. G., and Papacosta, O. (1992). Do maternal and intrauterine factors influence blood pressure in childhood? *Archives of Disease in Childhood*, 67, 1423–9.

Whincup, P. H., Cook, D. G., Adshead, F., Taylor, S., Papacosta, O., Walker, M., *et al.* (1996). Cardiovascular risk factors in British children from towns with widely differing adult cardiovascular mortality. *British Medical Journal*, 313, 79–84.

Wilson, A. C., Forsyth, J. S., Greene, S. A. *et al.* (1998). Relation of infant diet to childhood health: seven year follow-up of cohort of children in Dundee infant feeding study. *British Medical Journal*, 316, 21–5.

SECTION FOUR

CLINICAL CARE

CHAPTER SIXTEEN

Reproductive information and advice in primary care

Michael Modell and Bernadette Modell

Introduction

The objective of providing reproductive information if possible for couples rather than women alone, is to increase the chance of the birth of a healthy baby. The list below summarizes the areas to be covered in this chapter:

- before pregnancy:
    - need for referral to an obstetrician or reproductive endocrinologist because of a bad obstetric history or infertility
    - implications of advancing maternal age
    - implications of a family history of possible genetic disease
    - indications for genetic screening because of ethnic background
    - dangers of infections, and rubella immunization status
    - concern that smoking, alcohol, and diet may affect future pregnancies
    - desirability for folic acid supplementation *before* conception
    - possible consequences of maternal disease such as diabetes or epilepsy.

- during pregnancy:
    - the above, if not already done
    - worry about the effect of drugs taken at the time of conception
    - concern about the risk of miscarriage
    - concern about a fever in pregnancy
    - anxiety about X-rays in pregnancy
    - concern about an abnormal standard prenatal test result
    - the need to support couples (in collaboration with the obstetrician and/ or geneticist) when a fetal abnormality is found, by explaining the likely effect of the disorder on the child and supporting parents in their choice of action.

Reproductive counselling builds on the enormous advances in the primary prevention of fetal disease that have occurred during the last 30 years or so. For example, in developed countries, haemolytic disease of the newborn is becoming rare. In the past it led to a fatal outcome or residual brain damage in up to 3.5 per1000 births (calculation based on Bowman and Pollock 1965). In its most severe form, hydrops fetalis, it is now almost completely preventable. There has been a dramatic decrease in the incidence of congenital rubella following pre-pregnancy immunization. A more recent advance is the evidence that peri-conceptional folic acid supplements prevent neural tube defects.

Information may be offered spontaneously by the health professional; more often it is given in response to questions and worries raised by the mother. Ideally, this information should be provided *before* gestation for two main reasons: firstly, to minimize risk factors at the time of conception; and secondly, in the case of identified genetic risk, to provide couples with the full range of reproductive options, including whether or not to proceed with pregnancy.

It is relatively uncommon for couples to consult specifically for preconception advice. They generally prefer to concentrate first on getting pregnant; in addition, many pregnancies are not planned. A few enthusiastic family doctors have initiated preconception clinics. Unfortunately, the danger is not only that attendance will be biased towards the motivated, articulate, worried well, but also that the knowledge that the practice runs a special clinic will lead to the neglect of other opportunities for providing preconception care. Health professionals should ideally use any opportunity to provide information to women of child-bearing age. Particularly pertinent are consultations relevant to reproduction. These include visits for family planning advice, a cervical smear, or following a negative pregnancy test or a miscarriage. Even consultations unrelated to reproduction can be used to remind certain groups to report pregnancy as soon as a period is missed. These groups include: women over 35 years of age (an early ultrasound is advised to check for fetal viability), couples carrying specific recessively inherited diseases who may wish for prenatal diagnosis, and women with diabetes or on anticonvulsants. Many practices may wish to produce their own protocol and an information pack for providing reproductive information.

Even though pre-pregnancy information is the ideal, it is not too late to raise many of the issues discussed below when a woman first reports a pregnancy to her GP or midwife; on average at about eight weeks' gestation, four weeks before she first attends the hospital antenatal clinic (Harris *et al.* 1993), or even later in the first trimester. The booking consultation is also a good opportunity to arrange for an early ultrasound to check fetal viability when there has been bleeding in early pregnancy.

Reproductive advice and information may prevent fetal damage from infection, pre-existing maternal disease, drugs, and toxins, e.g. cigarettes and alcohol. It permits the offer of screening for carriers of several important inherited diseases, such as haemoglobin disorders and Tay–Sachs disease which involve specific ethnic groups. Screening for carriers of cystic fibrosis has become a reality, involving the whole Caucasian population. A brief family history can highlight some other genetic risks.

Poor obstetric history or infertility

Women often seek advice because of a poor obstetric history or because they are having difficulty in becoming pregnant. A detailed discussion of this field is beyond the scope of this chapter (but see Recurrent abortion, below). It is important that referrals for recurrent abortion are made to obstetricians with a special interest in infertility.

Implications of advancing maternal age

Couples may seek advice on when to start a family. There are two reasons for not postponing child-bearing too long. Maternal age is positively related both to the risk of miscarriage and to the birth of a child with a chromosomal abnormality. The general risk of miscarriage for recognized pregnancies is about 10% for women aged 20–35, about 20% in women aged 35–40, and at least 30% for women over 40 (Stein *et al.* 1980). These facts should be more widely known, especially to older women, as they can influence people's decisions about when to plan a pregnancy and their expectations during early pregnancy.

Most chromosomal disorders and congenital malformations cannot be predicted in advance; they occur at random when the ova and sperm are formed, or during development of the embryo. The commonest chromosomal abnormality is Down's syndrome (trisomy 21) which in the absence of prenatal diagnosis would occur in about one in 1000 births at age 30. The risk increases to about one in 400 at 35, and one in 100 at 40 years of age. Risks to younger women are significantly increased if the mother has had a previous Down's pregnancy. Paternal age can also be important. DNA mutations arise more often in the father's than the mother's germ cells, and the mutation rate increases with paternal age. The contribution of new mutations to the overall number of congenital malformations and infants with genetic disease is relatively small, but a 50-year-old father has six times the risk of a 30-year-old father of having a child with a new mutation (Modell and Kuliev 1990). The commonest such condition is the dominantly inherited achondroplasia.

Family history of possible genetic disease

A couple may be concerned about producing a child with a genetic disease or congenital disorder because of a problem in a previous child, or a family history of possible genetic disease. They should be referred for genetic counselling if there is any doubt about the inheritance of the disorder. Malformations such as congenital dislocation of the hip, cleft palate, or pyloric stenosis are thought to be the end result of the interaction of several genes and environmental factors. The feature of this so-called multifactorial inheritance is that there is an empirical 2–10% rate of recurrence in siblings and children of an affected person (Harper 1988). This rate is increased if more than one family member has been affected. The birth of a previous child with a significant malformation is an indication for an expert fetal ultrasound scan in succeeding pregnancies (check whether this is provided by the local obstetric unit).

A family tree is the key to identifying people who would benefit from referral to a clinical geneticist, or other specialist. In some practices the family history is already extensively used as a short-hand method of highlighting events of both emotional and genetic significance, and to help in understanding the dynamics of the family. Progressing from this basic family history to constructing a simple pedigree is the key to involving the family doctor in all other aspects of identifying genetic risk, besides reproductive counselling. The primary care family tree will usually only need to include first-degree relatives, unless genetic disease is already suspected in a family member. The registration examination provides a good opportunity for constructing a family tree, as do consultations concerned with reproduction. However, to make the task simple and quick, primary care workers need to be provided with tools, such as a simple computer program for drawing up a family tree which includes lists of genetic risk factors.

Health professionals may be alerted to the possibility of a genetically relevant family history because of:

- intrauterine death, stillbirth, or neonatal death. These are sometimes due to chromosomal abnormalities or inherited metabolic diseases

- unusually deep or prolonged neonatal jaundice (caused for example by the X-linked glucose-6-phosphate dehydrogenase deficiency, carried by about 7% of the world's population (WHO 1989))

- death in infancy. This can be caused by numerous genetic conditions of slightly later onset, such as sickle cell disease or metabolic disorders

- failure to thrive, repeated respiratory infections (cystic fibrosis), or specific symptoms such as a bleeding tendency in a male (haemophilia)

- severe learning difficulty (fragile-X syndrome), sensorineural deafness, or blindness.

Need for genetic screening tests because of ethnic background

Diseases with Mendelian patterns of inheritance make up only about 10% of all congenital disorders, but they are particularly important because they are often severe and involve a high, often predictable, and avoidable genetic risk for some families (Baird *et al.* 1988). This particularly applies to recessively inherited conditions. Carriers of a handful of recessively inherited conditions are common, i.e. each make up more than 1% of the population. Carriers of these disorders are common because they have an evolutionary advantage, for example increased resistance to certain diseases. Carriers of the haemoglobin disorders (sickle-cell disease and thalassaemia) are less vulnerable to falciparum malaria. This explains why these genes are very common in ethnic groups originating from Africa, Asia, and the Middle-East. Carriers of cystic fibrosis (the commonest inherited disease of Caucasians) probably have an increased resistance to infantile gastroenteritis.

Children who develop a recessively inherited disorder must have inherited a mutant gene from both of their healthy carrier parents. Since this situation depends on two carriers meeting by chance, there is rarely a family history except in communities with an exceptionally high proportion of carriers. When both parents carry the same abnormal recessive gene, on average 25% of their offspring inherit it from both and have the disease, 50% are carriers, and 25% inherit two normal genes. Fifty per cent of first-degree relatives of carriers are also carriers. Thus the identification of one carrier should alert the family doctor to the high probability of other carriers within that family, and the need to offer relatives the opportunity to be tested.

One of the objectives of reproductive counselling is to detect couples (usually without a family history) at risk of producing a child with a recessively inherited, or occasionally X-linked, condition, in time to offer them the possibility of prenatal diagnosis. If these couples are identified before pregnancy, or in the first two months of pregnancy, they have more time to decide what action to take. For example, unlike couples who are only identified via the antenatal clinic in mid-pregnancy, they are able to choose early prenatal diagnosis. Late prenatal diagnosis leading on to termination of an affected pregnancy, perhaps at around 20 weeks' gestation, is a particularly traumatic event. Prenatal diagnosis is mainly done by amniocentesis at 15–16 weeks' gestation or chorionic villus sampling from about 10 weeks' gestation. The objective of both is to obtain fetal cells which can then be analysed for a chromosomal, DNA, or metabolic abnormality. There is evidence that most couples at risk for a sickle-cell disorder are in favour of prenatal diagnosis, but *only* if this can be done in the first trimester. At present, many of these couples are not identified in time for prenatal diagnosis in the presenting pregnancy at all. It is, of course, essential to avoid pressurizing 'at-risk' couples into opting for prenatal diagnosis, and when they do choose this option to avoid pressure to terminate an affected pregnancy. A wanted child with a genetic disease is one successful outcome of counselling. It is possible to make a serious impact on the incidence of inherited diseases only if couples at risk can be detected and counselled before they start their family. Most north European couples do not have more than two children, so diagnosis and counselling of carrier couples after the birth of their first affected child can have very little effect on the total birth rate of affected children.

The birth incidence of homozygotes is directly related to the carrier frequency in the relevant population (Table 16.1).

Some ethnic groups from Pakistan, the Middle East, North Africa, and Turkey have a convention of consanguineous marriage. Close parental consanguinity increases the likelihood of recessively inherited disorders in the children, especially when there is a family history, because of common genes from a shared ancestor. If there is any suggestion of an inherited disease in the

Table 16.1 *Carrier frequency in different populations*

Population at risk	Carriers (% of population)	Number of people tested to detect a carrier couple
Indians: Hb disorders	3	1144
North Europeans: CF	4	650
Chinese: Hb disorders	8	169
African Caribbeans: Hb disorders	12	78
Cypriots: Hb disorders	17	40
Pakistanis	4.5	200
Sub-Saharan Africans: Hb disorders	25	20

Based on Modell and Anionwu (1996).

family it is desirable to refer such couples to a clinical geneticist. Health professionals should be supportive to these couples and not blame parental consanguinity for the problem. The custom has many social advantages in the groups where it is practised and these outweigh the increased genetic risks.

There is a strong case for offering carrier testing for haemoglobin disorders, Tay–Sachs disease (carried by 3–4% of Jews of Eastern origin), and cystic fibrosis before pregnancy (Modell and Modell 1992). Many members of ethnic minorities are already aware of their risk and request testing.

In females carriers of X-linked disorders, mutant genes carried on the X-chromosome usually have a recessive mode of inheritance and cause little clinical effect. As males have only one X chromosome, this gene is necessarily 'dominant' in males, which explains why it is males who usually suffer from X-linked disorders. Many carrier females are related to a known affected male, but some carry new mutations and some have inherited the abnormal gene in the female line, without a known affected male. One of the commonest of such disorders is the fragile-X syndrome, which accounts for about 10% of cases of children with severe learning difficulties. It is now possible, by DNA studies, to identify carriers of this syndrome. The GP may consider discussing this test with a woman who has a close relative with severe undiagnosed learning difficulty.

Rubella immunization status

It is not uncommon for a woman in early pregnancy, or who thinks she may be pregnant, to seek advice because she has been in contact with a child with a rash. It is impossible to make a definite diagnosis of German measles clinically, but most viral rashes are not due to rubella, and most women are immune. In 1993, about 6% of 13–14 year-old girls were reported to be susceptible to rubella, and there were 25 confirmed infections in pregnant women.This compares to 12 in 1991 and 2 in 1992 – a warning that there should be no relaxation in the rubella immunization programme (Miller *et al.* 1994). If non-immune women are identified before conception they can be offered immunization against rubella, and also against hepatitis B if they are in a group considered at risk (health professionals, drug addicts, transfusion-dependent individuals). The triple MMR (measles, mumps rubella) vaccine produces an antibody response to all three viruses in over 95% of people vaccinated, and as 92% of children aged 5–16 received the measles and rubella vaccine in 1994 (Cutts 1996), congenital rubella is likely to become a disease of the past when today's teenagers become mothers. Reassuringly, there is no evidence that rubella vaccine inadvertently given during the first trimester of pregnancy is teratogenetic.

Danger of infections

Maternal infection with rubella, toxoplasmosis, or cytomegalovirus is often asymptomatic, so even if the mother was well in pregnancy, congenital infection must be considered in the differential diagnosis of a sickly infant who fails to thrive, or has a neonatal infection or evidence of a congenital heart defect. In some cases, a problem may only become apparent after the neonatal period. In all three conditions, apparently unaffected infants may later develop hearing loss and various degrees of severe learning disability. On the other hand, all three infections can cause a clinically similar picture of acute infection at birth, including features such as low birthweight, hepatosplenomegaly, jaundice, petechiae, and purpura.

Rubella

Smithells *et al.* (1990), reporting on congenital rubella in the UK, noted that only half the mothers of affected infants had a history of a rubella-like illness, so the fetus may be affected whether or not there are maternal symptoms. Cataracts, malformations of the heart, and deafness are the best known complications of fetal rubella. Perceptive or sensorineural deafness is the commonest problem, and may occur alone. Hearing loss ranges from a severe disability, making normal schooling impossible, to a mild loss detectable only by audiometry. Central nervous system symptoms such as abnormal irritability, with or without occasional fits, and severe learning disorder can also occur.

Toxoplasmosis

Toxoplasma gondii is a protozoan intracellular parasite found in many animals, but sexual reproduction and spore production occurs only in the intestine of the cat. It is thought to be transmitted to humans (and other animals) through contact with cat faeces, or by eating undercooked meat. Congenital toxoplasmosis occurs in about 10% of cases (Mombro *et al.* 1995) and can cause miscarriage, neonatal disease, and severe ocular problems. There is a case for offering serological screening for toxoplasmosis to women before pregnancy, and advising those who are not immune to be particularly careful.

The risk of toxoplasmosis may be reduced if pregnant women cook meat carefully and wash their hands after handling raw meat. Those with pet cats should also cook the cat's meat well (tins seem to be safe) and wear gloves when cleaning up cat litter. The effectiveness of such advice has not been demonstrated. Another possibility might be to immunize pet cats against toxoplasma.

Infection in adults is sometimes overt and may mimic glandular fever, but most infections in immunocompetent people are asymptomatic. Spiramycin is usually recommended for the pregnant woman with suspected acquired toxoplasmosis, and has been shown to reduce the frequency of congenital disease in the baby (Matsui 1994). The most informative studies on the natural history, treatment, and prevention of toxoplasmosis come from France where about 1% of pregnant women become infected and screening is now common. By contrast, in the UK, a lower proportion of women become infected during pregnancy, and screening is not routine.

Cytomegalovirus

Cytomegalovirus (CMV), one of the herpes group of viruses, is a cause of Paul–Bunnell negative glandular fever (a fever with enlarged glands and hepato-and splenomegaly). Most postnatal infections are asymptomatic. Overt infections are particularly likely in the immunosuppressed. Fortunately, fetal damage from CMV is rare even if the mother is infected, as there is no obvious way to lessen the risk of maternal infection. Possibly the only effective approach for prevention will be by vaccinating non-immune young women prior to pregnancy, but the efficacy and safety of the vaccine will first have to be demonstrated.

It is important to have a high index of suspicion for CMV and toxoplasma if a pregnant woman has a glandular fever-like illness.

Human Immunodeficiency Virus (HIV)

The HIV-positive woman who is contemplating pregnancy has a difficult choice to make, as does the well HIV-positive woman who becomes inadvertently pregnant. There is no evidence that asymptomatic infection has a major effect on the course or outcome of the pregnancy. The estimated rate of vertical transmission of the virus to the fetus is 15–20% in Europe, increasing to 25–35% in Africa (Johnstone 1996). The assumption is that in most cases, fetal infection occurs around delivery, though the role of an elective Caesarean in preventing this is unclear. The virus is transmitted more frequently to the fetus when the disease is more advanced in the mother. Infected infants do not differ from the remainder at birth with respect to weight, length, head circumference, or frequency of malformations. Antiretroviral therapy and avoiding breastfeeding can reduce the risk of a congenital infection in babies of HIV-positive mothers by more than half (Johnstone 1996). This means that HIV testing in pregnancy can benefit the fetus, though many mothers-to-be will find it very difficult to cope with the implications of a positive test.

Anonymous neonatal screening has shown that one in 580 pregnant women in London are HIV positive – a suprisingly high figure (MacDonagh *et al.* 1996). Despite the universal offer of HIV testing to pregnant women, less than 10% of previously undiagnosed infected women accepted the test and were identified antenatally; perhaps lack of trained antenatal clinic counsellors provided with written information materials affected the level of uptake (MacDonagh *et al.* 1996).

Herpes simplex virus

Couples with a past history of genital herpes may worry about the possibility of the spread of the herpes simplex virus to the fetus or newborn baby. The main danger is neonatal infection, though the risk even when there is a history of recurrent genital herpes in the woman is low. 'Safe sex', i.e. the use of condoms, is advised throughout pregnancy if the man has had recurrent genital herpes but his partner has no history of infection. The current strategy for prevention is to carefully examine the vulva and cervix of all women entering labour. Women with active herpetic lesions are then offered a Caesarean section. Neonatal infection may lead to disseminated disease, encephalitis, and/or lesions limited to the skin, eye, or mouth. Even with antiviral therapy, the risk of death is significant.

Listeria

Listeria is a very common infection of animals, including shellfish, domestic and game fowl, sheep, cattle, and flies. It is caused by a widespread intracellular parasite, *Listeria monocytogenes*, a small gram-positive bacillus. Pregnant women seem to be particularly susceptible to listeriosis which, in the non-pregnant, usually causes only a mild influenza-like illness. In order to prevent infection, they are advised to avoid food that may be contaminated with *Listeria*. These include undercooked poultry or cooked chilled meals, pate, and soft cheese. Recognized disease in pregnant women is rare, with an incidence of 0.123 per 1000 births in one English city (Jones *et al.* 1994). If a mother is infected early in pregnancy, transplacental spread to the fetus can cause abortion or stillbirth. If infection occurs late in pregnancy, the baby may develop pneumonia, septicaemia, and widespread abscesses soon after birth. Early antibiotic treatment often results in a complete recovery.

Chickenpox

Chickenpox in the first 20 weeks of pregnancy is associated with a 2–4% increased risk of a fetus with congenital defects, such as limb hypoplasia (Pastuszak *et al.* 1994).

Measles

Measles in pregnancy may lead to an increased risk of loss of the fetus and prematurity, especially in the first two weeks after the onset of rash (Eberhart-Phillips *et al.* 1993).

Parvovirus infection

Parvovirus infection may be subclinical but can cause a fever followed by rash – 'slapped cheek' disease. In pregnancy it may cause fetal anaemia leading to a miscarriage or stillbirth.

Alcohol and smoking

About one third of the adult population smoke and more drink alcohol, at least socially. It is well known that cigarettes and alcohol can have a bad effect on the fetus, and mothers-to-be not infrequently reduce both to a minimum when trying to become pregnant, rather than waiting until pregnancy is confirmed. It is not yet possible to definitely identify a safe limit of drinking and smoking during pregnancy. Women who consume small amounts of alcohol (a unit a day) and smoke the occasional cigarette can be reassured. It is the combination of excess alcohol with smoking which is more potentially damaging to the fetus.

Alcohol

It has been suggested that 40 ml of ethanol daily begins to have an adverse effect on the child's future psychosocial development (Larroque *et al.* 1995). This is the amount contained in three glasses of wine or two pints of beer. It is not unusual to see a child who is small, and somewhat slow mentally and physically, come from a family where excess drinking is suspected. In these cases it is difficult to prove a direct relationship between maternal alcohol consumption and the child's stunted developmental progress, or to separate congenital from environmental factors. In fact, the effect of alcohol varies from no discernible harm with minimal intake to full-blown fetal alcohol syndrome (FAS) with high intake. The features of FAS include learning difficulties, poor growth, and various congenital abnormalities which may involve the face, limbs, heart, and nervous system. The incidence in the United States is estimated at 0.97 cases per 1000 live births and 4.3% among 'heavy' drinkers (Abel 1995). It will be necessary to point out to parents of an affected child that a high recurrence rate of FAS is to be expected.

Smoking

Several studies in the 1970s indicated that smoking in pregnancy was a risky business, the risk increasing with the number of cigarettes smoked. Smoking increases the chance of miscarriage, bleeding in pregnancy, and premature birth, with an increase in the perinatal morbidity. In addition, maternal antenatal smoking (and parental smoking after the birth) is a modifiable major risk factor for sudden infant death syndrome (Taylor and Sanderson 1995). Although tobacco smoke contains various compounds that can cause fetal hypoxia, there is no evidence that maternal smoking significantly increases the risk of congenital malformations. There is encouraging evidence that stopping smoking in early pregnancy will reduce the risk to the fetus and newborn baby (Ahlsten *et al.* 1993).

Maternal disease

Diabetes

Some women develop abnormal glucose tolerance during pregnancy which usually improves after delivery. Their infants do not have a detectable increase in congenital abnormalities. Neither do the offspring of the rare mother with non-insulin-dependent diabetes. However, in insulin-dependent diabetes there is an increased risk of stillbirth, or a sick and often overweight infant. There is also a threefold increase (to about 6%) in the incidence of congenital malformations in the children of frankly diabetic mothers (Willhoite *et al.* 1993), with a high proportion of fatal and multiple malformations, the risk being highest for mothers with diabetic vascular complications. The risk falls to around the normal 2% if the diabetes is well controlled around conception and in early pregnancy (Kitzmiller *et al.* 1991). Diabetic women contemplating pregnancy can be reassured that meticulous control of the blood sugar at the time of conceiving and throughout pregnancy minimizes maternal and fetal risks. Ideally, the family doctor should refer pregnant diabetic patients to an expert centre, if one is accessible. Tight control of the diabetes does increase the risk of hypoglycaemia so it is wise to check that the woman's family know how to give glucagon. Diabetic mothers should be offered expert fetal anomaly scanning in the second trimester of pregnancy.

Epilepsy

Anticonvulsant drugs are associated with an increased risk of congenital abnormalities. Women of child-bearing age taking this medication should automatically be warned of this, even if they are not obviously contemplating pregnancy at the time of the consultation. If they are planning a pregnancy, a specialist reassessment of medication may be indicated, with the aim of minimizing the number of different anticonvulsant drugs taken at the time of conception. Women taking carbamazepine and/or valproate have an increased risk of having a child with a neural tube defect and should be advised to take folic acid, for example 5 mg daily before conception. Like diabetic mothers, those on anticonvulsants should be offered expert fetal anomaly scanning.

Folic acid supplementation and vitamins in pregnancy

The Medical Research Council Vitamin Study of folic acid given to women who had had a previous baby with a neural tube defect (NTD) concluded that folic acid prevented 72% of NTDs and that 4 mg a day of peri-conceptional folic acid significantly reduced the risk of recurrence. Since then an Expert Advisory Group has recommended that ' all women who are planning a pregnancy should be advised to take 0.4 mg folic acid as a daily medicinal or food supplement from when they begin trying to conceive until the 12th week of pregnancy'. This is twice the average dietary intake. For those who don't wish to take tablets, the richest sources of folic acid are green leafy vegetables (lightly cooked), jacket potatoes, yeast and beef extracts, and cereals and cereal products fortified with folic acid. There is some debate at present as to whether flour should be routinely fortified with folic acid. The birth prevalence of NTD has in fact decreased in the UK, from about 4 to 0.3 per 1000 over the last 20 years, largely due to screening and selective termination of affected pregnancies (Cuckle *et al.* 1989).

Not all vitamins are good news in pregnancy and an excessive intake (more than 10 000 IU/day) of vitamin A or related compounds in the first two months of pregnancy appears to double the normal risk of congenital abnormality, typically causing facial dysmorphology, eye, ear, and palatal defects (Rothman *et al.* 1995). Liver normally contains a relatively large amount of vitamin A and it has been suggested that pregnant women should not take tablets containing Vitamin A, or eat more than 50 g of liver a week or 100 g of liver-sausage or pate.

Counselling in pregnancy

Many women have some concern that various events that happened to them around the time of conception may have adversely affected the baby. They can usually be reassured. For example, there is no evidence that common maternal infections during pregnancy, other than those discussed above, cause a significant increase in congenital abnormalities.

Drugs in pregnancy

Most medicines taken in normal doses are probably harmless though, as a general precaution, most drug sheets advise against taking the drug during pregnancy. Relatively few drugs have been definitely shown to cause congenital malformations. The most dangerous (apart from anticonvulsants) include cytotoxic drugs, acitretin, isotretinoin and vitamin A, lithium, and warfarin. The list does not include aspirin, paracetamol, penicillin, commonly taken antihistamines, and modern oral contraceptives. However, teratogenesis is not the only risk. Drugs taken after the first trimester may adversely affect fetal growth and functional development (British National Formulary 1997).

A comprehensive, regularly updated table of the effects of drugs taken in different stages of pregnancy and lactation is included in the British National Formulary, an essential reference source for anyone offering reproductive counselling. It offers the sensible advice that 'drugs should be prescribed in pregnancy only if the expected benefit to the mother is thought to be greater than the risk to the fetus, and all drugs should be avoided if possible during the first trimester. Drugs which have been extensively used in pregnancy and appear to be usually safe should be prescribed in preference to new or untried drugs; and the smallest effective dose should be used'.

Chance of a miscarriage

Many couples are reluctant to publicize their pregnancy in the first three months because they are aware that early miscarriages are frequent. Pregnant women commonly consult either to discuss their risk of miscarrying or because they have had a slight loss of red or brown blood. Ananth and Savitz (1994) combined the evidence from several mainly hospital-based studies and reported on the association between varying amounts of vaginal bleeding and the outcome of pregnancies that did not miscarry. They concluded that bleeding before 28 weeks was associated with about twice the normal risk of a preterm or low-birthweight birth or a child with congenital malformations, and about four times the normal risk of a stillbirth or neonatal death. However, most of these studies did not distinguish between light and heavy bleeding, making it very difficult to be certain that these findings are relevant to women who have only minimal blood loss.

Many conceptions fail before the fertilized ovum is implanted, and others abort shortly afterwards leading to a slightly prolonged 'period' which may not even be delayed, so the woman does not realize that conception occurred. Everett (1997) reported on the outcome of 550 recognized pregnancies in general practice. Bleeding occurred in 117 (21%), and 67 (12%) ended in a miscarriage. However, these figures do not include unsuspected loss in early pregnancy, or miscarriages in women who do not report their pregnancy to the practice. Thus about 15% of reported pregnancies end in spontaneous miscarriage. As previously stated, the older the mother, the higher the risk of miscarriage.

A miscarriage is by far the commonest genetic complication of pregnancy. It usually occurs because a pregnancy is non-viable. This may be because no embryo has developed in the gestation sac, or an embryo has started to develop but fails to progress (usually seen as an empty sac on ultrasound examination), or an embryo that appears to be developing normally dies. Miscarriage of a live embryo or fetus is relatively uncommon. Some couples may be comforted to know that miscarriage prevents the birth of most infants with chromosomal abnormalities, especially the more severe ones. At least 50% of early miscarriages, and more in mothers over 35, are chromosomally abnormal (Alberman and Creasey 1977), the commonest abnormality being 45 X, resulting from loss of the paternal X chromosome. The later in pregnancy a miscarriage occurs, the lower the chance that it is due to a chromosomal abnormality.

Usually, a number of weeks pass between failure of the pregnancy and miscarriage because placental tissue is nourished by maternal blood and can survive for weeks, even if the embryo is absent or dead. Therefore, though most miscarriages occur around 12 weeks' gestation, most non-viable pregnancies can be identified prospectively by ultrasound examination at

7–9 weeks' gestation. This gives the woman the opportunity to decide whether to wait for bleeding to start or to have a medical or surgical evacuation of the uterus at the time non-viability is diagnosed.

Recurrent miscarriage

Women who have had one or two miscarriages seem to be at a slightly increased risk of a third one. However, even after recurrent abortion, the chance of a successful outcome seems reasonably high, probably 60–70% (Katz and Kuller 1994). Referral for further investigations is usually indicated after two or three successive miscarriages. Possible causes include parental chromosomal abnormalities, a congenital or acquired disorder of the uterus or cervix (for example, an incompetent os), or a maternal disease such as diabetes, but no reason will be discovered in about half of women with recurrent abortion.

X-rays in pregnancy

Mothers-to-be are often concerned about the risk of inadvertent diagnostic radiology injuring their baby. Though it is advisable to restrict non-essential X-rays to the first few days following the onset of a period (10-day rule), the present risk of damage appears to be slight. It is sensible to consider postponing an abdominal or pelvic X-ray if the period is overdue. The main anxiety appears to be the danger of irradiation *in utero* increasing the risk of childhood cancer. According to Bury *et al.* (1995), exposure to 'the highest doses regularly achieved in diagnostic radiology' after the first missed period might double the risk of a fatal childhood cancer before the age of 15 to one in 1300. Diagnostic X-rays in pregnancy appear to have an insignificant effect on the incidence of other adverse affects on the fetus, such as congenital abnormalities. There is no evidence of harm from radiation from computers or video screens (Parazzini *et al.* 1993).

Standard prenatal tests

Ultrasound examination

It is unusual for a woman to get through pregnancy without at least a couple of ultrasound examinations, sometimes a cause of concern to a couple, perhaps because they associate ultrasound with X-rays. Ultrasound is a method of producing an image by reflection of sound waves, like deep-sea sonar. There is no convincing evidence that it is at all detrimental to the fetus, and parents-to-be are usually delighted to see a moving image of their developing child (Docker 1992) (Chapter 13). However, the results obtained can be the prelude to extremely difficult decisions about amniocentesis and possible late termination of pregnancy.

Maternal serum alphafetoprotein (AFP) estimation

The level of AFP in maternal serum can be used for screening for some fetal malformations that disrupt the continuity of the fetal skin. Maternal AFP screening can be organized through the hospital antenatal clinic or be done in collaboration with community midwives and general practitioners. A raised AFP is a cause of anxiety for a couple until it has been sorted out. Results are usually expressed as 'multiples of the median' (MoMs) for each centre rather than in absolute figures because normal values vary with method, ethnic group, and gestational age. The commonest causes are underestimation of the gestational age and multiple pregnancies. A maternal serum AFP of more than about 2.5 MoMs includes all pregnancies where the fetus has anencephaly and most where it has spina bifida in addition to non-viable pregnancies and growth-retarded fetuses (Wald and Cuckle 1992).

Initially, the next step when the maternal serum AFP was raised was amniocentesis to assay amniotic fluid AFP and enzymes specific for neural tube defects. However, careful ultrasound is replacing amniocentesis because it is safe, accurate (at least in expert centres), and will detect other congenital malformations.

Identification of chromosomal abnormalities

The longest established of prenatal diagnosis services is the offer to older mothers of amniocentesis (and later chorionic villus sampling) to identify the chromosomal make-up of a fetus (karyotyping). It is usually offered only to women with a more than one in 250 risk of having an affected child – giving an up to 99.5% false positive rate. Until recently, the only two groups of pregnant women who could be shown to have this level of risk were those over 35–37 years old and mothers who had already had a previously affected pregnancy. However, offering karyotyping to these groups alone would have a limited impact on the total birth incidence of infants with chromosomal disorders. Uptake of testing by *all* pregnant women over 35 could prevent the birth of 15–55% of Down's syndrome fetuses in different European countries, the figure being lowest in Eastern Europe where parents are predominantly young (Modell *et al.* 1991).

Screening now is much more efficient because of the discovery of several biochemical markers in the maternal blood. When the fetus has Down's syndrome the human chorionic gonadotrophin (hCG) is often relatively raised and the unconjugated oestriol is relatively low, as is the alphafetoprotein (the 'triple test'). In addition, the neutrophil alkaline phosphatase (NAP) can also be raised. These markers are measured at about 15–20 weeks' gestation and integrated with maternal age. It is then possible to give a statistical risk for every pregnant women that her fetus actually has Down's syndrome, prenatal diagnosis being offered to those couples with a risk of less than one in 250. The screening process would be most efficient if all pregnant women were offered the tests (about 60% of Down's pregnancies identified).

However, this may not be considered very cost-effective. Testing only women aged 25 years and older will reduce the workload by about one third, and lead to a 5% fall in the detection rate. Limiting the triple test to women aged 30 years and over means that only about 30% of pregnancies are tested, but only 43% of affected pregnancies are identified (Cuckle 1994).

It is important to explain to a couple that these tests are not a replacement for amniocentesis, chorionic villus sampling, or a detailed fetal anomaly scan. They will simply identify women at increased risk of having a child with a chromosomal anomaly. In fact, very few 'screen-positive' results mean an affected infant. It is also important to emphasize that a 'screen-negative' result does not exclude the possibility of the fetus being affected. Even with the best screening methods available, only about 60% of women bearing a Down's syndrome fetus will be identified; in the remainder, all the test results will be in the normal range (Wald *et al.* 1992).

It may soon be possible to diagnose a Down's syndrome fetus in the first trimester of pregnancy by ultrasound examination (increased thickness of the nape of the neck) and by the measurement of another placental product, the Pregnancy Associated Plasma Protein A (PAPP-A).

Conclusion

Information on maintaining the health of the mother-to-be and the fetus are part of mainstream primary care. It is provided most effectively by a team approach, involving the woman and her partner, midwife, GP, health visitor, and sometimes the practice nurse. Clearly written educational material is an invaluable back-up for the consultation. Much is available, for example booklets and leaflets on folic acid and the prevention of neural tube defects, the dangers of infections such as toxoplasmosis in pregnancy, and the reasons for testing for carriers of common recessively inherited diseases. Though pre-pregnancy advice is the ideal, many of the issues are also pertinent to early pregnancy.

References

Abel, E. L. (1995). An update on incidence of FAS: FAS is not an equal opportunity birth defect. *Neurotoxicol. Teratology*, 17(4), 437–43.

Ahlsten, G., Cnattingius, S., and Lindmark, G. (1993). Cessation of smoking during pregnancy improves foetal growth and reduces infant morbidity in the neonatal period: a population-based prospective study. *Acta Paediatrica*, 82(2), 177–81.

Alberman, E. D. and Creasey, M. R. (1977). Frequency of chromosomal abnormalities in miscarriages and perinatal deaths. *Journal of Medical Genetics*, 14, 313–15.

Ananth, C. V. and Savitz, D. A. (1994). Vaginal bleeding and adverse reproductive outcomes: a meta-analysis. *Paediatric and Perinatal Epidemiology*, 8, 62–78.

Baird, P. A., Anderson, T. W., Newcombe, H. B., and Lowry, R.B. (1988). Genetic disorders in children and young adults: a population study. *American Journal of Human Genetics*, **42**: 677–93.

Bowman, J. M., and Pollock, J. M. (1965). Amniotic fluid spectrophotometry and early delivery in the management of erythroblastosis fetalis. *Pediatrics*, 815–32, May 1965.

British National Formulary no. 32. (1997). British Medical Association and the Royal Pharmaceutal Society of Great Britain.

Bury, B., Hufton, A. and Adams, J. (1995). Radiation and women of child-bearing potential. *British Medical Journal*, **310**, 1022–3.

Cuckle, H. S. (1994). Down's syndrome screening: the use of models in risk calculation, formulating policy, informing users, and quality assessment. *Proceedings of the UK NEQAS Meeting*, **1**, 112–19.

Cuckle, H. S., Wald, N. J., and Cuckle, P. M. (1989). Antenatal diagnosis of neural tube defects in England and Wales. *Prenatal Diagnosis*, **9**, 393–400.

Cutts, F. T. (1996). Revaccination against measles and rubella. *British Medical Journal*, **312**, 589–90.

Docker, M. F. (1992). Ultrasound imaging techniques. In: *Prenatal diagnosis and screening* (ed. D. J. H. Brock, C. R. Rodeck, and M. A. Ferguson-Smith). Churchill Livingstone, London.

Eberhart-Phillips, J. E., Frederick, P. D., Baron, R. C., and Mascola, L. (1993). Measles in pregnancy: a descriptive study of 58 cases. *Obstetrics and Gynecology*, **82**(5), 797–801.

Ellwood, D. A. (1995). The role of ultrasound in prenatal diagnosis. In: *Handbook of prenatal diagnosis* (ed. R. J. Trent). Cambridge University Press, Cambridge.

Everett, C. (1997). Incidence and outcome of bleeding before the 20th week of pregnancy: prospective study from general practice. *British Medical Journal*, **315**, 32–4.

Expert Advisory Group (1992). *Folic acid and the prevention of neural tube defects*. Department of Health, London.

Hanshaw, J. B., Dudgeon, J. A., and Marshall, W. C. (1985). Viral diseases of the fetus and newborn. In: *Major problems in clinical pediatrics*, Vol. 17 (2nd edn). Saunders, New York.

Harper, P. S. (1988). *Practical genetic counselling* (3rd edn). Wright, London.

Harris, H., Scotcher, D., Hartley, N., Wallace, A., Craufurd, D., and Harris, R. (1993). Cystic fibrosis carrier testing in early pregnancy by general practitioners. *British Medical Journal*, **306**, 1580–3.

Hook, E. B. (1992). Prevalence, risks, and recurrence. In: *Prenatal diagnosis and screening* (ed. D. J. H. Brock, C. R. Rodeck, M. A. Ferguson-Smith). Churchill Livingstone, London.

Johnstone, F. D. (1996). HIV and pregnancy. *British Journal of Obstetrics and Gynaecology*, **103**, 1184–90.

Jones, E. M., McCulloch, S. Y., Reeves, D. S., and MacGowan, A. P. (1994). A 10-year survey of the epidemiology and clinical aspects of listeriosis in a provincial English city. *Journal of Infectious Diseases*, **29**(1), 91–103.

Katz,V. L. and Kuller, J. A. (1994). Recurrent miscarriage. *American Journal of Perinatology*, 11(6), 386–97.

Kitzmiller, J. L., Gavin, L. A., Gin, G. D., Jovanovic-Peterson, L., Main, E. K., and Zigrang W. D. (1991). Preconception care of diabetes: glycemic control prevents congenital anomalies. *Journal of the American Medical Association*, 265(6), 731–6.

Lachelin, G. C. L. (1985). *Miscarriage: the facts.* Oxford University Press, Oxford.

Larroque, B., Kaminski, M., Dehaene, P., Subtil, D., Delfosse, M. J., and Querleu, D. (1995). Moderate prenatal alcohol exposure and psychomotor development at preschool age *American Journal of Public Health*, 85(12), 1654–61.

MacDonagh, S. E., Masters, J., Helps, B. A., Tookey, P. A., Ades, A. E., and Gibb, D. M. (1996). Descriptive survey of antenatal HIV testing in London: policy, uptake, and detection. *British Medical Journal*, 313, 532–3.

Matsui, D. (1994). Prevention, diagnosis, and treatment of fetal toxoplasmosis. *Clinical Perinatology*, 21(3), 675–89.

Miller, E., Tookey, P., Morgan-Capner, P., Hesketh, L., Brown, D., Waight, P., *et al.* (1994). Rubella surveillance to June 1994: third joint report from the PHLS and the National Congenital Rubella Surveillance Programme. *Community Dis. Rep. CDR Rev.*, 4(12): R146–52.

Modell, B. and Kuliev, A. K. (1990). Changing paternal age distribution and the human mutation rate in Europe. *Human Genetics*, 86, 198–202.

Modell, B., Kuliev, A. K., and Wagner, M. (1991). *Community genetics services in Europe.* WHO Regional Office for Europe, WHO Regional Publications. European series no. 38.

Modell, B. and Modell, M. (1992). *Towards a healthy baby: congenital disorders and the new genetics in primary health care.* Oxford University Press, Oxford.

Modell, B. and Anionwu, A. (1996). Guidelines for screening for haemoglobin disorders: service specifications for low- and high-prevalence DHAs. In: *Ethnicity and health: reviews of literature and guidance for purchasers in the areas of cardiovascular disease, mental health, and haemoglobinopathies.* CRD Report 5, pp 127–224. NHS Centre for Reviews and Dissemination, York.

Mombro, M., Perathoner, C., Leone, A., Nicocia, M., Moiraghi-Ruggenini, A., Zotti, C., *et al.* (1995). Congenital toxoplasmosis: 10-year follow-up. *European Journal of Pediatrics*, 154(8), 635–9.

MRC Vitamin Study Research Group (1991). Prevention of neural tube defects: results of the Medical Research Council Vitamin Study. *Lancet*, 238, 131–7.

Olsen, J., Pereira, A. de C., and Olsen, S. F. (1991). Does maternal tobacco smoking modify the effect of alcohol on fetal growth? *American Journal of Public-Health*, 81(1), 69–73.

Parazzini, F., Luchini, L., La Vecchia, C., and Crosignani, P. G. (1993). Video display terminal use during pregnancy and reproductive outcome – a meta-analysis. *Journal of Epidemiology and Community-Health*, 47(4), 265–8.

Pastuszak, A. L., Levy, M., Schick, B., Zuber, C., Feldkamp, M., Gladstone, J., *et al.* (1994). Outcome after maternal varicella infection in the first 20 weeks of pregnancy. *New England Journal of Medicine*, 330(13), 901–5.

Rothman, K. J., Moore, L. L., Singer, M. R., Nguyen, U. S., Mannino, S., and Milunsky, A. (1995). Teratogenicity of high vitamin A intake. *New England Journal of Medicine,* **333**(21), 1369–73.

Smithells, R. W., Sheppard, S., and Holzel, H. (1990). Congenital rubella in Great Britain 1971–1988. *Health Trends,* **22**(2), 73–6.

Stein, Z., Kline, J., Susser, E., Shrout, P., Warburton, D., and Susser, M. (1980). Maternal age and spontaneous abortion. In: *Human embryonic and fetal death* (ed. E. B. Hook and I. H. Porter), pp.107–27. Academic Press, New York and London.

Taylor, J. A. and Sanderson, M. (1995). A re-examination of the risk factors for the sudden infant death syndrome. *Journal of Pediatrics,* **126**(6), 887–91.

Wald, N. J. and Cuckle, H. S. (1992). *Biochemical screening.* In: *Prenatal diagnosis and screening* (ed. D. J. H. Brock, C. R. Rodeck, and M. A. Ferguson-Smith). Churchill Livingstone, London.

Wald, N. J., Kennard, A., Densem, J. W., Cuckle, H. S., Chard, T., and Butler, L. (1992). Antenatal maternal serum screening for Down's syndrome: results of a demonstration study. *British Medical Journal,* **305**, 391–3.

WHO (1989). Glucose-6-phosphate dehydrogenase deficiency: report of a WHO working group. *Bulletin of the World Health Organization,* **67**, 601–11.

Willhoite, M. B., Bennert Jr, H. W., Palomaki, G. E., Zaremba, M. M., Herman, W. H., Williams, J. R., *et al.* (1993). The impact of preconception counseling on pregnancy outcomes: the experience of the Maine Diabetes in Pregnancy Program. *Diabetes-Care,* **16**(2), 450–5.

CHAPTER SEVENTEEN

New thoughts on the physiology of pregnancy

James J. Walker and Nigel A. B. Simpson

Introduction

Pregnancy produces considerable physiological changes in the mother to accommodate the developing baby, to allow growth and development to occur in a favourable environment, and to deliver the baby at the optimal time. These changes have traditionally been regarded in terms of the maternal response to the developing needs of her baby. However, the majority of physiological processes are determined and implemented well in advance of their needs and are driven separately by the mother's body and the placenta.

The mother prepares herself for the implantation of the embryo and the beginnings of pregnancy, then reacts to the presence of the embryo by protecting herself from the potential risks that pregnancy can bring, and finally prepares for delivery and postpartum life.

The placenta competes with the mother's body to produce the optimal intrauterine environment to allow the fetus to grow and develop, alters the mothers physiological control mechanisms to suit the demands of the growing baby, and prepares the mother for post-partum care of the newborn. The importance of the placenta as a controller of events has led to the placenta being labelled the third brain (Yen 1994).

It is this balance of fetal/placental demands and maternal response that decides the success or failure of the pregnancy. The baby wants the best environment possible but the mother must protect herself so she can survive to care for her baby and any future children. As far as the baby is concerned its survival is paramount. For the mother's body, however, it is not and any given pregnancy will be sacrificed if the demands on her are excessive or dangerous so she can try again.

In this chapter we shall examine the various stages of physiological change and the independent roles of the placenta and mother as they exert their separate influences during pregnancy. We will also discuss in five parts how knowledge of these processes can enable appropriate care during pregnancy:

(1) preparation for implantation and implantation

(2) early pregnancy changes

(3) later pregnancy changes

(4) labour and delivery

(5) post-partum changes.

Preparation for implantation and implantation

Preparation for implantation

The woman's body prepares for pregnancy every month with a regular cycle of developing follicle, endometrial growth, ovulation, and endometrial preparation for implantation. Other animal species either ovulate in response to intercourse or have estrous cycles that produce fertile seasons and times of inactivity when sexual intercourse is not permitted. Therefore, the human female is preparing for, and expecting the possibility of, pregnancy each month. Failure of implantation produces endometrial shedding and menstrual bleeding.

Each cycle, usually one follicle develops under the influence of follicle-stimulating hormone (FSH). As the follicle grows it produces oestradiol which stimulates new endometrial growth. When the follicle is about 20 mm in size, enough oestradiol is produced to stimulate the release of the luteinizing hormone (LH) from the anterior pituitary and ovulation follows within 24 hours. This 'follicular phase' determines the length of the menstrual cycle as, from the point of ovulation, the system is self-regulating. Following ovulation, the follicle converts into the corpus luteum which produces progesterone as well as continuing to produce oestrogen (luteal phase). The endometrium is converted to the secretory phase in preparation for implantation. This is crucial for a successful pregnancy. The time from ovulation to implantation is between five and seven days and only then is the endometrium receptive. Therefore, the endometrium must be ready when the embryo arrives and vice versa.

Fertilization and ovum transport

The released ovum can survive for 24–48 hours before fertilization, so the fertilized egg must be kept within the fallopian tube for at least five days until the endometrium is ready to receive it. Fertilization usually takes place at the ampullary end of the fallopian tube and the developing embryo travels slowly towards the uterine cavity over the next few days. It goes through symmetric cell division forming the morula (12–16 cell stage) and then the blastocyst. At this stage the conceptus is comprised of approximately 60 cells; it is defined by a well-demarcated eccentric inner cell mass, an acellular blastocystic cavity, and a single outer layer of cells. The inner cell mass – around 25% of the total – is destined to become the embryo; the outer layer – the majority of the blastocyst – at this time will demonstrate trophoblastic differentiation and act as the interface between the mother and her baby. When the blastocyst enters the uterine cavity, the process of implantation begins. Although these changes occur while in the fallopian tube, an active role for the mother in the development of the embryo at this stage is speculative. There must be some interaction between embryo and fallopian tube but there is no obvious maternal physiological response. When a tube is damaged by infection, ectopic pregnancy is more likely, suggesting that tubal cilia are involved in controlling the movement of the embryo towards the uterine cavity. In *in vitro* fertilization, where the embryo is inserted straight into the uterine cavity several days before it normally would arrive, successful implantation occurs. This suggests that the tube might aid in the controlling of the arrival of the embryo in the uterine cavity at the appropriate time but passage through the tube is not necessary.

Implantation

The processes of implantation and placentation, in which the trophoblast migrate into the decidua and myometrium, adapting the maternal vasculature, largely determine the future course of the pregnancy. Failure of this process accounts for a high proportion of both early and later pregnancy failure, fetal growth restriction, and hypertensive disorder (Bulmer 1992; Serle *et al.* 1994). It is believed that up to 50% of the embryos that reach this stage fail to successfully implant (Cross *et al.* 1994). Most of these losses occur prior to confirmation of the pregnancy by conventional tests but can be found if sensitive serum assays are performed.

Therefore, it is at this point that the maternal and fetal interaction is at its most critical. Around day seven since the LH peak, or day 21 of the menstrual cycle, the endometrium is most receptive to the implanting blastocyst. From this moment measurable levels of human chorionic gonadotrophin (hCG) are found in maternal serum. This hormone is secreted by trophoblast and primarily exerts its effect on the corpus luteum. Maintenance of this structure ensures a sustained production of progesterone, which at this stage is required for the continued decidualization of the endometrium and deferral of menstruation.

Therefore, from day 21 of the menstrual cycle, the mother's body is aware of the presence of the pregnancy and the normal menstrual cycle is interrupted leading to amenorrhoea – one of the first outward signs of pregnancy. As the embryo implants, the mother's physiology is taken over and the mother begins her reaction to it. Other early maternal signs that can occur before the first missed period are breast, particularly nipple, sensitivity and nausea. Both of these are due to increasing levels of pregnancy hormones.

Decidualization of the endometrium is really a continuation of the development seen in the luteal phase. The most important changes relate to the increase in the presence of immunocompetent cells, particularly large granular macrophages and lymphocytes (Sargent 1993). These cells appear to be important for the mother's ability to recognize the invading trophoblast and respond appropriately to it. This is a unique immunological event (Aplin 1996).

It used to be thought that there was a barrier between the fetal and maternal tissue, but it is now know that there is direct contact between the maternal cells, both decidual and blood, and the placental trophoblastic cells. These cells do not express the usual polymorphic class I and II MHC antigens that are responsible for the normal immune response (Sargent 1993; Schmidt and Orr 1993). Some of the cells do express a unique HLA-G-encoded class I MHC molecule and are believed to play a role in the maternal/fetal immune response (Sargent 1993; Schmidt and Orr 1993). There is also evidence of immunosuppression by the placental hormones which may result in a degree of maternal immunosusceptibility, particularly to viral infections. All these changes allow the trophoblastic cells to invade into the maternal tissues.

After implantation, the trophoblastic cells proliferate markedly and differentiate into villous trophoblast which form the placenta and non-villous trophoblast which invade the decidua and the maternal spiral arteries. It is the invasion of the decidua around and within the lumen of the maternal vessels that convert them into the classic funnel-shaped vessels which supply the intervillous space (Wells and Bulmer 1988). It is the failure of these changes that precede the placental insufficiency of later pregnancy.

There is a well-defined sequence of events starting with the development of the rudimentary intervillous space by the end of the second week post-conception, followed in the next two weeks by the invasion of the decidual (spiral) arteries. Initially, the trophoblast impedes flow within the spiral arteries, protecting the developing conceptus from excessively pulsatile flow until a functional uteroplacental circulation is established. Fetal heart activity can be seen by ultrasonographic studies at this time as well as flow within the umbilical vessels, indicating the establishment of the fetoplacental and uteroplacental components of the placental vasculature (Jauniaux 1996; Simpson *et al*. 1996).

By 10 weeks' gestation, the intervillous space has formed and is filled by maternal blood supplied from the developing uteroplacental arteries. The early placental villi develop within these spaces and fetal blood is brought into intimate apposition with maternal blood, only separated by maternal endothelium and fetal trophoblast.

Early pregnancy changes (0–12 weeks)

Embryogenesis

Even before implantation, there is a significant degree of organization with separation of the inner cell mass from the trophoblast. Any insult at this time tends to be absolute; in other words, either the embryo survives intact or is lost. By the time of implantation (day seven), the inner cell mass has begun to differentiate. Three separate layers are formed: the ectoderm that will form the nervous system and the skin; the mesoderm that will become the cardiovascular and urogenital systems, bone, muscle, and connective tissue; and the endoderm that will become the lungs and gastrointestinal tract.

Therefore, organogenesis begins at around the time of the first missed period and is largely complete by 12 weeks after the last menstrual period. Sex differentiation is complete by 16 weeks. If infection or drugs are to interfere with the development of the embryo, it must occur within this time scale. Damage can still occur after this time, but this will be to developed tissue.

The placenta

The syncytiotrophoblast has a variety of organelles which appear to be involved with both protein and steroid synthesis. Therefore, the syncytio-trophoblast represents the major site of hormone production within the placenta (Fox 1978). These hormones are largely responsible for many of the adaptive changes in maternal physiology. This is the mechanism through which the fetus and placenta can exert an influence at remote maternal sites and begin to direct the mother's physiology towards maintaining the pregnancy. The intention is to create an environment that will allow fetal growth and development in relative safety.

Maternal changes

The mother is the only source of nutrition and oxygen for the growing fetus and the only method of removal of carbon dioxide and nitrogen. There must be changes made in the maternal physiology to facilitate these functions. These changes must be present early and adequately enough so that, when demands are made on the mother's body, she has the capacity to respond. Therefore, the changes that are made happen early in the first trimester, long before the need and to a far greater degree than is usually necessary. It is the failure of these early responses that increase the chance of later pregnancy complications. The first half of pregnancy can be seen as the preparation for the growth seen in the second. The changes in the different systems will be taken in turn but it is important to remember that they do not occur in isolation.

Cardiovascular changes

The heart and circulation undergo extensive anatomic and functional changes during pregnancy (de Swiet 1991a). Haemodynamic changes include alterations in cardiac output, blood volume, and systemic vascular resistance resulting in changes in arterial pressure. Most of these changes occur in the first trimester, with lesser changes throughout the rest of pregnancy and further alterations during labour and the puerperium when the physiology returns to normal.

Cardiac output (CO) increases early in pregnancy from a non-pregnancy value of 4.9 l/min to 6.6 l/min by 12 weeks (Robson et al. 1989). Although both heart rate and stroke volume contribute to the increase, the earliest haemodynamic change associated with pregnancy is an increase in heart rate of 8 bpm by the end of the first trimester. This is believed to be the major contributor to the increase in CO.

To accommodate this increase in cardiac output, there is an accompanying increase in circulating blood volume from 4.5 litres to 6 litres. This is largely due to a rise in plasma volume and a lesser increase in the red cell mass. This produces the so-called 'physiological anaemia'. With the increase in red cell mass, the increased oxygen-carrying capacity is far greater than is generally required throughout pregnancy.

The increase in plasma volume, with a relative reduction of haematocrit, allows for an increased flow of blood to the tissues and a greater overall O_2 delivery to the developing fetus without a corresponding increase in whole blood viscosity. The increase in plasma volume is related to fetal size and greater increases are seen in women with larger babies and multiple pregnancy. The greater increase in plasma volume also enables a correspondingly improved removal of CO_2 as this is carried in the blood mostly dissolved in plasma.

This increase in blood volume will tend to increase the preload on the heart which in turn affects the stroke volume. The greater the preload, the greater the stroke volume. This further increases the cardiac output.

Conditions that interfere with the maternal ability to increase the cardiac output are particularly dangerous in pregnancy. These include stenotic valve lesions and left ventricular function defects. Both of these conditions produce symptoms of cardiac failure. Anyone presenting with breathlessness in early pregnancy should be investigated for potential pathology although the previously common mitral stenosis is now rare.

Generally, these changes produce an increased exercise tolerance in early pregnancy and women should be encouraged to continue their normal exercise programmes as long as they feel comfortable.

Venous pressure

If there is an increase in blood volume, there would normally be an increase in the venous pressure and a tendency to cardiac failure from circulatory overload. Although femoral venous pressure has been reported to be elevated, this reflects obstruction from the gravid uterus in later pregnancy. There is no evidence that central venous or pulmonary capillary wedge pressure is increased during pregnancy. Studies suggest that venous distensibility and capacitance are increased during pregnancy (Anumba *et al.* 1996).

These changes are most noticeable during the second trimester and this allows the increased blood volume to be accommodated without an increase in venous pressure. Venous pooling, particularly when standing up, probably contributes to the fainting of early pregnancy.

Arterial blood pressure

Systolic blood pressure changes little in pregnancy whereas diastolic pressure drops by up to 15 mmHg, reaching a nadir from 12–16 weeks' gestation, and thereafter rises to about pre-pregnancy values by term (MacGillivray *et al.* 1969). This relates to changes in peripheral vascular resistance.

As cardiac output increases and blood pressure (BP) falls during the first half of pregnancy, vascular resistance must fall to allow for this. The fall in systemic resistance reaches its lowest level by 20 weeks' gestation when values are 34% below those calculated prior to conception (Robson *et al.* 1989).

Therefore, the afterload is decreased during the first half of pregnancy due to the reduction in vascular resistance and blood viscosity. Towards the end of pregnancy there is an increase in both, leading to the rise in BP.

It is difficult to know how these changes come about, but they are probably interdependent. Arterial and venous vasodilatation are primary changes related to alterations in the control of vascular tone. This produces an increase in the heart rate to maintain blood pressure but also produces an 'underfill' situation where the mother responds with renal sodium and water retention with expansion of the extracellular and plasma volume compartments.

The mechanisms underlying the alterations in vascular resistance are unclear but are probably due to a reduction in vasoconstrictor response (Brown and Gallery 1994) and an increase in vasodilator activity by the vascular endothelium (Weiner *et al.* 1994; Anumba *et al.* 1996).

Structural changes in the heart

The ventricular wall thickens throughout pregnancy reaching values up to 50% above those in the non-pregnant state. These changes are similar to those seen after 12 weeks of exercise training. This may be the reason for the increase in exercise tolerance many women have in early pregnancy.

Valve diameters and areas also increase resulting in an increase in the incidence of regurgitant murmurs in pregnancy, particularly at the mitral valve.

Changes in organ blood flow

An increase in blood volume and cardiac output means a redistribution of blood to various organs. Although the uterus will take up to 25% of the cardiac output by the end of pregnancy, this is not true in the first trimester when most of the increase is seen.

Peripheral blood flow is increased substantially, primarily related to cutaneous vasodilatation with little or no change in muscle blood flow. The nasal mucosa becomes hyperaemic and congested causing the characteristic nasal 'stuffiness' of pregnant women and the increased risk of epistaxes. This increase in skin blood flow helps dissipate the extra heat generated by the fetus.

Cerebral blood flow is unchanged in pregnancy and mammary and coronary blood flow increase.

Renal blood flow rises in the first trimester and exceeds non-pregnant values by nearly 50%, coinciding with the changes in cardiac output.

Pulmonary blood flow also increases. This is achieved without an increase in right ventricular and pulmonary artery pressure which means that lung peripheral resistance is lowered, probably by dilatation of the pulmonary vasculature. This causes the ejection systolic murmur found in 92% of pregnant women.

Respiratory changes

The fetus requires the maternal respiratory system to adapt to meet two needs: the efficient removal of CO_2 and an increased O_2 requirement.

The non-pregnant values of arterial PCO_2 are generally between 35 and 40 mmHg. Levels start to fall in the first trimester of pregnancy and values are between 26 and 34 mmHg by term. This reduction in PCO_2 is mediated through a resetting of the respiratory centre, resulting in an increase in the minute ventilation. A lower level of PCO_2 enhances the passage of CO_2 from the fetus to the mother without embarrassing the maternal physiology (de Swiet 1991b). The decrease in PCO_2 results in a fall in plasma bicarbonate concentration as well as other plasma buffers but compensatory adjustments are made and the arterial pH values remain between 7.40 and 7.44.

There is an increase in oxygen consumption of between 15–20% during pregnancy. This is due to increased demands of both mother and fetus. In the first two trimesters, the mother produces most of the increases with demands from cardiac, respiratory, and renal function. In the third trimester, the uterus, placenta, fetus, and breasts contribute up to 50% of the increase.

The increase in minute ventilation may be expected to raise PO_2 but most studies have found little significant change. Because of the shape of the haemoglobin dissociation curve, any small increment in PO_2 will have little effect on haemoglobin saturation. The change in red cell mass is the major contributor to the increase in O_2 supply to the fetus. Since fetal haemoglobin has a greater affinity to O_2 than adult haemoglobin, O_2 transfers easily from maternal blood to the fetus.

Changes in minute ventilation

Since the respiratory rate remains unchanged in pregnancy, the increase in minute ventilation is largely due to the changes in tidal volume which increases from a non-pregnant value of around 500 ml to between 650 and 700 ml. Most of this change occurs by seven weeks of pregnancy. Although there is a small increase in the physiological dead space of about 60 ml, most of the increase in minute ventilation goes to increasing the alveolar ventilation which in turn reduces PCO_2.

The increased minute ventilation in pregnancy is achieved by breathing more deeply, not more frequently. There is an increase of the diaphragmatic movement and flaring of the ribs.

Anatomical changes

In pregnancy, there is a 4 cm upward displacement of the diaphragm which occurs early and is not due to pressure from the gravid uterus. To compensate for this, the circumference of the chest increases by approximately 15 cm. The internal volume of the thoracic cavity is unchanged.

Lung capacities, volumes, and pulmonary function

The changes in thoracic diameters would be expected to affect the various lung capacities. However, there is little change in the vital capacity apart from a small increase of 100–200 ml in late pregnancy. Similarly, there is only a small, progressive increase in the inspiratory capacity from a non-pregnant value to around 2200–2500 ml at term.

However, both residual volume and expiratory reserve decrease in pregnancy. This results in a reduced functional residual capacity of 2300 ml at term compared to 2800 ml when not pregnant. Hence the mother is more vulnerable to acute respiratory embarrassment.

There is no change in the forced expiratory volume (FEV_1) or the peak expiratory flow rate.

The effects of these changes

These changes, in conjunction with the cardiovascular ones, tend to increase the athletic performance of the mother in early pregnancy. They produce a significant degree of protection to the mother from the demands of chronic respiratory illness. Chronic lung diseases, such as cystic fibrosis, are not a contraindication to pregnancy as long as acute exacerbations can be controlled. It is usually an acute event (e.g. very severe asthma) which will compromise a pregnancy and susceptible mothers require appropriate surveillance.

Renal changes

The developing fetus requires an efficient maternal excretory system. This is achieved by an increase in the glomerular filtration, partially in response to the increased cardiac output. This results in an increased urine flow, manifest by urinary frequency in the first trimester. This, in itself, poses little risk, only inconvenience. The renal anatomy changes little although there is some dilatation of the renal pelvis and ureters, believed to be secondary to progesterone-induced relaxation. With the enlarging uterus there is increased pressure on the bladder which is seen in the first trimester when the uterus is a pelvic organ and again in late pregnancy from fetal head pressure. This also contributes to urinary frequency.

Functional changes

The increase in the glomerular filtration rate produces an increase in the loss of various substances usually found in the urine in small amounts. These are varyingly reabsorbed and/or excreted in the tubular system. Therefore, what is lost in the urine will depend on both the amount filtered by the glomerulus and the ability of the tubular system to control what passes through.

Nitrogen waste

The obvious consequences of these changes and the underlying reason for them is the increase, of around 50%, in creatinine and urea clearance. These changes begin in the luteal phase of the menstrual cycle and continue throughout the first trimester when most of the increase occurs. The systemic effect of this is a reduction in serum creatinine and urea as well as uric acid. This is important when assessing renal function in pregnancy as the normal levels are around half those seen in the non-pregnant. This has the effect of encouraging transfer of these waste substances from the fetus to the mother across the placenta.

Women with chronic renal failure also see an increase in renal function in pregnancy but, since their reserve may be reduced, they often run into problems in later pregnancy when the demands increase and should therefore embark on pregnancy only after appropriate counselling. There is no evidence, however, that any long-term further damage will occur if the pregnancy is successfully completed.

Glycosuria

A side-effect of these changes is the increase in the urinary loss of glucose and protein. Glycosuria is found in up to 60% of all pregnant women. The main reason for this is the increased glomerular filtration rate although there may also be some decreased tubular reabsorption. The glycosuria is usually sporadic and is a poor predictor of glucose intolerance but if it persists at the routine checks, tests for diabetes should be carried out. Because of this many centres have stopped the routine screening of urine at the antenatal clinic although others still value its use in screening for proteinuria.

Infection

Because of the structural changes in pregnancy, urinary tract infection is more common. About 6% of pregnant women will have asymptomatic bacteruria and around 1% will develop acute pyelonephritis (Peckham and Marshal 1983). Infections in the urine increase the incidence of preterm delivery (Schieve *et al.* 1994). If the bacteruria is treated, the incidence of frank infection can be reduced. Therefore, it is recommended that asymptomatic bacteriuria in pregnancy is treated in order to try and prevent progression to pylonephritis and premature labour (Grio *et al.* 1994). All women should have a routine urine culture at the beginning of pregnancy. Women with a structural or historical predisposition are particularly at risk. They should have regular MSUs and, if infection occurs, may benefit from prophylactic antibiotic treatment to prevent recurrence of infection.

Total body fluid

As well as the increase in blood volume, there is an increase in the interstitial fluid which demonstrates itself as tissue oedema in later pregnancy. This retention of fluid is associated with the softening and stretching of tissues and is partly responsible for the antenatal complaints of nasal stuffiness and joint laxity.

Approximately 40% of all pregnant women will demonstrate clinical oedema and, although a higher incidence is found in hypertensive pregnancies, it is of no clinical significance. The routine assessment of oedema in pregnancy should be abandoned although, if there has been a sudden apparent increase in swelling or body weight noticed by the woman or attendant staff, this should be investigated further.

Haematological changes

The haemoglobin levels fall in pregnancy due to the dilution effect and there is no change in corpuscular size or cellular haemoglobin concentration. Although the haematocrit can be increased if prophylactic iron is given, there is no evidence that this is necessary or desired. In fact, recent studies suggest that a haemoglobin of around 10 gm/dl is optimal (Steer *et al.* 1995) and increasing this may be harmful. As long as there are adequate maternal iron stores there should be no problem, and routine iron supplementation is not necessary and might be dangerous. Adequate iron must be available in the third trimester when fetal stores are accumulated to serve its needs for extrauterine life. Therefore if there are signs of anaemia, treatment in the third trimester is necessary.

Folic acid prophylaxis has taken on a new significance in recent years with the evidence of a reduction in the incidence of neural tube defect if supplementation is started some weeks prior to conception (Wald 1994). It was always advisable as megaloblastic anaemia in pregnancy is nearly always due to folate deficiency. It is thought that the pregnancy requirements are unlikely to be met from dietary folate alone, particularly in multiple pregnancy, and folic acid supplementation should be commenced by all women at least one month before conception. There is no convincing evidence that folate deficiency increases the risk of spontaneous miscarriage or abruptio placenta but because of other advantages, it is recommended for all pregnant women.

There is a marked increase in the white cell count in pregnancy which is largely neutrophils, with a relative reduction in lymphocytes (MacLean *et al.* 1992). This makes the use of the white blood cell measurement in pregnancy less valuable. These changes appear to be related to the general change in the immunological system and the importance of the neutrophil in pregnancy immunology (Billington 1992; Sargent 1993; Dejongh *et al.* 1996).

Coagulation factors

There are major changes in the coagulation system in order to protect the mother at delivery (Greer *et al.* 1992). Haemorrhage is traditionally the major cause of maternal mortality. There is an increase in the levels of the prothrombin complex, factors VII, X, and VIII, and fibrinogen. Fibrin degradation products (FDP) are also found in slightly increased amounts, suggesting that pregnancy activates the coagulation system. There is certainly an increased risk of thromboembolis which is now the main cause of maternal mortality. Any woman with a previous or family history of thromboembolism should be considered for anticoagulant prophylaxis, at least post-partum when the risk is greatest (Colvin *et al.* 1993). If there is a strong family history, familial thrombophilias should be looked for, such as Factor V Leiden abnormality or factor C or S deficiency (Greer *et al.* 1992).

Endocrine changes

The placenta produces many hormones which are similar to or mimic those normally produced by the mother. These substances act at various parts of the maternal body and produce most of the changes described. These include oestrogen and progesterone which act directly; human chorionic gonadotrophin (hCG) which is an LH-like substance which not only acts on the corpus luteum but has a mild thyrotrophin-releasing hormone (TRH) effect; corticotorphin-releasing hormone (CRH) which acts on the pituitary to increase adrenocorticotrophic hormone (ACTH) and melanin-stimulating hormone (MSH) release; human placental lactogen (hPL) which is a prolactin-like substance and is an insulin antagonist; placental growth hormone and other growth factors; and even a uteroplacental renin-angiotensin system.

The maternal effects range from a mild degree of hyperthyroidism that can occur in early pregnancy, the widely recognized insulin antagonism, salt and water retention, and an increased tendency to suntan (Yen 1994).

Gastrointestinal changes

Nausea and vomiting are very common in the first trimester. The degree to which this occurs varies considerably between individuals. Although it does appear to be related to hCG levels, the purpose of it is uncertain. It may simply be protective, discouraging the absorption of potential teratogens by allowing a limited oral intake during organogenesis. This feeling of nausea usually settles by 16 weeks, if not before, when hCG levels start to fall.

Later pregnancy changes (12–40 weeks)

After the first trimester, the pregnancy is established and the chance of fetal loss is only around 1–2%. Most of the major fetal structures have formed and the risk of damage, therefore, is lessened. The main aim for the fetus is to grow in an optimal environment. This requires further placentation and an adequate supply of nutrients and oxygen from the mother. The mother has prepared herself for fetal growth but must now ready herself for labour and delivery.

The placenta

During the second trimester there is continued invasion by the placental trophoblast leading to further modification of the uteroplacental vasculature. This is a critical time for the fetus as the extent of placental invasion will determine the growth potential *in utero* and even its long-term health, as low birthweight has been found to be correlated to the incidence of cardiovascular disease in later life (Barker 1995 in Chapter 15). The degree of invasion and membranous change is dependent on the maternal/placental interaction. The fetus is a passive participant in this process.

In early pregnancy there are few terminal villi and they have a simple structure covered with cytotrophoblast on the inside and then syncytio-trophoblast (Kingdom *et al.* 1994). From 10–20 weeks' gestation, the placenta rapidly increases in size and the villi become smaller but much more numerous and mature in appearance. There is a thinning of the syncytiotrophoblast, the cytotrophoblast becomes irregular and even absent in some villi, and the fetal capillaries within the villi increase in diameter. These changes increase the villous surface of the placenta and the capacity for exchange at a time when the fetal growth rate begins to exceed the placental growth rate. These changes continue with development of membranous and non-membranous areas that are almost certainly specialist sites of transfer and synthesis.

From approximately 20 weeks' gestation, there is a plane of cleavage established between placenta and decidua, such that delivery of the fetus will now be accompanied by that of the placenta and allow satisfactory contraction of the uterus. This allows the mother to survive even if the fetus does not. It also increases the chance of accidental separation.

Recent work has indicated the presence of a 'placental clock' which appears to predict and possibly determine the onset of labour. This is reflected in placental corticotrophin-releasing hormone production (Thorburn 1992). The precise mechanism is as yet not understood.

Cardiovascular changes

Although most of the cardiovascular changes have occurred by the end of the first trimester, there are some further changes and the cardiac output increases to around 7.1 l/min at 24 weeks' gestation (Robson *et al.* 1989). This represents a total increase of 45% over pre-pregnancy levels. Although previously believed, modern techniques have confirmed that there is no fall in CO_2 in the third trimester.

A greater percentage of the cardiac output goes to the uterus as pregnancy advances which mirrors the changes of plasma volume rather than cardiac output. The control of uteroplacental flow is not by autoregulation but by changes in blood volume and perfusion pressure. There is a direct relationship between uteroplacental blood flow and total conceptual size irrespective of gestational age.

Blood pressure rises gradually towards term to levels equivalent to the non-pregnant state. Since BP is a continuum, it is difficult to define an abnormal level. Most obstetricians would regard a BP of 140 mmHg systolic and 90 mmHg diastolic as the upper limit of normality. However, a rise in diastolic pressure to 90 mmHg is not uncommon but it might be a sign of developing pre-eclampsia and careful monitoring of the pregnancy is required with further investigations as to underlying cause (Walker 1994). In pre-eclampsia, the rise in blood pressure is associated with a fall in blood volume and cardiac output and a rise in peripheral vascular resistance; in other words, a return towards the non-pregnant values.

As the uterus enlarges there can be increasing pressure on the vena cava causing a reduction in cardiac return and hypotension when the pregnant woman lies on her back. A left lateral position can alleviate the problem.

Gastrointestinal changes

There is reduced acid secretion in mid to late pregnancy, explaining the relative rarity of peptic ulcer in this period. In fact, some of the gastric reflux in pregnancy is not due to acid but alkali from bile.

Reflux is aggravated by the generalized reduction in gut motility and incompetence of the cardiac sphincter. This can be extremely troublesome but can be relieved, at least in part, with simple measures such as sleeping propped up (Chapter 20).

The reduced motility in both the small and large intestine is thought to play some role in enhancing nutrient absorption from the gut, particularly iron. Absorption of water is also affected which can cause constipation.

Maternal weight gain in pregnancy

The average weight gain in pregnancy is 12.5 kg. However, neither a higher nor lower weight gain is necessarily associated with an abnormal outcome. In cases of pre-eclampsia, excessive weight can precede the onset of the disease, but this is due to fluid retention. There is no evidence that weight restriction will reduce the incidence of pre-eclampsia. Similarly, although women with a low weight gain tend to have lighter babies, regular weighing in pregnancy is a poor predictor of fetal problems. Therefore, apart from a booking weight to record the baseline, weighing at the antenatal clinic is not recommended in normal pregnancy. A booking weight of below 45 kg is associated with a higher incidence of premature delivery and intrauterine growth restriction. This would appear to relate to the past nutrition of the mother, as altered nutrition during pregnancy will not improve the outcome.

Maternal coagulation

Uterine contraction provides the primary mechanism for arresting blood loss from the uteroplacental vessels by crimping of these arteries. This initial process is quickly augmented by the subsequent thrombosis which is aided by the inherent thrombotic tendency observed in pregnancy. The same tendency predisposes to venous thrombosis and subsequent pulmonary embolus, particularly in the post-partum period (Colvin *et al.* 1993).

Nutrition in pregnancy

The pregnant woman demonstrates both tissue growth and fat deposition. The fat, which constitutes around 25% of the total weight gain, is deposited characteristically in the abdomen, buttocks, and thighs. This acts as an energy store, allowing the total pregnancy energy intake to be spread throughout the 40 weeks, and for preparation for breastfeeding the baby.

The necessary increase in daily energy intake is only 400 kcal. As long as a good balanced diet is taken there are no specific extra dietary needs. In recent years, dietary deficiencies are generally only seen in groups that are particularly deprived or subject themselves to abuse with drugs or alcohol (Chapters 11 and 12).

Studies of babies born during temporary starvation suggests that the effect on birthweight is maximal when it coincides with the second half of pregnancy. However, the infants are not shorter, just lighter by 300 g, and they catch up their anticipated weights within six weeks of delivery.

There is little evidence that vitamin supplementation is necessary or even desirable in pregnancy apart from folic acid. Asian mothers who may be at risk of developing vitamin D deficiency should receive 400 units/day supplementation.

Influences on nutrient exchange

The method of exchange of substances from the maternal blood to fetal blood varies. Some move by diffusion, dependent only on the total villous area available for exchange and the thickness of the trophoblastic barrier between the two circulations. This diffusion is dependent on the concentration gradients, the size of the substance, and the maternal blood flow. Others have active transport systems to encourage passage into the fetus.

The respiratory gases

These pass to and from the fetus by diffusion gradient. Oxygen is influenced by a lower fetal PO_2 and a higher affinity of fetal haemoglobin for it. CO_2 diffuses across the concentration gradient from fetus to mother, produced by the lower maternal PCO_2.

Nutrients

Glucose is the principal nutrient for the fetus and there is a specific glucose transport system that allows its preferential transfer (Schneider 1991).

Amino acids are also transferred by active transport and fetal plasma levels are generally higher than in maternal plasma. The only proteins transferred from mother to fetus are almost exclusively IgG which provide passive immunity *in utero* and in post-partum life (Landor 1995). All other proteins are synthesized by the placenta or fetus from transferred maternal amino acids (Hay 1991).

There appears to be free transfer of fatty acids across the human placenta although there is also some fetal synthesis (Hay 1991).

Water passes freely through all the tissues of the body and transport between mother and fetus occurs by bi-directional diffusion. The exchange of sodium tends to follow water. There may be a sodium–potassium (Na–K) pump in the syncytiotrophoblast which helps to protect fetal potassium levels. The transfer of chloride probably follows that of sodium.

Iron is actively transported across the placenta. The bulk of the transfer and the building of fetal iron stores occurs in the third trimester.

Intrauterine changes

Fetal growth

Fetal growth is largely determined by the efficiency of the maternal/placental exchange. If initial placentation is poor, there is reduced perfusion of the intervillous space leading to intrauterine growth restriction and reduced birth size. Also, failure of plasma expansion may restrict the nutrient supply by reducing placental perfusion. This form of growth restriction is not usually diagnosed until the third trimester and is asymmetrical as the fetal length and head circumference is not reduced. This is also termed as 'head sparing'.

The other main determinant of fetal growth is genetics. The body size and genetics of the mother largely determines the *in utero* growth. It is after birth that the paternal genes begin to act. Fetuses with major genetic or infective anomalies will demonstrate early growth restriction which is usually symmetrical.

From around 18 weeks, amniotic fluid is mostly produced by fetal urine (Lotgering and Wallenburg 1986). Differing amounts can be a sign of fetal compromise. Excessive production is associated with maternal diabetes and diminished amounts are seen in pregnancies where there is fetal growth restriction. Clinical assessment of liquor volume is an important part of any antenatal examination. This is done simply by assessing the softness and easiness of palpation of the fetus. If the fetal parts can be felt easily with plenty of fluid around it, this is adequate. If the uterus feels as if it is tight round the fetus with little room to move, the liquor is deficient. The fundal height is often found to be reduced in this situation as the uterine capacity is less. Fundal height measurements should be within 2 cm of the equivalent gestation, and serial measurements done by the same observer can show deficient growth trends. Extra ultrasound scans can clarify the situation.

Uterine changes

The uterus has two roles in the progressing pregnancy: it must ensure that it enlarges to accommodate the growing fetus and then prepare itself for labour and delivery.

Muscle fibres of the uterus undergo both hyperplasia and hypertrophy, leading to the uterine enlargement necessary to allow pregnancy growth. In the second and third trimester, the globular shape of the first-trimester uterus begins to change into an ovoid one, promoting a longitudinal lie. For reasons probably related to uterine shape, cephalic presentation is the most common at term and best suited for safe delivery.

Uterine quiescence and cervical competence are two essential features for fetal survival. The former is achieved by reduced myometrial cell contractility due to a lack of gap junctions and oxytocin receptors and increased resistance to oxytocin and prostaglandins. This is probably mediated by progesterone (Neulen and Breckwoldt 1994). If the rate of expansion of the pregnancy is too swift, such as in multiple pregnancy or polyhydramnios, these blocks are less effective and uterine contractions are likely.

The cervix remains competent largely due to its collagenous and uncompliant nature. The thick plug of mucus within the endocervical canal provides an effective barrier to the external environment (Calder 1994).

As term approaches, there is a rapid increase in the number of oxytocin receptors and myometrial gap junctions within the uterus, producing an increasing sensitivity and rapid spread of electrical stimuli between myometrial cells (Myers and Nathanielsz 1993). The increasing uterine activity towards term is most noticeable in the nights leading up to labour.

The cervix softens under the influence of prostaglandins and allows itself to dilate under pressure from the membranes and presenting part (Calder 1994; Neulen and Breckwoldt 1994).

Fetal changes

Preparation for labour and neonatal life occurs throughout most of the second half of pregnancy. Fetal lung maturity is usually complete by 36 weeks. Fetal gut similarly matures several weeks prior to delivery to be ready for oral feeding. Although still very dependent on its mother after birth, the fetus' physiological systems are ready for independent survival. These changes coincide with those of the uterus relating to the preparation for labour (Myers and Nathanielsz 1993).

Labour and delivery

The maternal changes seen in labour are due to the increased load on the maternal physiology and the effect of pain.

Cardiac output in labour

There is a further increase in cardiac output in the first stage of labour by as much as 2 l/min although effective analgesia will reduce this. Peak values as high as 10 l/min may occur during maternal pushing. Therefore, women with a reduced cardiac reserve can be helped by an epidural analgesia during labour, and by a short second stage.

The third stage of labour produces a dramatic increase in the right-sided cardiac return. This is aggravated by oxytocin administration. Women with a tight mitral stenosis are at particular risk. The venous capacitance will continue to provide some protection but, with the gradual loss of this after delivery, the risk of cardiac failure tends to increase to a peak at 18–24 hours post-partum.

Pulmonary function during labour

Ventilation

During painful contractions there can be significant hyperventilation which increases the oxygen consumption and causes a fall in PCO_2. These changes are greatly reduced with epidural analgesia. Therefore, the increased oxygen requirements in labour are due to the pain and not uterine work.

Gastric emptying

Since gastric emptying is further slowed both by labour and the use of narcotic analgesia, there is an increased risk of gastric acid reflux and aspiration. Antacids and, more recently, H_2 antagonists have been used to reduce this risk. Allowing maternal oral intake in labour has also been shown to reduce gastric acidity.

Post-partum changes

Cardiac output

The return to pre-pregnancy values does not occur at an even rate. The loss of venous capacitance occurs early before the blood volume decreases. This leads to an increase in peripheral oedema in most women before the natural diuresis starts from day two.

Although some functional adaptations appear to have returned to non-pregnant values by the sixth post-partum week, this does not apply to the stroke volume or the structural changes in the heart which can take some months. Many women athletes find that their performance is enhanced in this post-partum period.

Coagulation parameters

The coagulation factors do not return to normal at the same rate. Although most of the inhibitory factors disappear at delivery, the pro-coagulant changes can persist for some weeks. This produces an increased risk of thromboembolus (Colvin *et al.* 1993). Early mobilisation helps to reduce the possibility of thromboembolis but anyone at particular risk should be given anticoagulant prophylaxis.

Maternal/fetal interaction

Changes exerted by the placenta during pregnancy result in the development of the mother's breasts in preparation for milk production, so that the newborn baby receives adequate nutrition. After birth, the progesterone block to milk production is released and nipple stimulation and breast emptying provide the major stimulus for continued milk production. The milk is not 'sucked' from the breast, but nipple stimulation causes oxytocin release from the posterior pituitary, inducing contraction of the myoepithelial cells within the alveoli which ejects the milk into the babies mouth. This is also the source of the 'let-down' phenomenon (Chapter 24). The circulating oxytocin also produces the 'afterpains' which are due to uterine contractions.

Regular, repeated suckling is also associated with suppression of the pituitary–ovarian axis due to the release of prolactin. This reduces the chance of ovulation. By reducing the chances of further pregnancy, the baby increases the attention and support received from the mother without competition from a new sibling.

Summary

Physiologically, pregnancy can be seen as a competition between the mother and her baby. The baby demands changes that allow it to develop safely and grow and then survive the labour and delivery into extrauterine life. The mother's body makes sure that she has the reserve and the protective mechanisms in place to make sure she survives even at the cost of her baby's life.

Antenatal care should be targeted at looking for these changes and checking that the milestones are being achieved. An ultrasound scan in early pregnancy checks for successful implantation and fetal viability; mid-trimester examinations assess fetal normality; regular inquiry and investigation of maternal blood pressure and urine ensures that normal physiological changes are taking place; late pregnancy checks on fetal position make sure that preparations for labour are complete; simple regular assessments in labour ensure steady progression and fetal well-being; and finally, support after birth helps the new mother adapt to the physiological and psychological changes and cope with the demands of her offspring.

References

Anumba, D. O. C., Ford, G. A., Boys, R. J., and Robson, S. C. (1996).The role of nitric oxide in the modulation of vascular tone in normal pregnancy. *British Journal of Obstetrics and Gynaecology*, **103**, 1169–70.

Aplin, J. D. (1996).The cell biology of human implantation. *Placenta*, **17**, 269–75.

Barker, D. J. (1995).The fetal and infant origins of disease. *Europen Journal of Clinical Investigation*, **25**, 457–63.

Billington, W. D. (1992).The normal fetomaternal immune relationship. *Baillieres Clinical Obstetrics and Gynaecology*, **6**, 417–38.

Brown, M. A. and Gallery, E. D. M. (1994).Volume homeostasis in normal pregnancy and pre-eclampsia – physiology and clinical implications. *Baillieres Clinical Obstetrics and Gynaecology*, **8**, 287–310. *Baillieres Clinical Obstetrics and Gynaecology*, **6**, 461–86.

Calder, A. A. (1994).Prostaglandins and biological control of cervical function. *Australian and New Zealand Journal of Obstetrics and Gynaecology*, **34**, 347–51.

Colvin, B. T., Letsky, E. A., Rivers, R., Stevens, R. F., Walker, J. J., Machin, S.J .,*et al.* (1993).Guidelines on the prevention, investigation, and management of thrombosis associated with pregnancy. *Journal of Clinical Pathology*, **46**, 489–96.

Cross, J. C., Werb, Z., and Fisher, S. J. (1994). Implantation and the placenta: key pieces of the development puzzle. *Science*, **266**, 1508–18.

Dejongh, R., Jorens, P., Student, I., and Heylen, R. (1996).The contribution of the immune system to parturition. *Mediators of Inflammation*, **5**, 173–82.

de Swiet, M. (1991a). The cardiovascular system. In: *Clinical physiology in obstetrics* (ed.F. E. Hytten and G. Chamberlain), pp.3–38. Blackwell Scientific Publications, Oxford.

de Swiet, M. (1991b). The respiratory system. In: *Clinical physiology in obstetrcis* (ed. F. E. Hytten and G. Chamberlain), pp.83–100. Blackwell Scientific Publications, Oxford.

Fox, H. (1978). Placental structure. In: *Scientific basis of obstetrics and gynaecology* (ed.R. R. Macdonald), pp.28–42. Churchill Livingston, Edinburgh.

Greer, I. A., Walker, J. J., Lowe, G. D., and Forbes, C. D. (1992). Congenital coagulopathies in obstetrics and gynaecology. In: *Haemostasis and thrombosis in obstetrics and gynaecology* (ed. I. A. Greer, A. G. G. Turpie, and C. D. Forbes), pp.459–86. Chapman and Hall, London.

Grio, R., Porpiglia, M., Vetro, E., Uligini, R., Piacentino, R., Mini, D., *et al.* (1994).Asymptomatic bacteriuria in pregnancy – a diagnostic and therapeutic approach. *Panminerva Medica*, **36**, 195–7.

Hay Jr, W. W. (1991).The placenta. Not just a conduit for maternal fuels. *Diabetes*, **40**, 44–50.

Jauniaux, E. (1996).Intervillous circulation in the first trimester – the phantom of the color doppler obstetric opera. *Ultrasound in Obstetrics and Gynecology*, **8**, 73–6.

Kingdom, J. C., Macara, L. M., and Whittle, M. J. (1994). Fetoplacental circulation in health and disease. *Archives of Disease in Childhood: Fetal and Neonatal Edition*, **70**, 161–3.

Landor, M. (1995).Maternal–fetal transfer of immunoglobulins. *Annals of Allergy, Asthma, and Immunology*, **74**, 279–83.

Lotgering, F. K. and Wallenburg, H. C. (1986). Mechanisms of production and clearance of amniotic fluid. *Seminars in Perinatology*, **10**, 94–102.

MacGillivray, I., Rose, G. A., and Rowe, B. (1969).Blood pressure survey in pregnancy. *Clinical Science*, **37**, 395–407.

MacLean, M. A., Wilson, R., Thomson, J. A., Krishnamurthy, S., and Walker, J. J. (1992). Immunological changes in normal pregnancy. *European Journal of Obstetrics, Gynecology, and Reproductive Biology*, **43**, 167–72.

Myers, D. A. and Nathanielsz, P. W. (1993). Biologic basis of term and preterm labour. *Clinics in Perinatology*, **20**, 9–28.

Neulen, J. and Breckwoldt, M. (1994). Placental progesterone, prostaglandins, and mechanisms leading to initiation of parturition in the human. *Experimental and Clinical Endocrinology*, **102**, 195–202.

Peckham, C. S. and Marshal, W. C. (1983). Infections in pregnancy. In: *Obstetrical epidemiology* (ed. S. L. Barron and A. M. Thomson), pp.210–33. Academic Press, London.

Robson, S. C., Hunter, S., Boys, R. J., and Dunlop, W. (1989). Serial study of factors influencing changes in cardiac output during human pregnancy. *American Journal of Physiology*, **256**, 1060–5.

Sargent, I. L. (1993). Maternal and fetal immune responses during pregnancy. *Experimental and Clinical Immunoglobulins*, **10**, 85–102.

Schieve, L. A., Handler, A., Hershow, R., and Davis, F. (1994).Urinary tract infection during pregnancy – its association with maternal morbidity and perinatal outcome. *American Journal of Public Health*, **84**, 405–10.

Schmidt, C. M. and Orr, H. T. (1993).Maternal/fetal interactions: the role of the MHC class 1 molecule HLA-G. *Critical Reviews in Immunology*, **13**, 207–24.

Schneider, H. (1991). The role of the placenta in nutrition of the human fetus. *American Journal of Obstetrics and Gynecology*, **164**, 967–73.

Serle, E., Graham, R. A., Aplin, J. D., Seif, M. W., Li, T. C., Cooke, I. D., *et al.* (1994). Endometrial differentiation in the peri-implantation phase of women with recurrent miscarriage – a morphological and immunohistochemical study. *Fertility and Sterility*, **62**, 989–96.

Simpson, N., Nimrod, C., Devermette, R., Leblanc, C., and Fournier, J. (1996). Enhanced doppler ultrasound evaluation of intervillous flow in early pregnancy. *Journal of Physiology – London*, **494P**, P34–P35.

Steer, P., Alam, M. A., Wadsworth, J., and Welch, A. (1995). Relation between maternal haemoglobin concentration and birthweight in different ethnic-groups. *British Medical Journal*, **310**, 489–91.

Thorburn, G. D. (1992).The placenta, PGE2, and parturition. *Early Human Development*, **29**, 63–73.

Wald, N. J. (1994). Folic acid and neural tube defects – the current evidence and implications for prevention. *Ciba Foundation Symposia*, **181**, 192–208.

Walker, J. J. (1994). Day care assessment and hypertensive disorders of pregnancy. *Fetal and Maternal Medicine Review*, **6**, 57–70.

Weiner, C. P., Lizasoain, I., Baylis, S. A., Knowles, R. G., Charles, I. G., and Moncada, S. (1994). Induction of calcium-dependent nitric oxide synthases by sex hormones. *Proceedings of the National Academy of Sciences of the United States of America*, **91**, 5212–16.

Wells, M. and Bulmer, J. N. (1988).The human placental bed: histology, immunocytochemistry, and pathology. *Histopathology*, **13**, 483–98.

Yen, S. S. (1994). The placenta as the third brain. *Journal of Reproductive Medicine*, **39**, 277–80.

CHAPTER EIGHTEEN

Psychological health before, during, and after childbirth

Sarah Clement and Sandra Elliott

Pregnancy and childbirth are major life events which bring with them emotional challenges and the potential for psychological distress. Since women's contact with the health services is greater during maternity than at any other time in their lives, this period presents an ideal opportunity for promoting psychological health and preventing psychological problems (Royal College of Midwives 1987; Prince and Adams 1990; Royal College of General Practitioners 1995). The importance of pyschological care was also emphasized in *Changing Childbirth* (Department of Health 1993).

We begin by describing key aspects of the psychology of pregnancy, childbirth, and the early postnatal period. We then discuss possible strategies for promoting psychological health and for preventing and ameliorating psychological problems.

The psychology of childbearing

Becoming pregnant

The psychological context in which women become pregnant varies enormously. Reproductive decisions are embedded in a complex web of social, psychological, cultural, and pragmatic factors (Christopher 1991). Woollett (1991) has summarized evidence on what motivates people to want a child as a wish for the opportunity to express and receive love, the feeling of achievement and creativity from helping children grow, validation of adult status and identity, the anticipated enjoyment and fun that children may bring, and the opportunity of self-development and growth through parenting. The combination of motivational factors will vary between individuals, and less common motivations may also be present.

It is estimated that 30% of British pregnancies are unintended (Fleisig 1991). An unplanned pregnancy is not necessarily an unwanted one. Green and colleagues (1988) asked a large sample of pregnant women how they felt when they discovered they were pregnant. Nearly three quarters felt pleased or overjoyed, a quarter had mixed feelings or were unhappy. Although initial feelings can change quite markedly over the course of pregnancy (Wolkind and Zajicek 1981), initial negative feelings about the pregnancy can continue, and may be associated with low postnatal emotional well-being (Green *et al.* 1990).

Conception does not always follow the decision to conceive. There has been much debate about the role of psychological factors in infertility. Pre-existing personality does not appear to be an important factor (Edelmann and Connolly 1986). However, there is some evidence that psychological stress can contribute to reproductive failure (Edelmann and Golombok 1989).

Research suggests that women undergoing treatment for infertility may experience high levels of psychological distress (Wright *et al.* 1989). This results from the stress inherent in the diagnosis and treatment of infertility, although infertility is not experienced as a stressor for all couples it affects (Jones and Hunter 1996). When women with a history of infertility become pregnant it appears that they are no more likely to be anxious or depressed in pregnancy, or postnatally (McMahon *et al.* 1995). There is no evidence that previous infertility has any adverse effects on women's relationships with their children. Indeed, one study found that previously infertile parents expressed greater warmth towards their children and had a higher quality of interaction with them than other parents (Golombok *et al.* 1995).

Pregnancy

Green and colleagues (1988) report that the majority of women (68%) in their study felt reasonably cheerful most of the time during pregnancy, although a quarter reported mood swings. Riley (1995) lists five common positive responses to pregnancy: pleasure at fulfilment of reproductive role, increased status and attention from family and friends, successful transition to adulthood, increased feeling of well-being, and sharing an experience with one's own mother.

Pregnancy can also bring worries and anxieties. Controlled studies have found higher levels of reported anxiety in pregnant women than in non-pregnant women (Cox 1979). In early pregnancy, women's major worries appear to be the possibility of miscarriage, fears about fetal abnormality, and financial worries (Green 1990). Screening for fetal abnormality can be a major cause of anxiety (Roelofsen *et al.* 1993) which may persist even after tests have indicated that all is well (Marteau 1994).

There has been much research on the effects of stress and negative life events in pregnancy on outcomes such as preterm delivery and low birthweight. Although animal research provides quite strong evidence of the effects of maternal stress on fetal well-being (Newton 1988), the human research has tended to be contradictory. However, two large, prospective studies, controlling for confounding factors such as smoking, suggest that psychological distress, or social adversity in pregnancy, is associated with preterm delivery (Hedegaard *et al.* 1993; Peacock *et al.* 1995) but not with impaired fetal growth (Peacock *et al.* 1995; Hedegaard *et al.* 1996). However, trials of interventions designed to decrease stress in pregnancy through the provision of psychosocial support have tended to show little effect on preterm delivery or other clinical pregnancy outcomes (Hodnett 1995a).

There is also a body of research on the effects of anxiety and life events in pregnancy on postnatal psychological well-being. Several studies have shown anxiety in pregnancy to be an important predictor of postnatal depression (Riley 1995). The literature on adverse life events and postnatal depression is less clear (Elliott 1990; O'Hara and Swain 1996); however, some studies have found an increased number of negative life events during pregnancy in women depressed postnatally (Riley 1995).

A significant proportion of pregnant women will experience mental health problems. In a cohort study of 128 pregnant women, Watson and colleagues (1984) found that 13% experienced what could be classified as a psychiatric disorder, the main type of problem being affective disorders such as antenatal depression. When self-report measures of depression are used, women consistently report more depression in pregnancy than postnatally (Green and Murray 1994). In studies where the prevalence of depression has been assessed using recognized diagnostic criteria, findings are inconsistent (Green and Murray 1994), but two studies found that depression was more common antenatally than postnatally (Wolkind *et al.* 1980; Gotlib *et al.* 1989). Furthermore, antenatal depression appears to be an important precursor of postnatal depression for some women (O'Hara *et al.* 1991).

In other respects, pregnancy can have a positive effect on psychological well-being. Riley (1995) reports that panic disorder and obsessional–compulsive symptoms tend to improve during pregnancy. Pregnancy also has a dramatic protective effect against suicide (Appleby 1996).

Some pregnancies end not with the birth of a baby but with a miscarriage, an event which can have important and long-term psychological effects. Increased levels of anxiety and depression have been found three to six months after the loss (Neugebauer *et al.* 1992; Prettyman *et al.* 1993) and at one year (Robinson *et al.* 1994). The emotional legacy of miscarriage may also be carried forward into the next pregnancy (Statham and Green 1994). A variety of factors affect the level of distress women experience after miscarriage, including previous psychiatric history, lack of social support, and previous bereavement (Slade 1994). Perhaps surprisingly, Slade found that parity and gestation at miscarriage had little effect on psychological outcome.

Women's feelings about their babies is the final psychological aspect of pregnancy to be considered. Women vary in the extent to which they feel attached to their babies during pregnancy. Raphael-Leff (1991) believes that the degree of attachment depends on the mother's capacity to trust in a positive outcome. Women undergoing testing for fetal abnormality may delay attachment to their fetuses until the outcome of the test is known (Green and Statham 1996). Although women often report that having an ultrasound scan makes the baby seem more real, there is in fact very little research evidence to support the notion that scans increase maternal–fetal attachment (Clement *et al.* 1998).

Childbirth

Green and colleagues (1988) report that three quarters of women in their study found childbirth fulfilling, and when asked to give their birth experience a mark out of ten, two thirds gave their experience a score of 8, 9, or 10. However, a Norwegian study revealed that women can also experience negative or difficult emotions during childbirth with many women reporting that labour was 'very difficult', a third describing labour as intolerably painful, and one in five experiencing severe anxiety during labour (Thune Larsen and Moller-Pedersen 1988). Kitzinger (1987) has drawn attention to experiences of violation during childbirth, and reports that the words some women use to describe their birth experience are the same as those used by women who have been raped (Kitzinger 1992). Experiences in childbirth are not easily forgotten. In one study, women gave accurate and detailed accounts of their birth experiences 20 years after the event, with many accounts still being highly charged with emotion (Simkin 1991).

Many factors can influence women's experience of childbirth. Green *et al.* (1988) found that women were more dissatisfied with their birth experience if they did not have a choice about where to give birth, did not feel in control of what the staff did, received inadequate information, felt unsupported by care-givers, had a long labour, experienced obstetric interventions, and had labour pain that was different from that expected. In a study of women's experiences of caesarean childbirth, Clement (1995*a*) found that support from care-givers, involvement in decisions, and perceptions of necessity were the main factors influencing whether the caesarean was a positive or negative experience. Other research shows that being cared for by a midwife known during pregnancy is an important determinant of whether women enjoy labour (Hodnett 1995*b*).

The intensity of labour pain varies immensely. In one study, 8% of women reported having very little pain, and 16% rated their pain as being 'as bad as I could possibly imagine' (Niven 1992). Niven reported that it is not always easy for care-givers to estimate the amount of pain a woman in labour is experiencing, and that care-givers tend to underestimate the severity of pain. It is important to recognize that satisfaction in childbirth is not necessarily contingent upon the absence of pain. The crucial aspect appears to be whether women perceive their pain as bearable, and that is largely dependent on their sense of control over the process (Rajan 1996).

There has been much debate about the psychological effects of interventions in childbirth. Whilst the majority of researchers have found higher levels of intervention to be associated with lower levels of satisfaction with the birth experience (Oakley and Rajan 1990; Hillan 1992), findings have been contradictory for other psychological outcomes such as depression (Brown *et al.* 1994; Elliott *et al.* 1984). Methodological issues may account for much of this disparity as could sociodemographic (McIntosh 1989) or cultural (Sandelowski and Busamante 1986) differences between the various populations. Furthermore, differences in the way care was given, or the amount of involvement or control given to women, can influence their feelings about interventions (Green *et al.* 1988).

One factor that overshadows all other childbirth experiences is the death of a baby. The grief experienced after the loss of a baby at or after birth is now recognized to be as intense and long-lasting as that experienced after other forms of bereavement (Mander 1994). When a baby is born prematurely or is ill and has to receive care in a neonatal or special care baby unit, this can also be a traumatic experience for parents, and one which may have long-term psychological effects (McFadyen 1994).

After birth

In order to challenge postwar representations of mothers as contented housewives , women writers began to stress that depressed mood is as normal an experience in the puerperium as at other times, noting that childbirth brings losses with the gains and mothering brings stressful demands with the rewards (Oakley 1980; Sharpe 1984). This appears to have led to the opposite view that childbirth is a negative life event (Cox *et al.* 1986; Elliott 1990) and that it is normal to feel anxious or miserable when looking after a new baby (Whitton *et al.* 1996). Both perspectives appear to derive from the notion that pregnancy and childbirth somehow render women identical, whether via the power of biological (hormonal) changes or of psychosocial transitions. Conformity in emotional changes would render the task of delivering quality psychological health care, both antenatally and postnatally, much simpler. Unfortunately for those of us in health care provision, women remain as individual before and after childbirth as at other times (Elliott 1984,1990; Thorpe and Elliott 1998). An awareness of common themes related to physical vulnerability and psychological demands should not therefore replace sensitivity to individual needs and experiences.

An examination of the literature reveals the bases for the opposing views that women become more content and happy or more depressed and anxious following childbirth. The incidence of diagnosable depression is indeed higher in the first three to six weeks after birth (Cooper *et al.* 1988; Cox *et al.* 1993), so a number of women clearly experience sufficient increase in depressive symptomatology to cross the threshold into an emotional state which meets diagnostic criteria for depression. However, this is superimposed on an overall group trend which shows a postnatal decrease in self-report of negative symptomatology (Pitt 1968; O'Hara and Zekoski 1988; Elliott 1984; Green and Murray 1994), with most women feeling healthier and happier one month after than one month before childbirth.

In the first trimester of pregnancy more tiredness seems to be reported whereas in later pregnancy there is an increase in discomfort and worry about labour. There is a decrease in frequency of, and interest in, sex during pregnancy with a return of interest by three months after birth and a return of frequency by 12 months. There is a decrease in feeling bored and fed up from the month before to one month after the birth (Elliott *et al.* 1983). Smith (1989) found that the main worries reported by women four weeks after delivery related to fatigue, regulating demands, feeding the baby, emotional tension, and breast soreness. Women's feelings about their babies are generally positive. Green *et al.* (1991) found that the majority of women saw their babies as being alert, responsive, cuddly, contented, and fascinating, and only a minority described their babies as being draining, fretful, or unresponsive.

In the middle of this gradual transition from conception to the baby's first birthday is the birth and immediate aftermath. The tendency to emotional lability is well known with 50–70% of women experiencing mood swings, visible as tearfulness and generally referred to as the 'blues', between three to five days after birth (Stein 1982; Kennerley and Gath 1989). The fact that the 'blues' occur at a time of rapid hormonal change has led to speculation regarding a causal role but research has failed to confirm this (Riley 1995).

About 10% of women show elation and other features of hypomania in the first five days following childbirth, a phenomenon known as the 'highs' (Glover *et al.* 1994). Those who experience the 'highs' appear to be more likely to develop postnatal depression (Glover *et al.* 1994).

The prototypical woman therefore begins her pregnancy feeling tired and ends it in discomfort, worrying about the labour. The baby is delivered safe and well and she experiences brief elation before becoming emotionally labile and tearful around day three. Her emotions are generally positive and beginning to stabilize by one to three months after the birth. Whilst it is important to be aware of women whose emotional state goes against the trend, particularly postnatally, women and health care professionals should guard against overreacting. It is normal to feel depressed or anxious on occasion. Such feelings generally resolve spontaneously, or following talking issues through with someone demonstrating calm acceptance. Women who catastrophize low moods when they have a bad day are at increased risk of persistent depression (Teasdale 1985; Elliott 1989*b*). Only when depressed mood (or other difficulty) is persistent, severe, accompanied by other symptoms, and/or interfering with performance of daily life should sufficient concern be aroused to offer formal intervention.

Postnatal depression

Postnatal depression refers to a non-psychotic depressive episode that begins in or extends into the post-partum period (O'Hara and Swain 1996). It equates with the syndrome of depression as defined in psychiatric diagnostic protocols. Generally, a diagnosis of depression requires depressed mood to be accompanied by a specified minimum number of other symptoms (e.g. three from seven in ICD10 or four from eight in DSM-IV) for a specified minimum period, usually two weeks. These criteria are the same for men and women, both in and out of the puerperium. The ICD10 does include classifications specific to the puerperium, but these are intended only for use with syndromes which can not be classified elsewhere, with the implication being that the clinician has failed to gather sufficient information for the appropriate diagnosis (Cox 1994). Riley recommends that 'whatever the clinical coding given to puerperal patients, a further coding should be made under ICD10, category O99.3 – "Mental disorders and diseases of the nervous system complicating pregnancy, childbirth, and the puerperium" – so that future researchers can easily identify puerperal admissions' (Riley 1995).

In between happy and syndromal depression lies a continuum which passes through depressed mood and subclinical depression, which is unpleasant to experience but fails to meet diagnostic criteria. Confusingly, psychological studies utilizing self-reports of mood rather than diagnostic interviews may employ a numerical cut-off score then refer to high levels of symptomatology as postnatal depression. In this chapter we will use the titles 'Postnatal Depression' and 'Depression' to refer to diagnosed episodes and the term 'postnatal depression' and 'depression' (in lower case) to refer to the experience of measurable depressed mood.

Significant morbidity is identified utilizing either criteria. Consistent with prediction, more women report experiencing postnatal depression than would be formally diagnosed as experiencing Postnatal Depression. In a meta-analysis, self-report measures yielded a prevalence estimate of 14% compared to psychiatric interview diagnoses of 12% (O'Hara and Swain 1996). It is important not to assume that women not reaching diagnostic criteria do not have legitimate needs for additional health care since they may experience significant social morbidity (O'Hara and Swain 1996).

The discussion so far has considered how best to define and identify postnatal depression/Postnatal Depression – as a mood, symptom(s), or syndrome. Others contest the value of the concept itself.

Is it depression? Some have argued that to use the term depression is inappropriate because it is understood as a diagnostic label, thereby medicalizing experiences that are not a sign of individual pathology but are normal reactions to the social situation in which women mother (Oakley 1980). Although we recognize the importance of social context in unhappiness after childbirth, we use the term depression because it conveys the high level of distress women feel and the debilitating nature of the experience better than terms like unhappiness. Also, depression is the term that women themselves often choose to describe their experiences (Brown *et al*. 1994; Mauthner 1995).

Is it postnatal? In one study, a third of women classified as depressed eight months after childbirth said that the depression they were experiencing was not postnatal depression (Brown *et al*. 1994). This concurs with the evidence of a significant degree of overlap between antenatal and postnatal depression (Clement 1995*b*) and the fact that depression is a common experience for many women, regardless of their childbearing status. These women agreed that they had been depressed and did not deny that this had been in the postnatal period. Rejection of the term therefore implies that the women were operating a different definition to that of the researchers cited above. In the light of media coverage of Dalton's view that Postnatal Depression is a hormonal disorder specifically related to a drop in progesterone (Dalton 1971, 1980), it is likely that women considered that the diagnosis was dependent on presumed aetiology rather than timing.

Why has the term Postnatal Depression been retained by specialists in maternal mental health when it has been resisted by the committees who produce psychiatric diagnostic manuals, by sociologists and feminists, and by many mothers depressed after childbirth? What is the point of the term if it does not imply a specific aetiology? Why did the term not disappear when research demonstrated profiles and annual prevalence similar to that of non-childbearing women (Watson *et al.* 1984; Cooper *et al.* 1988; O'Hara *et al.* 1990; Cox *et al.* 1993)? Firstly, recent research did find a large peak in Depression in the first five weeks after childbirth (Cooper *et al.* 1988; Cox *et al.* 1993). Also, the factors associated with Depression appear to be different for women depressed in the postnatal period than for women depressed at other points in their life cycle (Murray *et al.* 1995). These findings may be accounted for by the existence of two subgroups, those with a first onset in the puerperium and those with a recurrence of Depression (Cooper and Murray 1995). It would not be helpful, however, for these to become known as 'real' Postnatal depression and routine Depression. Apart from the more stigmatizing connotations carried by the latter term, a pressing argument remains for the retention of a special term for all depression in the puerperium. This is quite simply the special nature of the puerperium itself as a context within which the depression is experienced. Depression at this critical point in the family transition poses a serious problem in that it is extremely distressing for the new mother who feels that she is missing an unrepeatable experience, and can have long-term effects on the emotional, behavioural, and cognitive development of the infant (Wrate *et al.* 1985; Cogill *et al.* 1986; Murray and Cooper 1996).

When postnatally depressed women are asked for the reasons for their depression, the main reasons they give are feeling unsupported, being isolated, tiredness, physical health factors, lack of time or space for themselves, and difficult material circumstances. Riley (1995) gives an overview of the many studies which have investigated factors associated with postnatal depression. These include poor social support, lack of a confiding relationship, stressful life events, marital disharmony, an unplanned or unwanted pregnancy, postnatal blues, previous postnatal depression, antenatal depression, and anxiety in pregnancy. A meta-analysis largely confirms the results of such narrative reviews but notes that the strength of relationships is weakened the wider the time frame for diagnosing the index group (O'Hara and Swain 1996). The meta-analysis can be used to create a tentative composite profile of the prototypical pregnant woman at risk for postnatal depression:

'She is most likely to occupy a lower social stratum but women representing middle and upper social strata will also be abundantly represented. She is very likely to have experienced stressors during pregnancy and may have had a more difficult than normal pregnancy or delivery. She will be experiencing marital difficulties and experience her partner as providing little in the way of social support. Compounding the life stress she is experiencing and her poor marital relationship will be her perception that others in her social network are not particularly supportive of her.

Finally, her history will show evidence of psychopathology, in most cases major depression or dysthymia, and she will show evidence of being at least mildly depressed and anxious, and excessively worried' (O'Hara and Swain 1996).

This profile omits mention of the woman's hormonal status. Hormone levels change so dramatically following childbirth that it seems obvious that they will play a role in vulnerability to postnatal depression. The difficulty is that although research is beginning to demonstrate the effects of ovarian hormones on cognitive functions and mood (Wieck 1996), it has so far failed to identify any differences in hormonal level or receptor activity between those who go on to be depressed and those who do not (O'Hara *et al.* 1991; Harris 1994), with the possible exception of the depression which accompanies other symptoms of thyroid disorder (Harris 1996). There is recent evidence that oestrogen can speed up the recovery from severe Depression after childbirth (Gregoire *et al.* 1996), but it is unclear whether this is via non specific psychotropic properties or via the 'cure' of an oestrogen deficiency.

It is probably unhelpful to take a polarized view that all postnatal depression is either socially or biologically caused (Thorpe and Elliott 1998). Most types of depression appear to be the result of an interaction between biological and psychosocial vulnerability (predisposing factors) combined with stressful life events, including stressful birth events, and biological changes (precipitating factors). Furthermore, it appears that stressful life events can become biologically encoded and actually cause the biological changes found to be associated with depression. For example, there is some evidence that girls who have been sexually abused have higher catecholamine functional activity (a psychobiological profile similar to that found in major depressive disorder) compared with controls (De Bellis *et al.* 1994). Perpetuating factors can therefore also be both biological (Harris 1996) and psychosocial, including attitudes of others to depression and personal 'Depression about Depression' (Teasdale 1985; Elliott 1989*b*; Whitton *et al.* 1996).

Puerperal psychosis

Around one in 500 women will experience a puerperal psychosis (Riley 1995). Puerperal psychoses typically have rapid onset within the first two weeks after delivery and are characterized by perplexity and confusion as well as one or more of the classic signs of psychosis such as delusions and hallucinations. Women who had a history of manic or depressive illness, were unmarried, having a first baby, and who had a caesarean section were found to be at greater risk of developing puerperal psychosis (Kendell *et al.* 1987). The debate continues as to whether there is a subgroup of psychotic depressions which is specific to the puerperium or whether all are manifestations of a lifelong vulnerability to psychoses which may reappear at other times (Kendell *et al.* 1987; Kumar 1989). The speed and timing of onset of puerperal psychoses lead most clinicians to suspect a biological aetiology specific to childbirth, at least for a subgroup (Brockington and Cox-Roper 1988), though again the nature of such underlying pathology has still to be identified (Riley 1995).

Post-traumatic stress syndrome

There have been recent clinical descriptions of postnatal-onset panic disorder and stress reactions resembling post-traumatic stress disorder (PTSD), with the traumatic event persistently re-experienced, avoidance of anything associated with the event, and increased arousal, following traumatic labour and delivery experiences (Bloor and Jones 1988; Metz *et al.* 1988; Moleman *et al.* 1992, reported in Riley 1995). Ballard *et al.* (1995) estimate the prevalence of PTSD in the puerperium to be 1% and identified themes in four case histories – these were threat to the baby's life, poor pain control, long or complicated labour, and a feeling of lack of control. Menage (1993) found that those with a history of fetal loss, and those who had previously undergone invasive obstetric or gynaecological procedures, were at risk. Pregnancy, birth, and parenting may also prove the triggers for reawakening past traumatic experiences such as childhood sexual abuse (Riley 1995).

Strategies for promoting psychological health and for preventing and treating psychological problems

Incorporating psychological care into routine maternity care

There is considerable scope for increasing the amount, or improving the quality, of psychological care within routine maternity care. One useful approach is to incorporate client-centred principles and basic counselling skills into all interactions between maternity care-givers and pregnant, childbearing, or postnatal women. Hunter (1994) gives a detailed account of how counselling skills derived from the approaches of Rogers (1961) and Egan (1990) can be used in maternity care.

Conveying empathy, genuineness, and respect

Historically, the organization of the maternity services has not been conducive to meeting women's needs for empathy, genuineness, and respect. There are examples of care-givers disregarding or disbelieving what women tell them, systematically disempowering women from their own experiences (Oakley 1980; Hunt and Symonds 1995).

One key element which has permitted and encouraged this type of depersonalized care has been the lack of continuity of carer. Controlled trials have suggested that increasing continuity of carer may have important psychological benefits, including greater feelings of control and enjoyment during labour, and feeling more able to discuss worries both antenatally and postnatally (Hodnett 1995*b*).

Psychosocial support

Psychosocial support is another important concept, but one which is hard to define. It may encompass practical support and emotional support through being with a woman, listening, reflecting back, encouragement, praise, and other strategies for enhancing self-esteem.

Psychosocial support should be built into every antenatal consultation. The amount of psychosocial support received during pregnancy may be related to the frequency of antenatal visits. If the number of routine antenatal visits is reduced without specific measures to maintain or increase the level of psychosocial support provided, this may result in poorer maternal psychosocial outcomes (Sikorski *et al.* 1996; Clement *et al.* 1997).

Support during childbirth can also have important effects on women's later emotional well-being since a trial in which labouring women received companionship from a lay labour companion showed that supported women had higher self-esteem and lower depression and anxiety ratings at six weeks after the birth (Wolman *et al.* 1993).

There needs to be an increased emphasis on psychosocial support in postnatal care. In a study comparing mothers' and midwives' perceptions of the needs of postnatal women, the mothers saw understanding their emotional needs as the main priority of postnatal care, but this did not appear at all in the top five priorities of midwives (Laryea 1989). Similar findings come from a study of general practitioners which showed that only one in seven saw the detection of worries or depression as a major benefit of the six-week postnatal check (Bowers 1985). However, professional attitudes may have changed since these studies were undertaken.

Choice, control, and decision-making

Giving women real choices about their maternity care is thought to be psychologically beneficial (Department of Health 1993), but enabling women to make informed choices is not always straightforward. It may be difficult for care-givers to accept women's choices when these conflict with their own beliefs about what is the best form of care. Choice carries responsibility, which some women may not wish to bear and which some care-givers may not want to relinquish. What is clear, however, is that withholding choice from women by undertaking procedures against their wishes (Clement 1994) or without explicit consent (Bergstrom *et al.* 1992) can result in feelings of violation (Kitzinger 1992) or post-traumatic stress disorder (Menage 1993).

The concept of choice is closely related to that of control. Strategies that may increase women's feelings of control include women holding their own notes (Hodnett 1995c) and the use of birth plans (Moore and Hopper 1995). Research by Green and colleagues (1988) highlighted the importance of control in childbirth as a mediator of postnatal emotional well-being. Green and colleagues found that women who did not feel in control of what the staff were doing to them or of their own behaviour during childbirth had lower postnatal emotional well-being. However, these researchers found no relationship between being involved in decision-making about the birth and postnatal emotional well-being, which suggests that control is not synonymous with involvement in decisions. Clearly, the concept of control is complex. Researchers are now beginning to unravel some of these complexities (Weaver 1998).

Asking about psychological health

Asking women about their psychological well-being should be a routine part of maternity care, beginning at the first antenatal visit. Psychiatric history is an important predictor of puerperal psychosis and postnatal depression. Women with a history of affective psychosis have a 50% risk of developing a puerperal psychosis (Marks *et al.* 1992). These women require careful monitoring in the weeks after childbirth, and preventive strategies should be considered. A history of severe depression increases the risk of developing Postnatal Depression threefold (Marks *et al.* 1992). Current screening systems are often haphazard and unsatisfactory (Kumar *et al.* 1994). Care-givers should also ask about women's current psychological well-being at each antenatal and postnatal visit. The postnatal check should include an assessment of psychological well-being since only a minority of depressed women seek professional help (McIntosh 1993; Whitton *et al.* 1996).

Strategies for providing additional psychosocial care

In this section we will consider approaches that involve the provision of psychosocial care in addition to that provided in routine maternity care and how care might be targeted at those in greatest need.

Individual approaches

A structured listening intervention, involving health visitors providing eight weekly 'listening' visits to women experiencing postnatal depression, has been shown to be an effective intervention, reducing the number of women still depressed at six months from 62% to 31% (Holden *et al.* 1989). Systems incorporating listening interventions are being implemented by many NHS trusts (Cullinan 1991; Gerrard *et al.* 1993; Thorpe and Elliott 1998) and a trainer training programme has been developed to support such initiatives (Gerrard *et al.* 1994).

There is also a case for using individual listening approaches in pregnancy as a possible strategy for preventing postnatal depression (Clement 1995*b*) since there is a significant overlap between antenatal and postnatal depression (Watson *et al.* 1984; Green and Murray 1994). Further evidence in support of individual listening approaches in pregnancy comes from trials of social support during pregnancy (Hodnett 1995*a*, 1995*d*). One such trial involved women receiving at least three supportive home visits and two telephone calls from research midwives during pregnancy (Oakley *et al.* 1990) Women who received this antenatal social support were less worried about their baby postnatally (Oakley *et al.* 1990), tended to be less depressed one year after the birth (Oakley 1992), and even seven years on, felt they were coping with life better and were more satisfied with life (Oakley *et al.* 1996). Listening visits during pregnancy, and the opportunities for referral such visits provide, may also help women with untreated psychological problems that predate the pregnancy, a client group which has previously received little clinical or research attention (Kumar *et al.* 1994). Any schedule of antenatal listening visits should also extend into the postnatal period to ensure continuity of care-giver during the often critical period after birth when women may be feeling particularly vulnerable. To withdraw a supportive relationship at the end of pregnancy may leave women feeling abandoned at a time when they may be in particular need of support (Elliott *et al.* 1988).

Another type of individual approach which may play an important part in the prevention of psychological problems after birth is postnatal debriefing, such as the Birth Afterthoughts Service (Charles and Curtis 1994). Such services enable women to talk through events in labour and delivery, and may help to prevent feelings of post-traumatic stress following childbirth. There may also be a case for incorporating debriefing into routine postnatal care (Ralph and Alexander 1994). However, further research is needed since the value of debriefing in general has yet to be demonstrated (Raphael and Meldrum 1995). Furthermore, if debriefing is undertaken in an inappropriate way, there is a danger of women being retraumatized by this process (Lyons 1998).

Individual approaches have also been shown to be effective for reducing psychological distress in women who have suffered a perinatal death (Forrest *et al.* 1982). Formal befriending approaches, such as the Homestart scheme in which specially trained volunteers make regular home visits to families experiencing difficulties, also appear to be beneficial (Harrison 1992).

Group approaches

Additional psychosocial care can also be provided in a group setting. Group approaches generally take up less professional time per woman helped, and women can receive support not only from the professional care-giver facilitating the group but also from the other women in the group.

Groups have a long history in antenatal education. In their traditional format, antenatal classes appear to offer little in the way of psychosocial support (Clement *et al.* 1997), but they have the potential for promoting psychological health if they are restructured to provide more informal supportive care throughout pregnancy. Thorley and Rouse (1993) have been running informal groups at their antenatal clinics, meetings being facilitated by a midwife, doctor, and sometimes a guest speaker with topics for discussion. New mothers often bring their babies to the group, and there is time for women to talk with each other and build up a cohesive support group. Another approach is to set up outreach pregnancy groups in the community. Such groups differ from traditional antenatal classes in that they run throughout pregnancy, are more informal with no structured teaching, and they aim to offer psychological support as well as preparation for birth and parenthood (Leap 1991).

Elliott and colleagues (1988) have demonstrated that antenatal groups for women with vulnerability factors for postnatal depression can help to prevent women becoming depressed postnatally. The groups met monthly from early pregnancy until six months after delivery and aimed to provide both social support and preparation for parenthood. The groups were effective with only 12% of the intervention group being diagnosed as depressed for two or more weeks in the first two postnatal months compared to 33% of the controls. Group interventions may need to be quite intensive since a similar trial involving just two antenatal group sessions and one postnatal group session for women vulnerable to depression failed to demonstrate any beneficial effect on postnatal emotional well-being (Stamp *et al.* 1995). Another group approach that has been shown to be useful is Newpin, which runs a series of home-like drop-in centres where women with young children can meet other women and are supported and befriended by trained volunteers. Women using Newpin became markedly less depressed (Pound and Mills 1985).

Targeting care

Interventions can be either universal, that is, directed at all pregnant and postnatal women, or selective, directed only at specific groups, such as those most vulnerable to postnatal depression. There is a case for universal approaches antenatally since it is not possible to predict accurately which women will experience postnatal depression, so if care is offered to all women then there is no danger of missing anyone. Universal approaches also avoid the problem of women who receive extra care feeling labelled and stigmatized (Elliott 1989*a*).

If care is to be targeted, the Edinburgh Postnatal Depression Scale (EPDS), developed by Cox and colleagues (1987), appears to be a useful tool for selecting postnatal women for additional psychosocial care. The EPDS is a 10-item questionnaire for screening for postnatal depression and is quite widely used by health visitors to select women for health visitor-provided listening interventions (Cullinan 1991; Gerrard *et al.* 1993; Thorpe and Elliott 1998). Such formal targeting is helpful since women do not always disclose depression or seek help. Research has shown that health visitors are unaware that women in their care are feeling depressed in up to 60% of cases (Holden 1994), and around two thirds of women who feel depressed postnatally will not seek any professional help (Brown *et al.* 1994). The use of the EPDS apparently gives women permission to talk about their feelings and to disclose negative mood (Holden 1994, 1996). Without a formal approach, care-givers may find it difficult to allocate extra time to women most in need. For example, researchers looking at the duration of postnatal home visits found that there was no relationship between the presence of social or emotional problems and the length of visits (Marsh and Sargent 1991). The introduction of psychological screening and listening visits might therefore be expected to improve the identification of women with depressive symptoms and the amount of listening time allocated to them. A structured approach is also likely to give midwives and health visitors increased confidence in their ability to offer constructive help (Holden 1994).

The EPDS could also be used as a screening tool in pregnancy (Clement 1995*b*) since it has been validated for antenatal use (Murray and Cox 1990). However, Appleby *et al.* (1994) found that previous or current treatment for depression was a much better antenatal predictor of postnatal depression than the EPDS. Vulnerability factors – relationship difficulties, previous psychiatric problems, previous postnatal depression, and anxiety in pregnancy – have been successfully used in a study on the prevention of postnatal depression through the provision of antenatal support groups for vulnerable women (Elliott *et al.* 1988; Leverton and Elliott 1989).

It is essential that any form of screening is well planned and undertaken with care (Elliott 1994). It is important that identification does not become an end in itself. There is little point in identifying women unless an effective intervention is to be offered; otherwise identification merely becomes an unhelpful label women have to carry with them during and after their pregnancy.

Pharmacological approaches

There are times when a pharmacological approach will be necessary. Unfortunately, research on the efficacy and side-effects of psychotropic drugs in pregnancy (Riley 1995) and during breastfeeding (Yoshida and Kumar 1996) is disconcertingly inadequate.

There appear to have been few controlled trials of antidepressant therapy specifically in the antenatal or postnatal periods. However, since depression before and after childbirth is very similar to depression occurring at other times, antidepressant therapy is likely to be as effective for antenatal or postnatal depression as it is for depression occurring at other points in the life cycle (O'Brien and Pitt 1994). Tricyclic drugs are used quite frequently, and the use of selective serotonin re-uptake inhibitors (SSRIs) is increasing. There are case histories of the amelioration of Postnatal Depression with SSRIs (Roy *et al.* 1993). A small randomized controlled trial comparing the effectiveness of fluoxetine (Prozac) and cognitive behavioural counselling in depressive illness in postnatal women found the two treatments to be equally effective, and both were better than placebo (Appleby *et al.* 1997). The researchers concluded that the choice of treatment may therefore be made by women themselves. There appeared to be no additional advantage in receiving both fluoxetine and cognitive behavioural counselling.

Hormonal approaches have also been advocated. Dalton (1971,1980) advocates progesterone injections or suppositories from the end of labour until the return of menstruation. This approach has never been tested in a double-blind randomized controlled trial, and without such a trial its effectiveness is unknown. Although there were some methodological deficiencies (Murray 1996), a randomized controlled trial has shown oestradiol patches to be significantly more effective than placebos in helping to lift postnatal depression (Gregoire *et al.* 1996). Harris and colleagues are undertaking a study of thyroxine as a prophylactic in thyroid antibody-positive women (Harris 1996).

At present, there are no nationally agreed guidelines or protocols for GPs prescribing for women who experience mental illness during the perinatal period. However, local guidelines are being developed by a number of centres.

Referral

Not all psychological problems can be prevented or treated successfully by midwives, GPs, or other primary health care workers. It is therefore vital that services are well coordinated, with good links between different members of the primary health care team and between primary and secondary care. Health care professionals need to come together locally to establish and clarify referral criteria. However, as a general rule, midwives and health visitors should consider recommending that women consult their general practitioner when they score high on the EPDS or similar instruments, when they describe a history of psychological problems, or simply when their clinical impression causes concern. Obstetricians and general practitioners should consider referral to the psychiatrist or community mental health team when pregnant or postnatal women meet diagnostic criteria, when they have had a diagnosis in the past which predisposes to a recurrence, when psychological or social needs are complex, or when they are concerned about mental state but unsure of the diagnosis or needs. Women with depression or anxiety disorders can be referred to a therapist, counsellor, or psychologist.

Concluding comments

It has been argued that since advances in medicine relating to the physical outcomes of child-bearing have apparently peaked, with maternal and perinatal mortality at an all-time low, it is appropriate that more clinical and research effort is devoted to psychological outcomes in the perinatal period (Elliott 1989*a*). Ideally, this will be led by the development of a subspecialty for the perinatal period in mental health services (Appleby *et al.* 1996; Oates 1996) and in mental health for obstetric and primary care professionals (Gerrard *et al.* 1994; Johnstone 1994; Thorpe and Elliott 1998).

We hope that we have been able to raise awareness about some of the important issues affecting women's psychological well-being before, during, and after childbirth, and that we have highlighted some of the strategies that community-based maternity care-givers might use to promote psychological health.

References

Appleby, L. (1996). Suicidal behaviour in child-bearing women. *International Reviews in Psychiatry*, 8, 107–16.

Appleby, L., Gregoire, A., Platz, C., Prince, M., and Kumar, R. (1994). Screening women for high risk of postnatal depression. *Journal of Psychosomatic Research*, **38**, 539–45.

Appleby, L., Kumar, R., and Warner R. (1996). Perinatal psychiatry. *International Review of Psychiatry*, **8**, 5–8.

Appleby, L., Warner, R., Whitton, A., and Saragher, B. (1997). A controlled study of fluoxetine and cognitive behavioural counselling in the treatment of postnatal depression. *British Medical Journal*, **314**, 932–6.

Ballard, C. G., Stanley, A.K., and Brockington I. F. (1995). Post-traumatic stress disorder (PTSD) after childbirth. *British Journal of Psychiatry*, **166**, 525–8.

Bergstrom, L., Roberts, J., Skillman, L., and Seidel, J. (1992). 'You'll feel me touching you, sweetie': vaginal examinations during the second stage of labour. *Birth*, **19**, 10–18.

Bloor, R. N. and Jones, R. A. (1988). Post-traumatic stress disorder and sexual dysfunction. *British Journal of Sexual Medicine*, **15**, 170–2.

Bowers, J. P. (1985). *The six-week postnatal examination*. In: *Proceedings of the 1984 Research and the Midwife Conference* (ed. S. Robinson and A. M. Thomson). Nursing Research Unit, King's College, London.

Brockington, I. and Cox-Roper, A. (1988). The nosology of puerperal mental illness. In: *Motherhood and mental illness 2*. (ed. R.Kumar and I. F.Brockington), pp.1–16. Wright, London.

Brown, S., Lumley, J., Small, R., and Astbury, J. (1994). *Missing voices: the experience of motherhood*. Oxford University Press, Oxford.

Charles, J. and Curtis, L. (1994). Birth afterthoughts: a listening and information service. *British Journal of Midwifery*, **2**, 331–4.

Christopher, E. (1991). Family planning and reproductive decisions. *Journal of Reproductive and Infant Psychology*, **9**, 217–26.

Clement, S. (1994). Unwanted vaginal examinations. *British Journal of Midwifery*, **2**, 368–70.

Clement, S. (1995*a*). *The Caesarean experience*. Pandora Press, London.

Clement, S. (1995*b*). Listening visits in pregnancy: a strategy for preventing postnatal depression? *Midwifery*, **11**, 75–80.

Clement, S., Sikorski, J., Wilson, J., and Das, S. (1997). Planning antenatal services to meet women's psychological needs. *British Journal of Midwifery*, **5**(5), 298–305.

Clement, S., Wilson, J., and Sikorski, J. (1998). Women's experiences of antenatal ultrasound scans. In: *Psychological perspectives on pregnancy and childbirth* (ed. S. Clement), pp.7–26. Churchill Livingstone, London.

Cogill, S. R., Caplan, H. L., Alexander, H., *et al.* (1986). Impact of maternal postnatal depression on cognitive development of young children. *British Medical Journal*, **292**, 1165–7.

Cooper, P. J., Campbell, E. A., Day, A., Kennerly, H., and Bond, A. (1988). Non-psychotic psychiatric disorder after childbirth: a prospective study of prevalence, incidence, course, and nature. *British Journal Psychiatry*, **152**, 799–806.

Cooper, P. J. and Murray, L. (1995). Course and recurrence of postnatal depression:

evidence for the specificity of the diagnostic concept. *British Journal of Psychiatry*, **166**, 191–5.

Cox, J. L. (1979). Psychiatric morbidity and pregnancy: a controlled study of 263 semi-rural Ugandan women. *British Journal of Psychiatry*, **134**, 401–5.

Cox, J. L. (1994). Introduction and classification dilemmas. In: *Perinatal psychiatry: use and abuse of the Edinburgh Postnatal Depression Scale* (ed. J. L.Cox and J. M.Holden), pp.3–7. Gaskell, London.

Cox, J. L., Kumar, R., Margison, F. R., and Downey, L. J. (1986). *Current approaches to puerperal mental illness*. Duphar, Southampton.

Cox, J. L., Holden, J. M., and Sagovsky, R. (1987). Detection of postnatal depression: development of the 10-item Edinburgh Postnatal Depression Scale. *British Journal of Psychiatry*, **150**, 782–6.

Cox, J. L., Murray, D., and Chapman, G. (1993). A controlled study of the onset, duration, and prevalence of postnatal depression, *British Journal of Psychiatry*, **163**, 27–31.

Cullinan, R. (1991). Health visitor intervention in postnatal depression. *Health Visitor*, **64**, 412–14.

Dalton, K. (1971). Prospective study into puerperal depression. *British Journal of Psychiatry*, **118**, 689–92.

Dalton, K. (1980). *Depression after childbirth*. Oxford University Press, Oxford.

De Bellis, M. D., Lefter, L., Trickett, P. K., and Putnam Jr, F. W. (1994). Urinary catecholamine excretion in sexually abused girls. *Journal of the American Acadmey of Child and Adolescent Psychiatry*, **33**, 320–7.

Department of Health (1993). Changing Childbirth: report of the expert maternity group. HMSO, London.

Edelmann, R. J. and Connolly, K. J. (1986). Psychological aspects of infertility. *British Journal of Medical Psychology*, **59**, 209–19.

Edelmann, R. J. and Golombok, S. (1989). Stress and reproductive failure. *Journal of Reproductive and Infant Psychology*, **7**, 79–86.

Egan, G. (1990). *The skilled helper*. Brooks/Cole, California.

Elliott, S. A. (1984). Pregnancy and after. In: *Contributions to medical psychology* (ed. S. Rachman),Vol. 3, pp.93–116. Pergamon, Oxford.

Elliott, S. A. (1989*a*). Psychological strategies in the prevention and treatment of postnatal depression. In: Psychological aspects of obstetrics and gynaecology (ed. M. R. Oates). *Balliere's Clinical Obstetrics and Gynaecology*, **3**, 839–56.

Elliott, S. A. (1989*b*). Postnatal depression: consequences and intervention. In: *Premenstrual, post-partum, and menopausal mood disorders* (ed. L. M. Demers, J. L. McGuire, A. Phillips, and D. R. Rubinow), pp.153–62. Urban and Schwarzenberg, Inc., Baltimore.

Elliott, S. A. (1990). Commentary on 'Childbirth as a life event'. *Journal of Reproductive and Infant Psychology*, **8**, 147–59.

Elliott, S. A. (1994). Uses and misuses of the EPDS in primary care. In: *Perinatal psychiatry: use and abuse of the Edinburgh Postnatal Depression Scale* (ed. J. L. Cox and J. M. Holden), pp.221–32. Gaskell, London.

Elliott, S. A. (1997). Post-partum depression. In: *Cambridge handbook of psychology, health, and medicine* (ed. A. Baum, C. McManus, S. Newman, J. Weinman, and R. West). Cambridge University Press, Cambridge.

Elliott, S. A., Rugg, A. J., Watson, J. P., and Brough, D. I. (1983). Mood changes during pregnancy and after the birth of a child. *British Journal of Clinical Psychology*, 22, 295–308.

Elliott, S. A., Anderson, M., Brough, D. I., Watson, J. P., and Rugg, A. (1984). Relationship between obstetric outcome and psychological measures in pregnancy and the postnatal year. *Journal of Reproductive and Infant Psychology*, 2, 18–32.

Elliott, S. A., Sanjack, M., and Leverton, T. J. (1988). Parents' groups in pregnancy: a preventive intervention for postnatal depression? In: *Marshalling social support: formats, processes, and effects* (ed. B. J. Gottleib). Sage, London.

Fleisig, A. (1991). Unintended pregnancies and the use of contraception: changes from 1984 to 1989. *British Medical Journal*, 302, 147.

Forrest, G. C., Standish, E., and Baum, J. D. (1982). Support after perinatal death: a study of support and counselling after perinatal bereavement. *British Medical Journal*, 285, 1475–9.

Gerrard, J., Holden, J. M., Elliott, S. A., *et al.* (1993). A trainer's perspective of an innovative programme teaching health visitors about the detection, treatment, and prevention of postnatal depression. *Journal of Advanced Nursing*, 18, 1825–32.

Gerrard, J., Elliott, S. A., and Holden, J. M. (1994). The management of postnatal depression: a manual for mental health trainers of primary care staff. Unpublished manuscript.

Glover, V., Liddle, P., Taylor, A., Adams, D., and Sandler, M. (1994). Mild hypomania (the highs) can be a feature of the first post-partum week. *British Journal of Psychiatry*, 164, 517–21.

Golombok, S., Cook, R., Bish, A., and Murray, C. (1995). Families created by the new reproductive technologies: quality of parenting and social and emotional development of the children. *Child Development*, 66, 285–98.

Gotlib, I. H., Whiffen, V. E., Mount, J. H. *et al.* (1989). Prevalence rates and demographic characteristics associated with depression in pregnancy and the post-partum. *Journal of Consulting and Clinical Psychology*, 57, 269–74.

Green, J. M. (1990). Is the baby alright and other worries. *Journal of Reproductive and Infant Psychology*, 8, 225–6.

Green, J. M., Coupland, V. A., and Kitzinger, J. V. (1988). *Great expectations: a prospective study of women's expectations and experiences of childbirth*. Centre for Family Research, University of Cambridge, Cambridge.

Green, J. M., Coupland, V. A. and Kitzinger, J. V. (1990). Expectations, experiences, and psychological outcomes of childbirth: a prospective study of 825 women. *Birth*, 7, 15–24.

Green, J. M., Richards, M. P. M., Kitzinger, J. V., and Coupland, V. A. (1991).

Mothers' perceptions of their six-week-old babies: relationships with antenatal, intrapartum, and postnatal factors. *Irish Journal of Psychology*, 12, 133–44.

Green, J. M. and Murray, D. (1994). The use of the Edinburgh Postnatal Depression Scale to explore the relationship between antenatal and postnatal dysphoria. In *Perinatal psychiatry: use and misuse of the Edinburgh Postnatal Depression Scale* (ed. J. L. Cox and J. M.Holden). Gaskell, London.

Green, J. M. and Statham, H. (1996). Psychological aspects of prenatal screening and diagnosis. In: *The troubled helix: social and psychological implications of the new human genetics* (ed. T. Marteau and M. Richards). Cambridge University Press, Cambridge.

Gregoire, A. J., Kumar, R, Everitt, B., Henderson A. F., and Studd, J. W. (1996). Transdermal oestrogen for treatment of severe postnatal depression. *Lancet*, 347, 930–3.

Harris, B. (1994). Biological and hormonal aspects of post-partum depressed mood. *British Journal of Psychiatry*, 164, 288–92.

Harris, B. (1996). Hormonal aspects of postnatal depression. *International Review of Psychiatry*, 8, 27–36.

Harrison, M. (1992). Linking with community and voluntary resources. In: *The prevention of depression and anxiety: the role of the primary care team* (ed. R. Jenkins, J. Newton, and R. Young). HMSO, London.

Hedegaard, M., Henricksen, T. B., Sabroe, S., *et al.* (1993). Psychological distress in pregnancy and preterm delivery. *British Medical Journal*, 307, 234–9.

Hedegaard, M., Henricksen, T. B., Sabroe, S., *et al.* (1996). The relationship between psychological distress during pregnancy and birthweight for gestational age. *Acta Obstetricia et Gynecologica Scandinavia*, 75, 32–9.

Hillan, E. M. (1992). Maternal–infant attachment following Caesarean delivery. *Journal of Clinical Nursing*, 1, 33–7.

Hodnett, E. D. (1995*a*). *Support from care-givers during at-risk pregnancy*. In: Pregnancy and Childbirth Module. Cochrane Pregnancy and Childbirth Database (ed. M. W. Enkin, M. J. N. C. Keirse, and M. J. Renfrew). The Cochrane Collaboration, Issue 2. Update Software, Oxford. Available from BMJ Publishing Group, London.

Hodnett, E. D. (1995*b*). *Continuity of care-givers during pregnancy and childbirth*. In: Pregnancy and Childbirth Module. Cochrane Pregnancy and Childbirth Database (ed. M. W. Enkin, M. J. N. C. Keirse, and M. J. Renfrew). The Cochrane Collaboration, Issue 2. Update Software, Oxford. Available from BMJ Publishing Group, London.

Hodnett, E. D. (1995*c*). *Women carrying their own casenotes during pregnancy* (revised May 1993). In: Pregnancy and Childbirth Module. Cochrane Pregnancy and Childbirth Database (ed. M. W. Enkin, M. J. N. C. Keirse, and M. J. Renfrew). The Cochrane Collaboration, Issue 2. Update Software, Oxford. Available from BMJ Publishing Group, London.

Hodnett, E. D. (1995*d*). *Support from care-givers for socially disadvantaged mothers*. In: Pregnancy and Childbirth Module. Cochrane Pregnancy and Childbirth Database (ed. M. W. Enkin, M. J. N. C. Keirse, and M. J. Renfrew). The Cochrane Collaboration, Issue 2. Update Software, Oxford. Available from BMJ Publishing Group, London.

Holden, J. M. (1994). Using the Edinburgh Postnatal Depression Scale in clinical practice. In: *Perinatal psychiatry: use and misuse of the Edinburgh Postnatal Depression Scale* (ed. J. L. Cox and J. M. Holden). Gaskell, London.

Holden, J. M. (1996). The role of health visitors in postnatal depression. *International Review of Psychiatry*, **8**, 79–86.

Holden, J. M., Sagovskym R., and Cox, J. L. (1989). Counselling in a general practice setting: a controlled study of health visitor intervention in the treatment of postnatal depression. *British Medical Journal*, **298**, 223–6.

Hunt, S. and Symonds, A. (1995). *The social meaning of midwifery*. Macmillan, Basingstoke.

Hunter, M. (1994). *Counselling in obstetrics and gynaecology*. British Psychological Society Books, Leicester.

Johnstone, M. (1994). *The emotional effects of childbirth*: Marce Society Distance Learning Pack., Marce Society, Doncaster.

Jones, S. C. and Hunter, M. (1996). The influence of context and discourse on infertility experience. *Journal of Reproductive and Infant Psychology*, **14**, 93–111.

Kendell, R. E., Chalmers, J. C., and Platz, C. (1987). Epidemiology of puerperal psychosis. *British Journal of Psychiatry*, **150**, 662–73.

Kennerley, H. and Gath,D. (1989). Maternity blues. *British Journal of Psychiatry*, **155**, 356–62.

Kitzinger, S. (1987). *Giving birth: how it really feels*. Gollancz, London.

Kitzinger, S. (1992). Birth and violence against women. In: *Women's health matters* (ed. H. Roberts), pp63–80. Routledge, London.

Kumar, R. (1989). Post-partum psychosis. *Balliere's Clinical Obstetrics and Gynaecology*, **3**, 823–38.

Kumar, R. C. and Robson, K. M. (1984). A prospective study of emotional disorders in childbearing women. *British Journal of Psychiatry*, **144**, 35–47.

Kumar, R. C., Hipwell, A. E. and Lawson, C. (1994). Prevention of adverse effects of perinatal maternal mental illness on the developing child. In: *Perinatal psychiatry: use and misuse of the Edinburgh Postnatal Depression Scale* (ed. J. L. Cox and J. M. Holden). Gaskell, London.

Laryea, M. (1989). Midwives' and mothers' perceptions of motherhood. In: *Midwives, research, and childbirth* (ed. S. Robinson and A. M. Thomson), Vol. 1. Chapman and Hall, London.

Leap, N. (1991). *Helping you to make your own decisions: antenatal and postnatal groups in Deptford, SE London*. VHS video.

Leverton, T. J. and Elliott, S. A. (1989). Transition to parenthood groups: a preventive intervention for postnatal depression? In: *The free woman* (ed. E. V. van Hall and W. Everaerd). Parthenon, Carnforth.

Lumley, J. M. (1982). Attitudes towards the fetus among primigravidae. *Australian Pediatric Journal*, **18**, 106–9.

Lyon, S. S. (1998). Post-traumatic stress disorder: causes, prevention, and treatment. In: *Psychological perspectives on pregnancy and childbirth* (ed. S. Clement), pp.123–43. Churchill Livingstone, London.

McFadyen, A. (1994). Special care babies and their developing relationships. Routledge, London.

McIntosh, J. (1989). Models of childbirth and social class: a study of 80 working class primigravidae. In: *Midwives, research, and childbirth*, (ed. S. Robinson and A. M. Thomson), Vol. 1. Chapman and Hall, London.

McIntosh, J. (1993). Post-partum depression: women's help-seeking behaviour and perceptions of cause. *Journal of Advanced Nursing*, **18**, 178–84.

McMahon, C. A., Ungerer, J. A., Beaurepaire, J., Tennant, C., and Saunders, D. (1995). Psychosocial outcomes for parents and children after *in vitro* fertilization: a review. *Journal of Reproductive and Infant Psychology*, **13**, 1–16.

Mander, R. (1994). *Loss and bereavement in childbearing*. Blackwell, Oxford.

Marks, M. N., Wieck, A., and Checkley, S. A. (1992). Contribution of psychological and social factors to psychotic and non-psychotic relapse after childbirth in women with previous histories of affective disorder. *Journal of Affective Disorders*, **29**, 253–64.

Marsh, J. and Sargent, E. (1991). Factors affecting the duration of postnatal visits.*Midwifery*, **7**, 177–82.

Marteau, T. (1994). Psychology and screening: narrowing the gap between efficacy and effectiveness. *British Journal of Clinical Psychology*, **33**, 1–10.

Mauthner, N. S. (1995). Postnatal depression:the significance of social contacts between mothers. *Women's Studies International Forum*, **18**, 311–23.

Menage, J. (1993). Post-traumatic stress disorder in women who have undergone obstetric and/or gynaecological procedures. *Journal of Reproductive and Infant Psychology*, **11**, 221–8.

Metz, A., Sichel, D. A., and Goff, D. C. (1988). Post-partum panic disorder. *Journal of Clinical Psychiatry*, **49**, 278–9.

Moleman, N.,van der Hart, O., and van der Kolk, B. A. (1992). The partus stress reaction: a neglected aetiological factor in post-partum psychiatric disorders. *Journal of Nervous and Mental Diseases*, **180**, 271–2.

Moore, M. and Hopper, U. (1995). Do birth plans empower women? Evaluation of a hospital birth plan. *Birth*, **22**, 29–36.

Murray, D. (1996). Oestrogen and postnatal depression. *Lancet*, **347**, 918–19.

Murray, D. and Cox, J. L. (1990). Screening for depression during pregnancy with the Edinburgh Postnatal Depression Scale (EPDS). *Journal of Reproductive and Infant Psychology*, **8**, 99–107.

Murray, D., Cox, J. L., Chapman, G., and Jones, P. (1995). Childbirth: life event or start of long-term difficulty? *British Journal of Psychiatry*, **166**, 595–600.

Murray, L. and Cooper, P. J. (1996). The impact of post-partum depression on child development. *International Review of Psychiatry*, **8**, 55–64.

Neugebauer, R., Kline, J., O'Connor, P., *et al.* (1992). Depressive symptoms in women in the six months after miscarriage. *American Journal of Obstetrics and Gynecology*, **166**, 104–9.

Newton, R. W. (1988). Psychosocial aspects of pregnancy: the scope for intervention. *Journal of Reproductive and Infant Psychology*, **6**, 23–39.

Niven, C. A. (1992). Psychological care for families: before, during, and after birth. Butterworth Heinemann, London.

Oakley, A. (1980). *Woman confined: towards a sociology of childbirth*. Martin Robertson, Oxford.

Oakley, A. (1992). Social support in pregnancy: methodology and findings of a one-year follow-up study. *Journal of Reproductive and Infant Psychology*, 10, 219–32.

Oakley, A. and Rajan, L. (1990). Obstetric technology and maternal emotional well-being: a further research note. *Journal of Reproductive and Infant Psychology*, 8, 45–55.

Oakley, A., Rajan, L., and Grant, A. (1990). Social support and pregnancy outcome. *British Journal of Obstetrics and Gynaecology*, 97, 155–62.

Oakley, A., Hickey, D., Rajan, L., and Rigby, A. (1996). Social support in pregnancy: does it have long-term effects? *Journal of Reproductive and Infant Psychology*, 14, 7–22.

Oates, M. R. (1989). Management of major mental illness in pregnancy and the puerperium. In: Psychological aspects of obstetrics and gynaecology (ed. M. R. Oates). *Balliere's Clinical Obstetrics and Gynaecology*, 3, 839–56.

Oates, M. R. (1996). Psychiatric services for women following childbirth. *International Review of Psychiatry*, 8, 87–98.

O'Brien, S. and Pitt, B. (1994). Hormonal theories and therapy for postnatal depression. In: *Perinatal psychiatry: use and misuse of the Edinburgh Postnatal Depression Scale* (ed. J. Cox and J. Holden), pp103–38. Gaskell, London.

O'Hara, M. W. (1994). *Post-partum depression: causes and consequences*. Springer-Verlag, New York.

O Hara, M. W. and Zekoski, E. M. (1988). Post-partum depression: a comprehensive review. In: *Motherhood and mental illness 2: causes and consequences* (ed. I. F. Brockington and R. Kumar). Wright, London.

O'Hara, M. W., Zekoski, E. M., Philipps, L. H., and Wright, E. J. (1990). Controlled prospective study of post-partum mood disorders: comparison of child-bearing and non child-bearing women. *Journal of Abnormal Psychology*, 99, 3–15.

O'Hara, M. W., Schlechre, J. A., Lewis, D. A., and Jarner. M. W. (1991). Controlled prospective study of post-partum mood disorder: psychological, environmental, and hormonal variables. *Journal of Abnormal Psychology*, 100, 63–73.

O'Hara, M. W. and Swain, A. M. (1996). Rates and risk of post-partum depression: a meta-analysis. *International Review of Psychiatry*, 8, 37–54.

Peacock, J. L., Bland, J.M., and Anderson, H. R. (1995). Preterm delivery: effects of socioeconomic factors, psychosocial stress, smoking, alcohol, and caffeine. *British Medical Journal*, 311, 53–6.

Pitt, B. (1968). Atypical depression following childbirth. *British Journal of Psychiatry*, 114, 1325–35.

Pound, A. and Mills, M. (1985). A pilot evaluation of Newpin: a home visiting and befriending scheme in South London. *Association of Child Psychiatry and Psychology Newsletter*, 7, 13–15.

Prettyman, R. J., Cordle, C. J. and Cook, G. D. (1993). A three-month follow-up of psychological morbidity after early miscarriage. *British Journal of Medical Psychology*, 66, 363–72.

Prince, J. and Adams, M. (1990). The psychology of pregnancy. In: *Antenatal care: a research-based approach* (ed. J. Alexander, V. Levy, and S Roche), pp.120–33. MacMillan, London.

Rajan, L. (1996). Pain and pain relief in labour: issues of control. In: *Modern medicine: lay perspectives and experiences* (ed. S. J.Williams and M. Calnan). UCL Press, London.

Ralph, K. and Alexander, J. (1994). Borne under stress. *Nursing Times*, **90**, 28–30.

Raphael, B. and Meldrum, L. (1995). Does debriefing after psychological trauma work? *British Medical Journal*, **310**, 1479–80.

Raphael-Leff, J. (1991). *Psychological processes of child-bearing.* Chapman and Hall, London.

Riley, D. (1995). *Perinatal mental health: a sourcebook for health professionals.* Radcliffe Medical Press, Oxford.

Robinson, G. E., Stirtzinger, R., Stewart, D. E., *et al.* (1994). Psychological reactions in women followed for one year after miscarriage. *Journal of Reproductive and Infant Psychology*, **12**, 31–6.

Roelofsen, E. E. C., Kamerbbek, L. I., and Tymstra, T. J. (1993). Chances and choices – psychosocial consequences of maternal serum screening: a report from the Netherlands. *Journal of Reproductive and Infant Psychology*, **11**, 41–7.

Rogers, C. R. (1961). *On becoming a person.* Houghton Mifflen, Boston.

Roy, A., Cole, K., Goldman, Z., and Barris, M. (1993). Fluoxetine treatment of post-partum depression. *American Journal of Psychiatry*, **150**, 1273.

Royal College of General Practitioners (1995). *The role of general practice in maternity care.* RCGP, London.

Royal College of Midwives (1987). *Towards a healthy nation: a policy for the maternity services.* RCM, London.

Sandelowski, M. and Busamante, R. (1986). Caesarean birth outside the natural childbirth culture. *Research in Nursing and Health*, **9**, 81.

Sharpe, S. (1984). *Double identity: the lives of working mothers.* Penguin, Harmondsworth.

Sikorski J., Wilson, J., Clement, S., Das, S., and Smeeton, N. (1996). A randomized controlled trial comparing two schedules of antenatal visits: the antenatal care project. *British Medical Journal*, **312**, 546–53.

Simkin, P. (1991). Just another day in a woman's life? Women's long-term perceptions of their first birth experience. *Birth*, **18**, 203–10.

Slade, P. (1994). Predicting the psychological impact of miscarriage. *Journal of Reproductive and Infant Psychology*, **12**, 5–16.

Smith, M. P. (1989). Postnatal concerns of mothers: an update. *Midwifery*, **5**, 182–8.

Stamp, G. E., Williams, A. S., and Crowther, C. A. (1995). Evaluation of antenatal and postnatal support to overcome postnatal depression. *Birth*, **22**, 138–43.

Statham, H. and Green, J. M. (1994). The effects of miscarriage and other 'unsuccessful' pregnancies on feelings early in a subsequent pregnancy. *Journal of Reproductive and Infant Psychology*, **12**, 45–54.

Stein, G. (1982). The maternity blues. In: *Motherhood and mental illness* (ed. I. F.Brockington and R. Kumar), pp.119–54. Wright, London.

Teasdale, J. D. (1985). Psychological treatments for depression: how do they work? *Behaviour Research And Therapy*, **23**, 157–65.

Thorley, K. and Rouse, T. (1993). Seeing mothers as partners in antenatal care. *British Journal of Midwifery*, 1, 216–19.

Thorpe, K. and Elliott, S. A. (1998). Emotional well-being of mothers. In: *Psychology of reproduction. Vol. 3: Current issues in infancy and parenthood* (ed. C. Niven and A. Walker). Butterworth Heinemann, Oxford.

Thune-Larsen, K. B. and Moller-Pedersen, K. (1988). Childbirth experience and post-partum emotional disturbance. *Journal of Reproductive and Infant Psychology*, 2, 61–78.

Watson, J. P., Elliott, S. A., Rugg, A. J., and Brough, D. I. (1984). Psychiatric disorder in pregnancy and the first postnatal year. *British Journal of Psychiatry*, **144**, 453–62.

Weaver, J. (1998). Choice, control, and decision-making in labour. In: *Psychological perspectives on pregnancy and childbirth* (ed. S. Clement), pp.81–99. Churchill Livingstone, London.

Whitton, A., Appleby, L., and Warner, R. (1996). Maternal thinking and the treatment of postnatal depression. *International Review of Psychiatry*, **8**,73–8.

Wieck, A. (1996). Ovarian hormones, mood, and neurotransmitters. *International Review of Psychiatry*, **8**, 17–26.

Wolkind, S., Zajicek, E., and Ghodsian, M. (1980). Continuities in maternal depression. *International Journal of Family Psychiatry*, 1, 167–82.

Wolkind, S. and Zajicek, E. (1981). *Pregnancy: a psychological and social study*. Academic Press, London.

Wolman, W. L., Chalmers, B., Hofmeyr, G. J., and Nikodem, V. C. (1993). Post-partum depression and companionship in the clinical birth environment: a randomized controlled trial. *American Journal of Obstetrics and Gynecology*, **168**, 1388–93.

Woollett, A. (1991). Having children: accounts of childless women and women with reproductive problems. In: *Motherhood: meanings, practices, and ideologies* (ed. A. Phoenix, A. Woollett, and E. Lloyd). Sage, London.

Wrate, R. M., Rooney, A. C., Thomas, P. F., *et al.* (1985). Postnatal depression and child development: a three-year follow-up study. *British Journal of Psychiatry*, **146**, 622–7.

Wright, J., Allard, M., Lecours, A., and Sabourin, S. (1989). Psychosocial distress and infertility: a review of controlled research. *International Journal of Infertility*, **34**, 126–42.

Yoshida, K. and Kumar, R. (1996). Breastfeeding and psychotropic drugs. *International Review of Psychiatry* , **8**, 117–24.

Further reading

Brown, S., Lumley, J., Small, R., and Astbury, J. (1994). *Missing voices: the experience of motherhood*. Oxford University Press, Oxford.

Clement, S. (ed.) (1998). *Psychological perspectives on pregnancy and childbirth.* Churchill Livingstone, London.

Cox, J. L. and Holden, J. M. (ed.) (1994). *Perinatal psychiatry: use and misuse of the Edinburgh Postnatal Depression Scale.* Gaskell, London.

Hunter, M. (1994). *Counselling in obstetrics and gynaecology.* British Psychological Society Books, Leicester.

Niven, C. and Walker, A. (ed.) (1996). *Psychology of reproduction Vol. 2: Conception, pregnancy, and birth.* Butterworth Heinemann, Oxford.

Niven, C. and Walker, A. (ed.) (1998). *Psychology of reproduction Vol. 3: Current issues in infancy and parenthood.* Butterworth Heinemann, Oxford.

O'Hara, M. W. (1994). *Post-partum depression: causes and consequences.* Springer-Verlag, New York.

Raphael-Leff, J. (1991). *Psychological processes of child-bearing.* Chapman and Hall, London.

Riley, D. (1995). *Perinatal mental health: a sourcebook for health professionals.* Radcliffe Medical Press, Oxford.

Resources

Marce distance learning pack
Available from:
The Marce Society
7–9 Duke Street
DONCASTER
DN1 1ED

Trainer training courses
Details available from:
Diane Jackson
North Staffordshire Medical Institute
HARTSHILL
Stoke on Trent
ST4 7NY

CHAPTER NINETEEN

Latest views on antenatal care programmes

Janet Tucker and Marion Hall

The aims of antenatal care

In defining the aims of antenatal care two main elements are repeated in health service literature: clinical monitoring of the pregnancy with appropriate intervention, and psychosocial support for the woman and her family. For example, James (1995) says that antenatal care should achieve the following:

- 'prevent, detect, and manage those problems and factors that adversely affect the health of the mother and her baby

- provide an ongoing screening programme (clinical and laboratory based) to confirm that the woman continues not to be at risk

- deal with the minor ailments of pregnancy

- provide advice, reassurance, education, and support for the woman and her family.'

These same elements appear in government policy and guideline documents over the last 20 years and in the Cumberlege Report (1993). However, the relative emphasis given to the two elements of care do vary. They may vary according to the author's perspective; for example, obstetricians may emphasize the monitoring of pregnancy to prevent or detect clinical abnormalities whereas midwives may put more emphasis on the supportive and educational role to ensure psychosocial well-being. Over the last 15 years growing emphasis has been placed on meeting women's individual and psychosocial needs. Following the publication of the Patient's Charter in particular (Department of Health 1991), the policy documents of England and Wales and Scotland over the last four years (Cumberlege Report 1993; Scottish Office Home and Health Department 1993, 1995) have underlined the importance of meeting women's expectations and require-ments of contemporary maternity services, and recognize that all women want a healthy baby but not necessarily the same kind of care. Priority areas identified as requiring improvement are information-giving and communication, as well as choice and continuity of care, but the safety of the mother and child to remain paramount.

The tension inherent in the two main aims of antenatal care arose from the increased development of technological intervention in antenatal and maternity care over the last 40 years as a growing number of women felt that their experience of child-bearing was marred by the very use of such interventions (Chapter 13). But as Oakley (1991) said:

'Whilst the consumer movement will not go away, neither will other important influences on the shape of maternity care. We live in a world which values technology, and which has relinquished control over many aspects of our lives to professionals.'

In addition to the pressures from women, some clinicians have questioned both the clinical elements of antenatal multiphasic screening and how the care is delivered. The potential and actual efficacy and efficiency of antenatal care was first raised 15–20 years ago (Chng *et al.* 1980). It was suggested that there was oversurveillance of many women and that productivity of antenatal care was low. More recently, Cumberlege (1993) suggested that antenatal care was 'not focused in the most appropriate or consistent manner'.

To allow development and implementation of new models of care, the views and attitudes of care-givers also have to be understood (Wraight *et al.* 1993; Sikorski *et al.* 1995*b*; Turnbull *et al.* 1995). Table 19:1 summarizes the dimensions of care programmes which should be evaluated to provide results to fully inform policy and decision-making. It should be noted that these dimensions are not independent of each other. The staff might dislike a style of care in spite of the fact that women like it, or might practise a style of care they dislike if they considered it to be the safest.

A review of contemporary models of antenatal care

International comparisons

International comparisons of antenatal care in developed countries have shown differences not only in how much antenatal care women are

Table 19.1 *Evaluation of antenatal services*

Dimension of care	Basic research question
Clinical effectiveness	How safe is it?
Views of women and measures of their satisfaction	Do the women like it?
Views, measures of satisfaction, and effect on workload of staff	Do the staff like it?
An economic evaluation	What are the comparative costs and benefits of the two styles of care?

recommended to receive but in the professional groups who deliver that care. Blondel et al. (1985) reported that the recommended number of antenatal visits in 13 European countries ranged from three or four in Switzerland to 14 in Finland. They noted that northern European countries tended to recommend many more visits than Belgium, Switzerland, France, and Luxembourg and that the relative roles played by midwives, general practitioners, and obstetricians also varied. They concluded that there were wide differences in the models of antenatal care delivered in countries with very comparable perinatal mortality outcomes. Similar conclusions were reached in 1985 by the World Health Organization study *Having a baby in Europe* (WHO 1985). This study also reported that, according to responses given by member governments, the relative professional roles of obstetricians, general practitioners, and midwives in antenatal care showed an increasing role for the obstetrician in the routine care of uncomplicated pregnancies and a general trend to transfer medical tasks from midwives to physicians. Furthermore, there were marked criticisms that perinatal technology was out of control and that widely held beliefs in the overall efficacy of antenatal care should be critically examined. However, these international comparisons of reported models of care may not accurately describe the actual practice in different countries, nor do they always take into account changes which have occurred through time. Kaminski et al. (1993) criticized inaccurate use of statistics and incomplete data in some studies, noting that in a comparison of perinatal outcomes and care during pregnancy and childbirth in England and Wales and France (Mascarenhas et al. 1992) the latest data used were from 1988, and that the authors failed to take account of a subsequent modification of French antenatal care regulations when the minimum number of visits required changed from three to seven for women to be eligible for state maternity benefits. Kaminski et al. (1993) concluded that the previously reported wide difference in antenatal visit number between France and England and Wales may have narrowed as the recommendations are no longer as disparate.

Similar uncertainty about the appropriate content of antenatal care was shown in a study which involved 10 European Community (EC) countries (Heringa and Hendrik 1988). There was limited agreement between 67 university/training hospitals in their *self-reported* use of 30 defined antenatal screening investigations. Although there was agreement over the traditional tests, e.g. blood pressure, glycosuria, blood group, and rhesus checks, there was no such agreement over more recent techniques with the exception of ultrasound scans.

A recommendation of five visits for low-risk multiparous and eight for primiparous women with a specific function for each visit was made by a working party of the Royal College of Obstetricians and Gynaecologists on antenatal and intrapartum care (RCOG 1982). This also recommended the use of shared care between obstetrician and GP/midwife, and that midwives should play a greater part in the provision of care of normal pregnant women. Information about actual antenatal care visits, supervision, content, and location is not routinely collected in Scotland, nor in England and Wales (Macfarlane *et al.* 1995), so the extent to which these recommendations had been implemented was unclear.

A population-based observational study of antenatal care in Scotland

In a retrospective cohort study of maternity case records at 15 representative hospitals in Scotland in the last quarter of 1989 (Tucker *et al.* 1994), the antenatal care delivered to a series of 4069 women was analysed to examine the number of visits, content, location, and supervision of women according to their risk category. The findings of this observational study showed that 97% of 3547 women had obstetrician-led shared care by agreement of the obstetric consultant and the general practitioner, with the majority of visits at GP clinics or health centres. This was in close agreement with the RCOG 1982 recommendations. However, although 81% were at low risk of pregnancy complications at the outset of their pregnancy and 64% remained at low risk throughout, there was little evidence of differentiation of care by risk category of the women.

The average number of antenatal visits was 14 per woman. Allowing for the 'preterm delivery bias' (Tyson *et al.* 1990), we showed there was little consistency in the differences in antenatal visit number between risk categories. Women who were outset high risk or changed to high risk during pregnancy tended only to have around one visit more than low-risk women and their increased requirement for specialist care appeared to be met by more admissions and in-patient care rather than more specialist-supervised clinic visits. The observed pattern of visits followed the traditional timing of that laid down in 1929 (Ministry of Health 1929), with four-weekly visits until 28 weeks, fortnightly visits to 36 weeks and weekly visits until term. Around 87% of all antenatal contacts were routine visits. Of those, at 98% of visits blood pressure checks occurred, at 93% maternal weight checks and urine analysis occurred, at 90% abdominal palpation occurred, and at 80% the fetal heart/movement was checked. There was little variation between hospitals or hospital types in the regular use of these checks. However, significant variations were found between the 15 hospitals in the use of alpha-fetoprotein tests (range 47–93% of mothers presenting before 20 weeks with at least one test) and in the use of ultrasound examinations before 20 weeks for attending women (range 79–99%).

Overall, general practitioners supervised the majority of visits – 43.5% (range 31–67%) compared to 36% (range 25–55%) attributed to hospital doctors and 12% (range 4–34%) to midwives – but there were differences in who supervised the antenatal visits between the hospitals and hospital categories. The results of this study led us to conclude that in Scotland at that time there was little evidence that a reduced schedule of visits for women with normal pregnancies had been implemented. Rather, the results showed a blanket application of a traditional schedule of shared antenatal care. It is not known whether this occurred because obstetricians and general practitioners did not accept the 1982 RCOG recommendations or whether there was simple duplication of visits because of shared care. Only a few units had a significant proportion of visits supervised by midwives.

Developing models of community antenatal care

There have been many studies and reports which identified shortcomings in the content and the delivery of shared antenatal care. These include fragmentation, centralized hospital clinics often a considerable distance from where women lived, long waiting times, lack of privacy, and lack of facilities for small children. Community-based schemes of maternity care were developed to try to overcome some of these difficulties. There are two main characteristics to consider about the re-emergence of community antenatal care. In addition to the obvious issue of placing care in local settings, there is also the question of who delivers the care.

Peripheral specialist clinics

The establishment of peripheral hospital specialist clinics in more local settings was one form of community care. At a time of mainly centralized, hospital antenatal clinics, Baird (1969) described an early example of peripheral specialist clinics in 1967 in Aberdeen. By the early 1980s very similar schemes to that described by Baird were reintroduced as peripheral specialist clinics of the Queen Mother's Hospital, Glasgow (at Drumchapel) and of Glasgow Royal Maternity Hospital (placed in a corporation house in Easterhouse). This latter initiative was evaluated by a randomized controlled trial (Reid *et al.* 1983). Results showed that the pregnancy outcomes were similar for the two groups but that the women who attended the peripheral clinic were more satisfied with how their care was provided. GPs had no prescribed role in either of these peripheral clinic initiatives in Glasgow, and who provided the care was not at issue.

Integrated specialist input in community settings

Models of community antenatal care reported later in the 1980s aimed to integrate more closely the professional groups who delivered care by having obstetric specialists attend general practice or health centre clinics. One study reported the benefit of an obstetrician at specific general practice clinics in a socially deprived locality as facilitating early booking visits of women and reducing referral delays (Robson *et al.* 1986). Further studies of integrated community antenatal care programmes were at Sighthill in Edinburgh, Huntington and East Barnwell near Cambridge, Balsall Heath in Birmingham, and Hackney and Lambeth in London (Wood 1991). The evaluations of integrated community antenatal care were observational studies which indicated improved quality of service in terms of access, continuity of care, and communication between women and professionals with clinical outcomes as good as traditional models of care.

Devolving care to primary carers in community settings

Marsh (1985) put forward a protocol for debate of a devolved model of community antenatal care for GP/midwife care. He suggested that around 75% of all women would be at low risk of pregnancy complications, eligible, and benefit from such a programme. He advocated reduced visit numbers from around 15 to eight for primiparous women and six for multiparous women and gave specific functions for each visit.

An evaluation of a community antenatal care programme was reported from West Berkshire (Street *et al.* 1991) as part of a new extended community obstetric service. GPs and midwives accepted full and legal responsibility for women who met the eligibility criteria and such women were not given the choice of consultant care. The audit showed that the number of visits to GPs and midwives nearly doubled whereas attendance at consultant antenatal clinics fell by around 20%. Of those women booked for GP/midwife care, 31% transferred antenatally to consultant care mainly because of post-maturity. They concluded that community obstetric care seemed to be a satisfactory solution for most women and that this model of care had replaced traditional shared care in West Berkshire.

Hill *et al.* (1993) also describe a comparative study in Oxford of a policy of fewer antenatal visits to obstetric specialists. They compared over 1000 women in each group who received either the reduced number of specialist visits from consultant group A or the traditional model from consultant group B in a study designed to control for any confounding concurrent changes in service over the study period. Selected, low-risk women were not randomized but allocated as referred by their GPs to consultants in groups A or B. The results showed a reduction of numbers of hospital antenatal visits for those allocated to the reduced specialist visit group, but no concurrent improvement in hospital clinic waiting times. There were no undiagnosed complications of pregnancy in the experimental group with reduced specialist visits.

These reports of community antenatal services suggested gains in women's satisfaction and some increased efficiency with no evidence of reduced effectiveness of care. However, there were still two main areas of controversy:

(1) is there good evidence to support the recommendation that a woman with a normal pregnancy can have routine care delivered wholly in community settings by GPs and/or midwives? Or do *all* women routinely need to see an obstetrician? (James 1995; Walker 1995)

(2) what is the evidence that a reduced schedule of antenatal visits will ensure that women with normal pregnancies receive appropriate and effective care? (Sikorski 1995*a*)

The evidence of the relative clinical effectiveness of different treatments or interventions as described by observational studies must be viewed with caution because of difficulties attributing observed differences to the intervention rather than many other possible confounding factors. Experimentally derived data are far more robust in assessing the relative efficacy of different interventions.

Recent randomized controlled trials of different organizational models of antenatal care

A number of pragmatic randomized controlled trials (RCTs) in the UK and elsewhere recently addressed the two main questions of *how much* routine antenatal care should be delivered *and by whom* in order to maximize efficiency, effectiveness, and acceptability.

These trials are of interest not only because of the rigour of the methodology but also because they have several design characteristics in common and allow comparison and possibly some amalgamation of results. Women eligible for the trials were at low risk of pregnancy complications. Measures of clinical effectiveness used both process variables and morbidity as indicators of quality of care because sample size needed for the primary outcome measures of maternal or perinatal mortality is so large as to be all but impracticable. When the intervention in a trial is a multiphasic screening process rather than comparison of one clinical component (e.g. comparing two drug therapies) then the duration of the intervention may be longer and the sample attrition greater as events of the pregnancy evolve. It was expected that some women would develop conditions during pregnancy which would require amplification of the basic care package as defined in the trial protocol. The analyses were by intention to treat.

Two trials have been reported recently to compare GP/midwife (Tucker *et al.* 1996) and midwifery (Turnbull *et al.* 1996) routine antenatal care with obstetrician-led shared care.

A multicentre randomized controlled trial of routine antenatal care delivered to low-risk women by GPs and midwives in community settings compared to obstetrician-led shared care (Tucker *et al.* 1996)

Fifty-one general practices with a total of 224 GPs and 45 community midwives were linked to nine hospital centres throughout Scotland. Of all 3826 women presenting in 1993/4 to participating GPs, 69% had none of the exclusion high-risk characteristics shown in Table 19.2, and were referred to the trial as being at low risk of pregnancy complications.

The trial protocol included care guidelines and a minimal model of antenatal visits and investigations for both arms of the trial which were to be amplified according to individual women's requirements (Table 19:3).

Definitions of complications arising during pregnancy were listed, each with the appropriate clinical response (Table 19:4).

Information about the care women had received was collected from medical records after delivery and a postnatal consumer questionnaire sent out six weeks post-partum.

Table 19.2 *Exclusion characteristics identifying ineligible women who were at high risk of antenatal complications and needed to see an obstetric specialist*

Previous obstetric conditions	Medical conditions	Current pregnancy
Previous perinatal/neonatal loss	Diabetes mellitus	Multiple pregnancy
≥ 3 spontaneous abortions	Essential hypertension	Age < 16 or > 35 years
Last birth preterm (< 34 weeks)	Cardiac disease	Haemoglobin < 10 g/dl
Last baby (< 2500 g)	Renal disease	Isoimmunization
Severe pre-eclampsia with proteinuria	Substance abuse	
Serious reproductive tract surgery	Weight problems	
Previous Caesarean section	Other serious medical conditions such as coeliac disease or ulcerative colitis	

Table 19.3 *Antenatal care schedule and content for women at low risk of complication*

Gestation (weeks)	Main purpose of visit
16–18	BP; urinanalysis (and weight as per local protocol); baseline weight; prenatal diagnosis
26	BP; FH; urinalysis (and weight as per local protocol); fundal height; identify risk of IUGR; rhesus check if applicable
30	BP; FH; urinalysis (and weight as per local protocol); fundal height
34	BP; FH; urinalysis (and weight as per local protocol); fundal height; identify risk of IUGR; rhesus check if applicable
36	**Primigravida (and multipara with previous hypertension)** BP; FH; urinalysis (and weight as per local protocol); fundal height; discussion of delivery and infant feeding
38	BP; FH; urinalysis (and weight as per local protocol); fundal height; check for malpresentation
40	**Primigravida (and multipara with previous hypertension)** BP; FH; urinalysis (and weight as per local protocol); fundal height
41	**Primigravida (and multipara with previous hypertension)** BP; FH; urinalysis (and weight as per local protocol); fundal height
41–42	BP; FH; urinalysis (and weight as per local protocol); fundal height; review need for induction

Of 2167 women still eligible after booking, 82% consented to join the trial and were randomized to the experimental GP/midwife group or to the control obstetrician-led shared care group. There were complete clinical data for 1674 women who consented (834 in the GP/midwife group and 840 in the shared care group with no differences in the baseline demographic characteristics) and a 78% response rate to the postnatal consumer questionnaire. The two aspects of clinical care evaluated were:

(1) measures of health service use (both routine and non-routine care)

(2) indicators of quality of care (such as rates of antenatal diagnosis of maternal and infant morbidity, failures to adhere to the care protocol, undiagnosed conditions at admisssion in labour, and intrapartum characteristics and outcomes).

Table 19.4 *Care guidelines for risk factors arising during pregnancy*

Risk factor	Plan
Hyperemesis	Admit if ketotic for IV
Hepatitis B or HIV +ve	Specialist consultation
Weight gain 16–26 weeks < 0.4 kg/week	Check IUGR risk (refer to check-list)
Weight gain 26–34 weeks > 0.8 kg/week	Weekly BP from 34 weeks
Fundal height 3 cm less than mean (mean = cm = weeks of gestation after 20 weeks)	Check IUGR risk after checking gestation (refer to check-list)
Fasting glycosuria	Spot blood sugar and refer if > 6 millimoles/litre; arrange GTT
Antibodies (rhesus or otherwise)	Refer to specialist
Hb < 100 g/l	Treat and FBC
Deep vein thrombosis	Admit for anticoagulation
Minor haemorrhage < 26 weeks	Rest; refer at 30/52 for scan; BPD/ placental site
Any haemorrhage > 26 weeks (or significant < 26 weeks)	Admit
Recurrent haemorrhage at any gestation	Admit; check growth
Polyhydramnios	Specialist consultation
Reduced fetal movements	Check fundal height and movement; specialist consultation
Intrauterine death	Admit
Diastolic BP > 90 mmHg	Domiciliary recheck; refer if confirmed
Proteinuria (trace or +)	Check for vaginitis; check MSSU
Proteinuria (++)	Admit
Haematuria	Check MSSU – treat infection; refer if persists
Abnormal presentation after 36 weeks	Refer to specialist
Preterm ROM (< 37 weeks)	Admit
Term ROM (rupture of membranes)	Admit for syntocinon if not in labour in 24 hours
Prolonged pregnancy (after T + 7)	Refer to specialist's next clinic

Check-list of risk features for IUGR
If any three of these features are present refer to specialist
Height < 1.52 m (5')
Weight equivalent to < 50 kg at 20 weeks
Weight gain 16–26 weeks < 0.4 kg/week
Smoking 10 cigarettes per day
Fundal height 3 cm less than mean*

---

* Fundal height 3 cm less than mean on three occasions would be an indication for specialist consultation even if no other factors were present.
Note: Routine biochemical screening for risk of fetal anomaly/gestational diabetes should be performed by primary carers according to local procedures with action on abnormal results triggered by consultant action.

Measures of health service use

The trial successfully shifted routine antenatal care visits from obstetric specialist to GPs and midwives in community settings and showed gains in the GP/midwife group of:

* improved continuity of care-giver (median number of care-givers was 5 vs 7)
* fewer non-attendances
* fewer antenatal admissions
* fewer day-care episodes at designated day care facilities
* fewer routine visits (10.9 vs 11.7)
* multiparae had fewer visits than primiparae (as suggested in the care plan)
* women without complications had fewer visits than those with complications
* fewer inductions of labour.

Indicators of quality of care

There were no significant differences between the two trial groups in *undiagnosed* conditions (including hypertension) at admission in labour, nor

Table 19.5 *Causes (%) of referrals in the GP/midwife and shared-care groups*

Condition	GP/midwife referrals	Shared-care referrals
Post dates/at term	110 (20%)	40 (10%)
PIH (+ queried)	38 (7%)	72 (18%)
Reduced fetal movements	43 (8%)	36 (9%)
Abdominal pain	39 (7%)	32 (8%)
Contracting (+ queried)	28 (5%)	33 (8%)
Vaginal bleed	28 (5%)	32 (8%)
SGA (queried)	45 (8%)	19 (5%)
Malpresentation/breech	49 (9%)	18 (4%)
Spontaneous rupture of membrane	23 (4%)	20 (5%)
Raised AFP (genetic queries)	18 (3%)	11 (3%)
Vomiting/diarrhoea	7 (1%)	7 (2%)
Accidents/falls	4 (1%)	7 (2%)
Queried gestation	5 (1%)	8 (2%)
Vaginal discharge	8 (2%)	5 (1%)
Headaches/dizzy/fainting	3 (1%)	2 (0%)
Other	76 (14%)	57 (14%)
Not known	19 (4%)	6 (2%)
Total number	543	405
Total %	100	100

in undiagnosed fetal abnormalities or newborn morbidity. Similarly there were no differences in reported morbidity during pregnancy except in the area of hypertensive disease where *fewer* women in the GP/midwife group had pregnancy-induced hypertension, proteinuria, or pre-eclampsia. This finding was unexpected and is unexplained. There were no other differences in the secondary intrapartum events, such as the use of pain relief and mode of delivery, and very few deviations from the care protocol.

Referrals and changes in style of care from that predetermined by the trial

Over half the women in both groups developed at least one antenatal complication, although the seriousness of the conditions varied. Following every self-referral, referral, or admission, the cause and its subsequent effect upon the woman's care was recorded. The recorded causes of referrals and self-referrals are detailed in Tables 19.5 and 19.6.

Following such events, any change from the style of care predetermined by the trial was noted. All non-routine events and any subsequent changes in style of care are summarized in Figure 19:1, but women in the shared-care group already had scheduled specialist visits whereas queries about problems experienced by women in the GP/midwife group would be referred for a

Table 19.6 *Causes (%) of self-referrals for women in the GP/midwife and shared-care groups*

Condition	GP/midwife self-referrals	Shared-care self-referrals
Contracting (+queries)	93 (22%)	89 (22%)
Abdominal pain	62 (15%)	54 (14%)
Vaginal bleed	44 (11%)	57 (14%)
Spontaneous rupture of membrane	50 (12%)	48 (12%)
Reduced fetal movements	29 (7%)	31 (8%)
Falls/accidents/violence	13 (3%)	16 (4%)
Vomiting/diarrhoea	13 (3%)	12 (3%)
Vaginal discharge	12 (3%)	11 (3%)
Urinary tract infection (+ queries)	15 (4%)	5 (1%)
Headaches and fainting	6 (1%)	8 (2%)
Pregnancy-induced hypertension (+ queries)	3 (1%)	9 (3%)
Preterm labour	4 (1%)	5 (1%)
Backache	11 (3%)	4 (1%)
Other	42 (10%)	34 (8%)
Not known	19 (4%)	16 (4%)
Total number	**416**	**399**
Total %	**100**	**100**

specialist opinion. Women in either group could have been changed to specialist or hospital-only care. As expected, the results showed more women in the GP/midwife group had more referrals and changes in their predetermined pattern of antenatal care in response to similar levels of morbidity in the two groups throughout pregnancy.

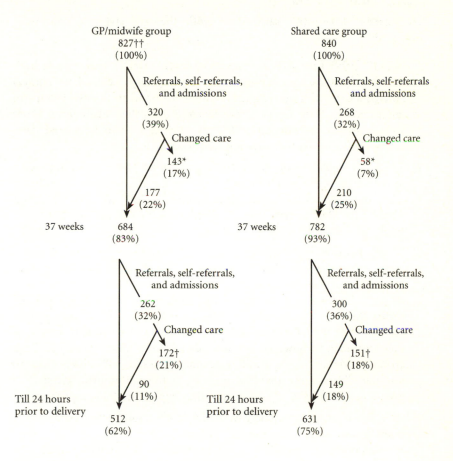

$^*\chi^2$ (with Yates correction) = 41.4, dfl, p < 0.001

$^†\chi^2$ (with Yates correction) = 8.7, dfl, p < 0.01

††(original seven withdrawals from the trial omitted in this analysis)

Figure 19.1 *Number (%) of women in GP/midwife and shared-care groups who changed their style of care at < 37 weeks and before delivery.*

An excess 10% of all referred women in the GP/midwife group had referrals because they were post-dates (110/543 (20%) vs 40/405 (10%) for the shared-care group) and changed their style of care only at this time, but the distributions of gestation at delivery did not vary for the two trial groups.

There were differences in neither rates of self-referral between the groups nor in the causes of self-referral (Table 19:6). These results did not suggest that women in the GP/midwife group were particularly anxious to see a specialist hospital doctor.

Women's views of their care

Five aspects of women's satisfaction with the two styles of care were compared:

(1) *Overall satisfaction with their antenatal care.* Overall, there was a high degree of satisfaction expressed by both groups with their clinical antenatal care, with no significant difference between the two groups in satisfaction with the medical care received from their main carer. More women in GP/midwife care, 70% vs 63% of women in shared care, unreservedly agreed that they enjoyed their care.

(2) *Satisfaction with the way that service was provided.* The majority of women in both arms of the trial were satisfied with the arrangement of antenatal visits they had experienced. More women in the GP/midwife group would have liked to have seen a hospital doctor but the numbers were small (8% (55) vs 5% (33), p < 0.02).

(3) *Their experience of attending clinics and relationships with staff.* Significantly more women in the GP/midwife group reported that they got on very well with their main carer (71% vs 67%) rather than 'well' or 'not at all well'. In all other items about the experience of attending antenatal clinics there were no significant differences between the groups in their evaluation of the GP clinics and hospital clinics. A consistent feature of their evaluations, however, are that significantly more women in both groups attributed more positive characteristics to GP clinics than to hospital clinics. Note that the women in the GP/midwife group had experience of hospital clinics only if they experienced a complication.

(4) *Provision of information.* There were high levels of satisfaction expressed by both groups about information provided on a range of care topics. Women in the GP/midwife group were more likely to say that advice was consistent most of the time, and significantly more likely to be given unsolicited advice without asking at both GP clinics and at hospital clinics.

(5) *Continuity of care.* Significantly more women in the GP/midwife group reported that it was important for them to see the same person each time (29% vs 17%) than agreed with other statements which indicated acceptance of increasing numbers of carers.

The conclusion from this trial was that there was no benefit to low-risk women from *routine* antenatal visits to specialists and that care by GPs and midwives appeared to be as safe as shared care. The women with GP/midwife care were referred appropriately as required by the protocol and received specialist care according to their need. Women's views of GP/midwife care appeared very positive in a few items but did not differ widely from those of women experiencing shared care. The economic evaluation (Ratcliffe *et al.* 1996; Ryan *et al.* 1996) which is described elsewhere (Chapter 8) showed that GP/midwife care incurred lower costs both to the NHS and to the women.

A randomized controlled trial of a midwifery-managed programme of care compared to obstetrician-led shared care (the Midwifery Development Unit at Glasgow Royal Maternity Hospital) (Turnbull *et al.* 1996)

The aim of this trial was to compare routine maternity care wholly delivered by midwives in an integrated midwifery service with obstetrician-led shared care in a large urban teaching hospital. Of the 1586 low-risk women who were eligible, 1299 consented (82%) and were equally randomized to the two trial arms. There was consistency in the direction of the results with those described by Tucker *et al.* (1996). Clinical evaluation (Turnbull *et al.* 1996) indicated that midwifery-led antenatal care was as clinically effective as shared care. For example, women in the experimental midwifery group had fewer antenatal routine visits (9.4 vs 10.2) and no differences in the use of antenatal out-patient tests. There were also no differences in the measures of non-routine care such as admissions, in-patient tests and treatments, and day-care attendances. As with the GP/midwife group in the multicentre trial, fewer women in the midwifery-led group had recorded hypertension, and fewer had labour induced compared with obstetrician-led shared care.

Descriptions of changes in styles of care from that predetermined by the trial are not directly comparable with those of the multicentre antenatal care trial. Only one third of the original women remained within the experimental midwife-care group throughout *all* their maternity care. A further 33% transferred temporarily for investigations or treatments outside the scope of the midwives' practice. The final third had permanent transfers from the midwifery model of care to obstetrician-led shared care and most of those occurred during the antenatal period: 116/648 (18%) changed their style of care during pregnancy. The overall continuity of carer during pregnancy was improved for the midwifery group who had a mean of 2.5 care-givers (standard deviation 1.5) compared with 5.4 (sd 2.4) per woman in the shared-care group (McGinley and Cheyne, personal communication).

Postal consumer questionnaires were sent out at 34–36 weeks' gestation and six weeks and seven months post-partum. The response rates varied from over 80% for the antenatal questionnaire to around 60% at seven months post-partum. The results showed that both groups of women tended to report high levels of satisfaction with the style of care that they had experienced. A number of Likert-scale items were used to measure five defined dimensions of care:

(1) general satisfaction

(2) information transfer

(3) social support

(4) choices and decision-making

(5) interpersonal relationships.

Women in both groups consistently had positive satisfaction scores in every dimension of care, but the women with midwifery care scored significantly more highly (p < 0.00001 in each dimension).

The results of this trial are entirely consistent with those of Tucker *et al.* (1996) but indicate that the primary care component of antenatal care for low-risk women *can* be provided mainly by midwives.

How much care?

Although an observational (before/after) study showed no increase in undiagnosed hypertension with reduced visit frequency (Hall *et al.* 1985), the major argument against reducing the number of antenatal visits has been that by increasing the intervals between visits, opportunities to detect hypertension prior to onset of severe disease will be missed (Redman 1988). Thus the following trials in the UK (Sikorski *et al.* 1996), USA (McDuffie *et al.* 1996), and Zimbabwe (Munjanja *et al.* 1996) appropriately used successful detection of hypertension and/or incidence of Caesarean delivery due to hypertension as outcome measures along with other process and quality of care variables.

A randomized controlled trial comparing two schedules of antenatal visits : the Antenatal Care Project (Sikorski *et al.* 1996)

This randomized controlled trial in South East London aimed to compare the clinical and psychosocial effectiveness of a reduced schedule of antenatal routine visits for low-risk women with the traditional schedule. There was a 74% consent rate and of 3252 women enrolled to the trial, complete data were available for 2758 (85%). Response rates to the antenatal and postnatal postal questionnaires were 70% and 63% respectively.

The traditional schedule of 12 visits was compared with a new reduced schedule (six for primparous and five for multiparous women) based on the Royal College of Obstetricians and Gynaecologists' working party recommendations (1982). The observed numbers of visits in the two trial groups showed that whereas women with the traditional schedule had fewer visits than intended (10.8 (observed) vs 12 (intended)) those with the reduced schedule had more (8.6 (observed) vs 5 or 6 (intended)). The magnitude of the difference in the experimental factor (visit number) was not as marked between the two trial groups as was intended by the trial design. The primary outcome measure of the clinical evaluation was the rate of Caesarean section deliveries for hypertensive disease. The hypothesis tested was that such a reduced schedule might be associated with an increased number of Caesarean sections due to an excess number of missed cases of pregnancy-induced hypertension in the reduced schedule. The results showed no difference between the groups in the number of Caesarean sections for pregnancy-induced hypertensive conditions (14/1369 (1% for the traditional schedule) vs 11/1359 (0.8% for the reduced schedule)). All the indicators of quality of care measured indicated that the reduced schedule was as clinically effective as the traditional schedule. Measures of health service use showed some positive attributes such as improved continuity of carer, less conflicting advice, and less day care.

However, measures of consumer satisfaction and measures of psychosocial well-being were reported as less good for the women in the reduced schedule group who expressed more dissatisfaction with the low frequency of visits, felt it more likely that they were not remembered by their carer at visits, showed a greater tendency to use negative words about the baby, worried more about fetal well-being, and felt less able to cope after delivery. However, more of them said they would prefer the reduced schedule in a future pregnancy.

Effect of frequency of the prenatal care visits on perinatal outcome among low-risk women (McDuffie *et al.* 1996)

A randomized controlled trial in Colorado, USA aimed to compare the reduced schedule of routine antenatal visits as recommended by the Public Health Service Expert Panel on the Content of Prenatal Care (1989) (nine visits for primiparous and eight visits for multiparous women) with the traditional more frequent schedule of 14 visits.

Fifty-nine per cent of all women were eligible and at low risk of pregnancy complications. Of those eligible, 68% consented to join the trial with 84% complete cases at follow-up. The response rates of the consumer surveys were low at 51%. The comparison of the two schedules included measures of health service process and maternal morbidity, including mild and severe pre-eclampsia, Caesarean section, low birthweight, and preterm delivery rates as indices of effectiveness. The number of visits in the experimental group (12) were still higher than the new recommended reduced number but significantly lower than the control group's traditional schedule number (14.7).

There were no differences between the trial groups in any clinical evaluation measures of effectiveness. Consumer surveys used Likert four or three-point scale items to measure consumer satisfaction with their allocated care schedule. The dimensions of women's evaluations included:

- quality of care
- quality of educational materials
- views on the timing of their visits.

The results of the six-week post-partum questionnaire showed no differences between the two trial groups in any of the dimensions of satisfaction with their care. The authors concluded that both perinatal outcome and patient satisfaction were maintained in the reduced schedule.

Randomized controlled trial of a reduced-visits programme of antenatal care in Harare, Zimbabwe (Munjanja *et al.* 1996)

In this randomized controlled trial clinics rather than individual women were randomized. The reduced-visit programme consisted of six goal-orientated visits, and was compared with traditional care (officially 14 visits but in practice only seven prior to the trial because of late booking). The average number of visits by the women in the experimental arm was four compared with six in the control arm. Even with the large sample size of this trial the power was insufficient to use mortality (maternal or perinatal) as an outcome measure, but results were reassuring as there was no evidence at all of failure of early diagnosis of hypertensive disease. Women's satisfaction was not specifically measured but compliance was good in both arms of the trial.

Conclusions

Who can deliver the care?

The evidence strongly supports the recommendation that routine antenatal care can be delivered by midwives and GPs in community settings to the benefit of many women with normal pregnancies and that no *routine* specialist visit is necessary. Much has been made of the unreliability of risk categorization to identify which women might most benefit from this style of care. It is clear that a proportion of women who appear at low risk at the outset of their pregnancy will go on to develop some problems. However, with agreed care guidelines and protocols for referrals within an inter-disciplinary maternity service, women were referred appropriately for specialist care or opinion in both the trials in Scotland. Of the women with GP/midwife and midwife-only care, the overall majority remained within their allocated style of antenatal care. Both the midwifery and GP/midwife antenatal care programmes allowed more focused, more individualized care with all component parts based on current best evidence. They could be offered as choices to similar groups of women. Furthermore, there is no reason that the methodology of using care guidelines, as in the Scottish multicentre trial, should not be used to develop care guidelines for particular 'high-risk' conditions. This would help make explicit the fact that current evidence of best practice is used as a basis for the interventions, and would ensure that high-risk women do not lose the potential benefit of enjoying a similar 'core' of routine care from the community-based primary maternity team.

How much care?

There is evidence that in approaching the recommended reduced schedules of routine antenatal visits in the UK, USA, and Zimbabwean trials, effective care for women was maintained. In the UK and USA trials the number of visits observed per woman in the reduced schedule groups exceeded that intended but were still significantly fewer than in the control groups. The evaluations of clinical effectiveness, and in particular measures designed to show any excess failures in the detection of hypertensive disease, showed no differences in any of these trials. Issues of cultural differences and expectations, and the comparability and reliability of questionnaire tools (Hansson and Rosling 1996), need to be considered in the interpretation of women's satisfaction with reduced visit schedules.

We recommend that the antenatal care schedule detailed in Table 19.3, used in conjunction with the referral protocols (Table 19.4), is appropriate for women at low risk (as defined in Table 19.2), though the detailed content is bound to evolve.

Looking forward

Looking forward to the next millennium it is to be hoped that providers, users, and those who fund maternity care will all be agreed that it must be evidence based, but that assessment of health gain must take full account of the views of individual pregnant women. Most women are, after all, healthy and well informed and likely to become more so. However, it is also incontrovertible that pregnant women with complaints and/or serious medical problems will need frequent access to midwifery and medical (usually obstetric) care, but there are wide variations in the management of common problems such as pre-eclampsia and diabetes, and many programmes and interventions have not been fully evaluated.

What is more surprising is that apparently normal women are still offered a resource-intensive screening programme which is not based on the usual principles of screening. The first principle, that the adverse outcome being sought should be common and/or serious, is certainly met for many conditions, e.g. iron-deficiency anaemia or pre-eclampsia, but others, such as clinically insignificant problems detected on scan, would be more doubtful. For rational screening early diagnosis should be of proven benefit and whereas this is clearly true for iron deficiency, it is often not the case for malpresentation. Tests should have high sensitivity and specificity and be reproducible, cheap, and non-invasive. For screening to be worthwhile there should be an effective therapeutic intervention or further test for those screening positive, which ideally should do no harm to false positives. These criteria may not apply to amniocentesis which carries a risk of miscarriage and causes psychological problems for couples awaiting results. Neither do they apply to screening for growth retardation where no clearly beneficial intervention exists and again many false positives are identified. Lastly, there is a need for clear thinking upon whether all screening tests should be applied to all women or only to those at higher risk. In turn then this depends upon the reliability of the identified risk factors. Such uncertainty is illustrated by the problem of pre-eclampsia which can be mild or very severe, can have a slow evolution or be a fulminating process with no prior warning, and can present early in pregnancy though late onset is much more common. Traditional antenatal care consists of blanket frequent blood pressure screening of all women; a rational alternative is to offer close surveillance only to high-risk groups, including primigravidae and those with multiple pregnancies. In the future, biochemical and biophysical tests may allow even better discrimination.

In many fields of health care rapid progress is being made towards increasing the proportion of care which is evidence based. Better utilization of meta-analysis of trials should ensure that the content of care of pregnant women improves at the same rate. What may be more difficult to achieve is optimal organization for the delivery of such agreed best elements of care. Vested interests and strongly held beliefs have sometimes impeded change but can also lead to change which is soundly based. Fortunately, moves towards devolving care for low-risk women to the primary care sector have been retrospectively validated by the recent trials described in this chapter, though there are still uncertainties because it is not yet possible to be sure what the impact of such changes will be upon perinatal mortality. It is also not known what the ideal mix of midwifery and general practitioner care is, nor whether the benefits of primary care for low-risk women could also be enjoyed to some extent by women with problems. It is essential that the care plans and referral protocols should be developed jointly by those who refer and by the obstetricians to whom the women will be referred. The results of trials devolving care to primary carers may not always be reproducible in routine normal practice and careful audit and quality assurance will be necessary as new styles of care become widespread.

There is scope for basic clinical and health services research to contribute to improvement in antenatal care with the active participation of women themselves.

References

Baird, D. (1969). An area maternity service. *Lancet,* I, 515–19.

Blondel, B., Pusch, D., and Schmidt, E. (1985). Some characteristics of antenatal care in 13 European countries. *British Journal of Obstetrics and Gynaecology,* **92**, 565–8.

Chng, P .K., Hall, M. H., and MacGillivray, I. (1980). An audit of antenatal care: the value of the first antenatal visit. *British Medical Journal,* **281**, 1184–6.

Cumberlege Report (1993). *Changing childbirth: the report of the expert maternity group.* HMSO, London.

Department of Health (1991). *Patient's charter.* HMSO, London.

Hall, M., McIntyre, S., and Porter, M. (1985). *Antenatal care assessed: a case study of an innovation in Aberdeen.* University Press, Aberdeen.

Hansson, G. and Rosling, H. (1996). Culture and the antenatal first visit. *Lancet,* **348**, 1103.

Heringa, M.P. and Hendrik, H. (1988). Antenatal care: current practice in debate. *British Journal of Obstetrics and Gynaecology,* 95, 836–40.

Hill, A.M., Yudkin, P.L., Bull, D.J., Barlow, D.H., Charnock, F.M., and Gilmer, M.D.

(1993). Evaluating a policy of reduced consultant antenatal clinic visits for low-risk multiparous women. *Quality in Health Care*, 2, 152–6.

James, J. K. (1995). Controversies in management. Should obstetricians see women with normal pregnancies? Obstetricians should focus on problems. *British Medical Journal*, 310, 37–8.

Kaminski, M., Blondel, B., and Breart, G. (1993). A comparison of antenatal (*sic*) outcome, antenatal and intrapartum care between England and Wales and France [letter]. *British Journal of Obstetrics and Gynaecology*, 100, 1067.

McDuffie, R. S., Beck, A., Bischoff, K., Cross, J., and Orleans, M. (1996). Effect of frequency of prenatal care visits on perinatal outcome among low-risk women. *Journal of the American Medical Association*, 275, 847–51.

Macfarlane, A., Mugford, M., Johnson, A., and Garcia, J. (1995). *Counting the changes in childbirth: trends and gaps in national statistics.* National Perinatal Epidemiology Unit, Radcliffe Infirmary, Oxford.

Marsh, G.N. (1985). New programme of antenatal care in general practice. *British Medical Journal*, 291, 646–8.

Mascarenhas, L., Eliot, B. W., and Mackenzie, I. Z. (1992). A comparison of perinatal outcome, antenatal and intrapartum care between England and Wales and France. *British Journal of Obstetrics and Gynaecology*, 99, 955–8.

Ministry of Health (1929). *Maternal mortality in childbirth. Antenatal clinics: their conduct and scope.* HMSO, London.

Munjanja, S. P., Lindmark, G., and Nystrom, L. (1996). Randomized controlled trial of a reduced-visits programme of antenatal care in Harare, Zimbabwe. *Lancet*, 348, 364–9.

Oakley, A. (1991). The changing social context of pregnancy care. In: *Pregnancy care in the 1990s* (ed. G. Chamberlain and L. Zander). Parthenon, Carnforth, Lancs.

Public Health Service Expert Panel on Prenatal Care (1989). *Caring for our future: the content of prenatal care.* Public Health Services, US Department of Health and Human Services, Washington, DC.

Ratcliffe, J., Ryan, M., and Tucker, J. (1996). The costs of alternative types of routine antenatal care for low-risk women:shared care vs care by general practitioners and community midwives. *Journal of Health Service Research and Policy*, 1, 135–40.

Redman, C. W. G. (1988). Screening for pre-eclampsia. In: *Effectiveness and satisfaction in antenatal care* (ed. M. Enkin and I. Chalmers). Spastics International Medical Publications/Heinneman, London.

Reid, M. E., Gutteridge, S., and McIlwaine, G. M. (1983). *A comparison of the delivery of antenatal care between a hospital and a peripheral clinic.* Social and Paediatric Research Unit, University of Glasgow, Glasgow.

Robson, J., Boomla, K., and Savage, W. (1986). Reduced delay in booking for antenatal care. *British Journal of the Royal College of General Practitioners*, 36, 274–5.

Royal College of Obstetricians and Gynaecologists (1982). *Report of the RCOG working party on antenatal and intrapartum care.* RCOG, London.

Ryan, M., Ratcliffe, J., and Tucker, J. (1996). Using willingness to pay to value alternative models of antenatal care. *Social Science and Medicine*, 44, 371–80.

Scottish Office Home and Health Department (1993). Health policy and public health directorate. *Provision of maternity services in Scotland: a policy review*. HMSO, Edinburgh.

Scottish Office Home and Health Department (1995). *CRAG/SCOTMEG Working Group on Maternity Services. Antenatal care*. SOHHD, Edinburgh.

Sikorski, J. (1995a). The frequency of antenatal visits. *Diplomate*, 2(3), 180–6.

Sikorski, J., Clement, S., Wilson, J., Das, S., and Smeeton, N. (1995b). A survey of health professionals' views on possible changes in the provision and organization of antenatal care. *Midwifery*, 11, 61–8.

Sikorski, J., Wilson, J., Clement, S., Das, S., and Smeeton, N. (1996). A randomized controlled trial comparing two schedules of antenatal visits: the antenatal care project. *British Medical Journal*, 312, 546–53.

Street, P., Gannon ,M. J., and Holt, E. M. (1991). Community obstetric care in West Berkshire. *British Medical Journal*, 302, 698–700.

Tucker, J., Florey, C. du V., Howie, P., McIlwaine, G., and Hall, M. (1994). Is antenatal care apportioned according to obstetric risk? The Scottish antenatal study. *Journal of Public Health Medicine*, 16, 60–70.

Tucker, J. S., Hall, M. H., Howie, P. W., Reid, M. E., Barbour, R. S., Florey, C. du V., *et al.* (1996). Should obstetricians see women with normal pregnancies? A multicentre randomized controlled trial of routine antenatal care by GPs and midwives compared with shared care led by obstetricians. *British Medical Journal*, 312, 554–9.

Turnbull, D., Reid, M., McGinley, M., and Shields, N. R. (1995). Changes in midwives' attitudes to their professional role following the implementation of the midwifery development unit. *Midwifery*, 11, 110–19.

Turnbull, D., Holmes, A., Shields, N., Cheyne, H., Twaddle, S., Gilmour, W.H., *et al.* (1996). Randomized controlled trial of the efficacy of midwife-managed care. *Lancet*, 348, 213–18.

Tyson, J., Guzick, D., Rosenfeld, C. R., Lasky, R., Gant, N., Jiminez, J., *et al.* (1990). Prenatal care evaluation and cohort analyses. *Pediatrics*, 85, 195–204.

Walker, P. (1995). Controversies in management. Should obstetricians see women with normal pregnancies? Obstetricians should be included in the integrated team. *British Medical Journal*, 310, 36–7.

Wood, J. (1991). A review of antenatal care initiatives in primary care settings. *British Journal of General Practice*, 41, 26–30.

World Health Organization (1985). Public Health in Europe No. 26. *Having a baby in Europe: report on a study*. WHO Regional Office for Europe, Copenhagen.

Wraight, A., Ball, J., Seccombe, I., and Stock, J. (1993). *Mapping team midwifery: a report to the Department of Health*. The Institute for Employment Studies, University of Sussex, Brighton.

CHAPTER TWENTY

The prevention and treatment of illness in pregnancy

David White, Frances Griffiths, Patrick O'Neill,
and Ann Jackson

Introduction

The invitation to contribute a chapter with the above title came as something of a surprise. We have worked together in a primary health care team for the last eight years providing general medical and maternity care with access to GP intrapartum care in a nearby GP/consultant delivery suite, but apart from AJ, who is a midwife, we have no special interest in maternity care. Having said that, the practice has been involved in education and research for many years, with one former partner responsible for numerous publications, including an audit of maternity care spanning 26 years (Marsh and Channing 1985a; 1985b; 1989). Our main motivation for writing the chapter has been to describe the 'craft' of general practice maternity care, what we see, and what we do. We do not intend this to be a systematic review, although we have drawn on such evidence where appropriate and available. We hope that this will stimulate readers to review their own practice, perhaps even to realize that many of the problems that present to us concern matters about which there is as yet no evidence. There is undoubtedly a need for good research to be carried out in a general practice setting to assist GP obstetricians making clinical decisions in the future.

In our practice, routine antenatal care is provided by midwives who are professionally responsible and have a statutory requirement to attend all deliveries. Communications between GPs and midwives is given an extremely high priority. GPs and midwives provide medical and obstetric care throughout the antenatal, intrapartum, and puerperal periods except for women with complications where the care is shared with an obstetrician who undertakes responsibility for the delivery. Care for pregnant women may be provided in the course of midwife-run antenatal clinics in our medical centre or in separate consultations with the GP either in routine surgeries or in the woman's home. We have access to an integrated GP unit at the local maternity hospital, which also provides all laboratory facilities.

Prevention of harm to the woman and fetus in pregnancy

The major aim of medical and especially midwife care is to prevent harm to the woman and fetus during pregnancy. Pregnancy provides an opportunity for sharing information about health and the prevention of illness. Continuity of carer and frequency of patient contacts can lead to a trusting, relaxed relationship between the pregnant woman, the midwife, and her GP. The following topics are commonly discussed with our patients. We mention them only briefly – we know there are omissions but we believe that by focusing on these conditions, the woman's attention is drawn to a need for taking care of herself during the pregnancy and adopting a healthier lifestyle. If this persists after birth, then this is a bonus.

Medication

Most pregnant women are aware of the potential risk of teratogenesis from some drugs but it is useful to remind them about checking any that they buy as well as those prescribed. Paracetamol is considered safe and this information can relieve anxiety in women who have used it before they realized that they were pregnant.

Smoking

Maternal smoking is associated with lower birthweight as is passive smoking (Lumley and Astbury 1989). We advise women to stop whilst acknowledging that this is difficult for some. The best results appear to come from a behavioural approach (Lumley 1994). We suggest that their partners join with them in their initiative. The baby once born will benefit from a smoke-free atmosphere.

Alcohol

High levels of alcohol in pregnancy can damage the fetus (Halliday *et al.* 1982). Lack of evidence makes advising on upper limits difficult. One study found no adverse outcome associated with drinking less than two units of alcohol a day (Lumley and Astbury 1989). We advise women that drinking one or two units of alcohol two to three times a week would probably not cause the fetus any harm, explaining that the medical evidence is unclear. Heavy drinkers are advised to reduce their intake and are offered help from drug and alcohol counsellors if necessary.

Travel

The risks and benefits of any immunization should be carefully discussed and where malaria prevention is needed it is important to refer to data on current malaria resistance and drug guidelines (Department of Health 1995). When travelling to countries where drinking tap water is not recommended, a pregnant woman should use bottled water, peel fruit, and avoid salads washed in tap water. Airlines have varying regulations regarding gestation limits, minimal age for neonates, and insurance so women should seek individual advice.

Back pain

Giving the pregnant woman verbal permission to 'slow down', 'rest more', and ' make more time for herself' may reduce stress and help prevent back pain. GP, midwife, and physiotherapist can work together to give advice on good posture, including avoiding high-heeled shoes. 'Bend from your knees rather than the waist' prevents back strain.

Varicose veins

Women should be advised to avoid prolonged periods of standing and can be shown simple ankle exercises to promote venous return. Support stockings and tights help to relieve aching.

Heartburn

Heartburn is common (see p. 364) and can be very distressing, often interfering with sleep. Smaller more frequent meals taken while sitting up straight and avoiding particular foods, including those fried or highly spiced, is suggested (Health Education Authority 1996). Heartburn at night can be helped by sleeping well propped up.

Rubella

Preventive measures should be taken whenever possible through preconception testing of immune status followed by immunization where appropriate. Prior to 16 weeks' gestation, the very few pregnant women known not to be immune to the virus should be advised to avoid people who have it or have been in contact with it.

Varicella

Pregnant women should avoid contact with known cases of varicella unless they are sure they have immunity.

Prevention of *Candida*

Much of the advice given to pregnant women about preventing thrush is folklore rather than evidence based. We seem to agree on the following common sense approach and proffer it:

- avoid scented soap and bath essences
- wear loose cotton underwear
- treat the woman's partner to avoid reinfection.

Toxoplasmosis

To avoid infection, women should be advised to cook meat well and wash fruit, vegetables, and salads thoroughly. Hands must be washed after handling animals. Sick cats should never be handled. Gloves must be worn when cleaning cat-litter trays and when gardening. Sheep should be avoided at lambing time (Health Education Authority 1996).

Listeria

The causative organism, *Listeria monocytogenes*, has the unusual ability to multiply at low temperatures, such as those found in refrigerators. Since cooking kills listeria, the greatest risk arises from foods which are eaten raw, undercooked, or are precooked and then subsequently eaten cold or inadequately reheated.

The worried well, who are anxious solely on account of having recently consumed 'high-risk' food, do not require prophylactic antibiotics nor examination of the food. They should be advised to contact their doctor or midwife if they have pyrexia or 'flu-like' symptoms. Advice about avoiding 'high-risk' foods and the importance of good hygiene when handling food should be reinforced. No extra precautions are required in subsequent pregnancies for those patients who have a past history of infection. A proportion of the population transiently carry *Listeria* species in the vagina or the gut but there is no evidence that this increases the risk of contracting listeriosis.

'High-risk' foods are:

- soft ripened cheeses such as Brie, Camembert, and blue-vein types
- all types of pate
- cook–chill meals and ready-to-eat poultry, unless reheated to 'piping hot'.

  Advice about hygiene should include the following:
- meat and poultry should be well cooked
- keep foods for as short a time as possible and observe 'use by' dates on the labels
- wash salads, fruit, and vegetables that will be eaten raw
- make sure the refrigerator is working properly; store cooked foods away from raw foods and cheeses
- when reheating food ensure it is piping hot all the way through; do not reheat more than once. Throw away leftover reheated food
- cooked food not eaten straight away should be cooled as quickly as possible and then stored in the refrigerator (Department of Health 1992*a*).

Salmonella

Ensure eggs are cooked thoroughly and avoid foods containing raw eggs such as mousses and some mayonnaise (Department of Health 1996*a*).

Vitamins

To reduce the risk of fetal spina bifida, a daily supplement of folic acid 400 mcg is recommended (Department of Health 1992*b*). Vitamin A may cause birth defects so pregnant women should avoid eating liver and using vitamin supplements containing vitamin A (Department of Health and Social Security 1990).

Genital herpes

It is important for the midwife to ask about a history of genital herpes at the first antenatal visit (see p. 375).

Haemoglobinopathy

Appropriate populations should be screened early in pregnancy so management can be planned (see p. 375).

The 'top 10' intercurrent medical problems in pregnancy

We now focus on 10 of the most common medical problems reported by women during pregnancy (Box 20.1).

Box 20.1 *The 'top 10' medical problems brought to the general practitioner**

1. Urinary tract infection
2. 'Thrush'
3. Upper respiratory tract infection
4. Abdominal pain
5. Headaches
6. Back pain
7. Depression
8. Verucca
9. Haemorrhoids
10. Mastitis

*Based on 301 GP contacts with 109 women delivered in 12 months in 1995–96 (excludes women who miscarried or who were already pregnant on registering with the practice. Gastro-oesphageal reflux, nausea, and vomiting omitted – see text).

Because we record all consultations on computer in our practice and have done for a few years, we have been able to count retrospectively the problems dealt with by women receiving antenatal care at our medical centre. We thus revealed our 'top 10' problems. These problems far outweigh the more serious and rare conditions which receive headline treatment in newspapers and many pages in obstetric texts. Nevertheless, these are the conditions which make the lives of women miserable, often recurrently so, during their pregnancies. We believe community midwives and GPs have a unique expertise in treating them although the 'evidence basis' is frequently minimal and sometimes lacking altogether. There is an inordinate need for research into the management of these common problems. We realize that what we do may not ultimately be proven to be correct or as effective as it could be, but it is what we do and other practices will be interested to compare notes. Some of the problems such as 'thrush' open the way to our discussing other causes of vaginal discharge and their treatment. In the final part of this chapter we do discuss other medical problems which although less common, need to be remembered. But in our day-to-day practice they are frequently totally absent and always dwarfed in importance by our 'top 10' conditions.

Gastro-oesophageal reflux, nausea, and vomiting

Our computer search for the top 10 conditions did not pick up these problems. We believe that they were so common in our antenatal clinics – almost the norm – that we did not formally record them! We have developed our own informal management protocol within our primary health care team. For gastro-oesophageal reflux, an antacid, commonly magnesium trisilicate or Gaviscon, is used. The latter has been found to be no more effective but is more palatable for some women. We manage nausea and vomiting with explanation, encouragement, frequent fluids and, if using drugs, promethazine theoclate or prochlorperazine in tablet or suppository form.

Urinary tract infection

Acute cystitis and acute pyelonephritis each occur in about 1% of pregnancies. Some cases can be prevented by treatment of asymptomatic bacteriuria discovered when we take a booking mid-stream urine (MSU), although a significant number will have had negative screening cultures. We treat symptomatic bacteriuria with seven days' antibiotics (Smaill 1994a).

Acute cystitis with frequency, dysuria, strangury, suprapubic discomfort, haematuria, and little or no fever is most commonly caused by *Escherichia coli* (*E. coli*). We commence treatment with a first-generation cephalosporin or ampicillin/amoxycillin whilst a culture and sensitivity results are awaited. Cephalexin is the cephalosporin of which there is most experience and is the drug of choice since about half the common gram-negative bacteria causing urinary tract infections are resistant to ampicillin (Wise 1995). Nevertheless, there is no evidence of any difference in outcome between penicillin and cephalosporin (Smaill 1994b). Following the results of microbiological sensitivity, treatment can be modified. Nitrofurantoin should not be used during the last weeks of pregnancy as it may precipitate haemolytic anaemia in the newborn. Trimethoprim is not recommended for use in the first trimester since it is a folic acid antagonist. Nevertheless, it is used extensively and is probably safe but it should not be a drug of first choice (Davison and Bayliss 1995). Treatment of cystitis should be for seven days (Smaill 1994c) with the aim of abolishing symptoms and preventing pyelonephritis.

Acute pyelonephritis may have a causal role in initiating premature labour and GPs should be vigilant in diagnosis and thorough in management. Acute pyelonephritis often presents with frequency and dysuria but fever, malaise, abdominal and loin pain indicate involvement of the upper urinary tract. The differential diagnosis includes other causes of pyrexia and acute abdominal pain. It is important to send an MSU sample for culture and sensitivities testing before antibiotics are commenced. GPs must therefore know the arrangements for their laboratory regarding receipt of urine samples at different times of day, at weekends, and during statutory holidays, the more so if management is to be undertaken outside hospital.

Two standard texts (Wise 1995; Wang and Smaill 1989) state that antibiotic treatment should be undertaken in hospital although we believe that some cases can be managed satisfactorily without admission and we do so. There is evidence that oral and intravenous therapy produce similar outcomes (Smaill 1994d). E. coli is the most common organism and the same treatment principles as for cystitis should be followed but should continue for two or three weeks (Wise 1995).

Treatment of asymptomatic bacteriuria, cystitis, and pyelonephritis should be followed by a test of cure by culture of an MSU specimen one week after the conclusion of therapy. This is an important difference between the management of urinary tract infection in the pregnant and non-pregnant woman since the former is liable to failure of treatment, relapse, or recurrence. It is prudent after asymptomatic bacteriuria, cystitis, and pyelonephritis to take urine cultures at all subsequent antenatal visits (Wise 1995). There is no evidence that continuous antibiotic prophylaxis is necessary (Smaill 1994e).

Vaginal discharge

A woman's normal vaginal discharge can change when pregnant and this can sometimes be difficult to distinguish from vaginal discharge caused by infection. Colonization of the vagina with Candida is more frequent in pregnant than non-pregnant women (Wang & Smaill 1989), but there is no evidence that treating asymptomatic Candida is of benefit to the woman or the neonate (Young 1994a).

Vaginal candidiasis can cause discharge and irritation but assessment of symptoms and clinical examination are not reliable in diagnosis (Wang and Smaill 1989). Treatment should be with an imidazole applied vaginally since this is more effective than nystatin (Young 1994b). The safety of oral treatment in pregnancy is not known (Enkin et al. 1995); we avoid it.

Our approach to a woman presenting for the first time in pregnancy with symptoms suggestive of vaginal candidiasis is to treat with a single dose vaginal pessary such as clotrimazole 500 mg. There have been no trials of this treatment in pregnancy but for many women it seems to work and relieves their symptoms rapidly (Enkin et al. 1995). We try to bear in mind sexually transmitted disease when treating vaginal discharges even though these are rare. If symptoms recur, we take a high vaginal swab to confirm the diagnosis of *Candida* and to establish whether there is infection with *Trichomonas*, *Gardnerella*, or *Streptococcus*. As a more general rule, when the vaginal swab is taken the GP or midwife should consider whether to take a swab for chlamydia based on the local incidence and guidelines and an assessment of the particular patient's risk of infection through sexual transmission. Sometimes a referral to the genito-urinary clinic is advisablefor testing for other sexually transmitted infections and contact tracing.

If the swab confirms *Candida*, a four to seven-day course of an imidazole cream should clear the infection (Young 1994*c*, 1994*d*), although we often use a three-day course of clotrimazole 500 mg pessaries and find this is usually successful. A woman's partner can be advised to use an imidazole cream.

Trichomonas can cause symptomatic vaginitis in pregnancy but whether its presence has an effect on pregnancy outcome is unclear. Where symptoms are present, treatment should be with metronidazole 400 mg twice a day for seven days to both the woman and her sexual partner to clear the infection. However, this should be avoided in the first trimester because of possible teratogenic effect on the fetus, although this has never been reported (Wang and Smaill 1989).

If *Gardnerella* is identified on a vaginal swab, this can be treated with metronidazole 400 mg twice a day for seven days. The vaginal flora and pH can take time to return to normal which makes the woman prone to reinfection (van Royen 1993).

Swabs sometimes reveal the presence of Group B streptococci in the vagina. At delivery this carries a risk of overwhelming sepsis in the neonate so the woman needs intrapartum antibiotics to prevent this risk (Smaill 1994*f*). Treatment during pregnancy does not influence outcome (Smaill 1994*g*).

Maternal infection with *Chlamydia trachomatis* can give rise to inclusion conjunctivitis and pneumonia in the newborn. The mother may be asymptomatic. Alternatively, she may have salpingitis, mucopurulent cervicitis, or the urethral syndrome. Prevalence estimates range from 2% to 37% with higher rates being found in young women, black women, those from lower socio-economic groups, and those attending inner-city antenatal clinics. The diagnosis is made either by culture of the organism from an endocervical specimen or by the identification of chlamydial antigens directly in endocervical smears. The value of screening routinely will depend on the prevalence of the condition in the population being screened, and is probably not justified if this is less than 6%. Erythromycin 250 mg four times a day for seven days is currently the drug of choice and the sexual partner also needs treatment (Wang and Smaill 1989).

Upper respiratory tract infections and flu-like symptoms

The advice we give to a pregnant woman with an upper respiratory tract infection (URTI) or flu-like illness is the same as for the non-pregnant woman, including sympathy, reassurance, rest, increased fluids, and symptom relief with paracetamol. Such illnesses, albeit minor, may feel like 'one too many things to cope with', particularly if the woman is having a difficult pregnancy and/or working and looking after other children. A GP's advice to rest can justify her taking time out of her other responsibilities and thus improve her well-being. The question 'when is the flu not the flu' must be considered. GPs may well know the symptoms of the viral illnesses prevalent in their community and this can provide some guidance; careful thought as to alternative diagnoses is essential. We have listed a practical guide (Box 20.2) and consider the management of the rarer but important conditions towards the end of this chapter.

Box 20.2 *Practical points for a general practitioner faced with a pregnant woman with a flu-like illness*

- Does she have any symptoms or signs that might suggest a simple, obvious explanation for her symptoms, e.g. frequency, dysuria, and loin pain; cough productive of purulent sputum; sore throat with tonsillar exudate and cervical lymphadenopathy; diarrhoea and vomiting; offensive vaginal discharge; relevant travel history?

- Has she got or had any rash suggestive of a viral infection (varicelliform or rubelliform) or has she had any recent contact with anybody suffering from varicella or rubella?

- Has she handled or eaten any raw/undercooked/reheated foods likely to contain *Listeria* or *Toxoplasma*?

- Does she have a fever? If persistently more than 38C for 48 hours, consider arranging blood cultures to exclude listeriosis.

- Does she or her neighbours have any cats? Does she garden a lot and does she wear gloves when she does? Consider testing for toxoplasmosis if her answers suggest an increased risk.

Abdominal pain

From our clinical experience it seems that the majority of abdominal pains occurring in pregnancy are idiopathic or non-specific. It may be that such patients who often have enduring recurrent persistent pain remain in our minds because our pragmatic symptomatic treatment is ineffective. Hence we may forget those patients with clearer-cut diagnoses who receive appropriate definitive therapy.

The differential diagnosis of abdominal pain in pregnancy includes, probably in order of prevalence:

- non-specific abdominal pain
- mechanical abdominal pain due to anatomical change
- urinary tract infection

- referred pain from the lumbar spine

- gastrointestinal disorders, e.g. gastro-oesophageal reflux, gastroenteritis, irritable bowel syndrome

- gynaecological emergencies, e.g. torsion of ovarian cysts, pelvic inflammatory disease, necrobiosis of a uterine fibroid

- obstetric emergencies, e.g. ruptured uterus, placental abruption

- surgical emergencies, e.g. appendicitis, biliary colic.

Our approach is similar to that for abdominal pain in the non-pregnant woman, relying on a careful history with appropriate examination and tests. However, we have a lower threshold for arranging MSU culture and for admission to hospital to clarify the cause of pain and maintain the well-being of the fetus.

Special mention must be made of ectopic pregnancy which, in the years 1991 to 1993 in the UK, had an incidence of 9.6 per 1000 pregnancies with nine deaths occurring in approximately 30 000 ectopic pregnancies. These nine deaths represented 4.2% of all maternal deaths and compared with 15 deaths in the previous three years. Eight of the nine were directly due to rupture of the ectopic pregnancy and were considered to be associated with substandard care, three involving failure of diagnosis by GPs. So GPs must consider the diagnosis of ectopic pregnancy in any woman presenting with abdominal pain and amenorrhoea with or without vaginal bleeding (Department of Health 1996b).

We are fortunate to have available a clinic operating five days a week for ultrasound examination of emergencies in early pregnancy. This is in line with the Royal Colleges of Radiologists and Obstetricians and Gynaecologists' recent guidance (1995). Ultrasound scanning and laparoscopy remain the cornerstone of diagnosis and if ectopic pregnancy is likely then vaginal examination is best deferred until the woman is in hospital (Department of Health 1996b).

Spontaneous abortion may cause symptoms similar to ectopic pregnancy. Evidence is accumulating that following ultrasound diagnosis of a non-viable fetus, surgical evacuation of the uterine contents does not always confer benefit (Forbes 1995). Prior to the development of ultrasound for diagnosis, admission was not arranged by GPs (Everett *et al.* 1987). Since its use we are currently admitting virtually all our patients to hospital for definitive action.

Anti-D immunoglobin should be administered to Rhesus-negative women following bleeding in the first trimester. This can present practical problems as occasionally a woman's blood group will not yet be known, Anti-D immunoglobin has to be given within 72 hours of the first bleed, and it has to be obtained from the local district general hospital. We sometimes have to do some running around! The risk of sensitization is lower during the first trimester than subsequently and up to 13 weeks of pregnancy a dose of 50–75 ug of Anti-D gammaglobulin is sufficient to ensure adequate protection. In the second trimester we use the standard post-partum dose of 250 units up to 20 weeks and 500 units beyond that (Enkin *et al.* 1995).

Headache

The assessment of a pregnant or post-partum woman with headache is the same as for the non-pregnant woman except that hypertension must always be borne in mind. So we almost automatically reach for the sphygmomanometer to measure the blood pressure before considering other problems. A normal blood pressure is reassuring, even more so if it is similar to the woman's blood pressure early in pregnancy. If the latter is not available, arrangements may be needed for earlier follow-up. A normal urinalysis completes the exclusion of hypertension of pregnancy and should be arranged as soon as practicable. If there is definite hypertension of pregnancy, we admit the woman to hospital. If the blood pressure is borderline, the woman can be monitored by the midwife whilst resting at home; many women settle uneventfully in this way.

Anxiety, tension, cervical spine disorders, URTI, sinusitis, and migraine can all cause headache and can affect the pregnant as well as the non-pregnant. For symptom relief we use paracetamol. Stronger analgesics containing opiates, such as codeine, are apparently safe except around the time of delivery. We check other drugs in the *British National Formulary* or equivalent texts. Women on migraine prophylaxis should ideally discuss the risks and benefits of its use before conception, but at least at the earliest possible opportunity during pregnancy.

Back pain

During pregnancy mechanical forces in the back change and this may lead to back pain. Our management is based on history and examination and we avoid X-rays. Advice on posture and lifting can be helpful and the analgesic of choice is paracetamol. Non-steroidal anti-inflammatory drugs can be used but should be avoided in the third trimester as they may interfere with closure of the ductus arteriosus in the fetus. Physiotherapy departments provide varying degrees of service for pregnant women ranging from input in antenatal and parentcraft sessions to individual sessional treatment. We are experimenting with NHS-funded osteopathy after 16 weeks of pregnancy. There is also a possible role for transcutaneous electrical nerve stimulation (TENS) machines during pregnancy.

An occipito-posterior position appears to us to be a frequent cause of back pain. Following abdominal palpation, explanation of the fetal position can at least alleviate concern about the pain.

Depression and anxiety

Pregnancy and childbirth are major life events and can precipitate depression of all severities (Chapter 18). Women should be asked about any stresses they may be undergoing as well as worries concerning the pregnancy, labour, and child care. Attitudes to the pregnancy can be explored, particularly in those who seem to be under stress. Social support during and after pregnancy can often be lacking and should be discussed. We look back in our records and ask the woman about previous depression associated with pregnancy, and possible past relevant experiences such as stillbirth, miscarriage, termination, or sexual abuse. We may well have been involved in previous episodes.

Treatment needs to take into consideration the context of pregnancy, breastfeeding, and a new baby to care for. Any drug treatment should be checked in the *British National Formulary* or equivalent texts for its safety in pregnancy or while breastfeeding.

The midwife may be able to offer extra psychological support and the health visitor can be invited to become involved preferably before delivery, particularly if she is likely to be the main professional providing support after the baby is born. The health visitor may also be able to help secure nursery places for older children and home help to relieve pressure on the mother.

For more intensive counselling or therapy, provision varies widely. There may be a practice-based counsellor or an attached community psychiatric nurse able to provide this service; we are fortunate to have both. The GP and the midwife may feel able to provide support and counselling and often have the advantage of having known the woman before this episode of depression. Referral to a psychiatrist or clinical psychologist may be needed for more severe depression or sometimes to secure appropriate services.

Counselling or other therapy, in particular after birth, will need to be arranged at times which are practical for the woman, for example when she can leave her baby with family or other carers. If postnatal depression is severe enough to require hospital admission, the GP should seek a unit where both mother and baby can be admitted (Chapter 18).

Verucca

This was number eight in our 'top 10' and reminded us that pregnant women get mundane conditions. The basic principles of whether treatment should be different in managing the condition in pregnancy should be considered. For veruccas, podophyllin is contraindicated (teratogenic). But in the majority of coincidental minor pathologies such as this, our management is identical to that in the non-pregnant.

Haemorrhoids

Pregnancy and childbirth can precipitate haemorrhoids and these can become very uncomfortable, particularly for mothers who are breastfeeding. Fortunately, they shrink fairly rapidly so only short-term treatment is needed. The midwife can advise on alternative feeding positions. Sitting on something cold such as frozen ice-pops or a packet of frozen peas can ease the discomfort. If in great pain, an ointment that includes a local anaesthetic can provide temporary relief. There is a risk of sensitization but as use is usually brief we take that risk. Where the haemorrhoids are not causing distress, reassurance and explanation that they will shrink down is usually sufficient. All mothers should increase their fluid intake to help ease any constipation.

Mastitis

Women are predisposed to infective mastitis antenatally and postnatally. We usually use flucloxacillin or, if allergic to penicillin, erythromycin for the traditional signs of redness, warmth, pain, and swelling. If the mother is breastfeeding, feeding should continue with both the affected and unaffected breast (see Chapter 24 for management of mastitis in breastfeeding women).

The unusual but important

The remainder of this chapter is about conditions that we very rarely see and hope not to. What follows is what we understand of the theory and a guide as to what we would do. In addition to what we have written, we would almost certainly be looking up the problem in the latest text – probably in the small print – or ringing up obstetricians or microbiologists for advice.

Some of these infections have particular significance in pregnancy because of their effect on both mother and baby. Many present in non-specific ways with a flu-like illness and the midwife or doctor has to decide 'when is the flu not the flu?', basing their assessment on specific clinical features that prompt them to order the microbiological tests to clarify the diagnosis (Box 20.2).

It is important that there is good communication with the local pathology laboratory to ensure that the appropriate specimens are taken at the correct times and transported in a suitable medium. Full details of the clinical condition of the woman are helpful to the laboratory.

Varicella zoster infection

Overall, there are no studies showing a conclusively higher mortality rate for pregnant compared to non-pregnant women. Nevertheless, varicella is more severe in adults in general and women who are pregnant are more susceptible to developing varicella pneumonia because of their reduced pulmonary ventilation. Tests are available for the rapid determination of a woman's immune status which then guides treatment. For pregnant women with no clear past history of varicella infection (for example women who do not think they have had chickenpox or have poor memory of illness) and who have been exposed to infection, testing of immune status should be arranged.

Two thirds will turn out to have immunity, and those who do not should receive the varicella zoster immunoglobulin (VZIG). This is likely to attenuate but not necessarily prevent infection, even if given within 72 hours, but is effective up to 10 days after exposure. For those women who develop symptomatic infection, especially those with symptoms of pneumonia, admission to hospital is indicated, and systemic acyclovir would be the drug of choice (Banatvala 1996).

The incidence of congenital varicella syndrome is about 1.6 per 100 000 births, and in England and Wales one would expect about 10 cases per year (Venkatesan 1996). A joint British and German study identified the syndrome in 0.4% of maternal varicella infections between 13 and 20 weeks of pregnancy, the period of greatest risk (Enders *et al.* 1994). Manifestations of the syndrome include cicatricial skin lesions, limb paresis and hypoplasia, microcephaly, and chorioretinitis.

There is a high risk of neonatal varicella if the rash develops in the mother within the period from four days before delivery to two days after delivery, during which time the infant can be born incubating the virus without the protection of maternal varicella zoster antibodies.

Infants born to mothers who develop varicella (but not zoster) from seven days before to a month after delivery should receive VZIG. Early treatment with intravenous acyclovir is recommended for infants if a mother develops chickenpox four days before to two days after delivery. VZIG is also recommended in non-immune infants exposed to chickenpox or herpes zoster in the first 28 days of life (Department of Health 1996c). All in all, varicella around the time of birth needs to be taken very seriously.

Listeriosis

Materno–fetal listeriosis is an extremely rare disease. In 1990 there were only 24 confirmed cases associated with pregnancy in over 700 000 births in England and Wales. Clinical manifestations of infection include a range of symptoms, from a mild flu-like illness (fever, headache, myalgia, and back pain which can mimic urinary tract infection) to occasional gastrointestinal symptoms to fatal septicaemia and meningoencephalitis. The incubation period may vary from two days to over six weeks.

Neonatal listeriosis presenting in the first week of life has a high mortality and late-onset disease at one to four weeks of life usually presents as meningoencephalitis in a baby who was initially healthy.

The diagnosis rests on the history and blood cultures as there are no pathognomonic signs. Recent travel, the woman's occupation, and appropriate dietary exposure are all important points in the history. Other causes of febrile illness need exclusion. Although listeriosis is more likely in those who have eaten high-risk foods, the diagnosis should still be considered in those without this history. The absence of illness in other members of the family who have eaten the same food is of no diagnostic value.

Faced with a pregnant woman with a pyrexia of 38C or over which does not resolve within 48 hours and which cannot be confidently attributed to some other cause (e.g tonsillitis, urinary infection, etc.), we would feel blood cultures were necessary and probably admit the woman to hospital. Vaginal swabs taken for some other reason and reported to have grown *Listeria* should be interpreted with caution because a positive isolation is at best only consistent with, and not pathognomonic of, infection. Microbiological examination of foodstuffs is not useful in making the diagnosis in an individual but the public health department may wish to examine them later should a diagnosis be confirmed.

If we did keep the woman at home because she did not seem particularly toxic, we would give oral amoxycillin 500 mg three times daily, or erythromycin 500 mg four times daily, for five to seven days, pending the results of our blood cultures (Department of Health 1992*a*).

Rubella and parvovirus 19

The success of the rubella immunization programme has meant that only 2–3% of women are susceptible to rubella in pregnancy (Banatvala 1996). The effects of intrauterine infection, particularly in the first trimester, are severe, including fetal death, low birthweight for gestational age, deafness, cataracts, jaundice, purpura, hepatosplenomegaly, congenital heart disease, and mental retardation. A two-year follow-up study found that nine infants infected before the 11th week had significant cardiac disease and deafness, but no defects were found in the 63 children infected at 16 weeks (Wang and Smaill 1989). Prenatal screening should be carried out on all women who have no documentation of immunity and vaccination given following either delivery or abortion. The diagnosis of rubella infection in pregnancy can be difficult as the pattern of antibody response to acute infection and reinfection will vary according to the assay method used, so close liaison with the local laboratory is essential. Where maternal infection is diagnosed in the first 16 weeks of pregnancy, termination should be discussed. Although the routine use of immune serum globulin for post-exposure prophylaxis of rubella is not recommended, it may have a role where maternal rubella occurs and termination is not an option (Wang and Smaill 1989).

Parvovirus 19 can also produce a rubelliform rash, associated with a flu-like illness with arthralgia, but the symptoms are milder than in rubella. In contrast to rubella, congenital malformations have not been reported, although if infection occurs during the second and third trimesters, fetal hydrops may occasionally occur. Pregnant women with parvovirus 19 infections would be monitored by ultrasonography for evidence of fetal hydrops.

Cytomegalovirus

Most of the children born to mothers who are infected with cytomegalovirus during pregnancy are apparently healthy at birth, but follow-up studies show that about 10% develop sensorineural deafness or some degree of psychomotor retardation later in life. Infection does not usually therefore constitute grounds for termination of pregnancy. Screening programmes in pregnancy have little or no value (Banatvala 1996).

Toxoplasmosis

Maternal infection with the protozoan parasite *Toxoplasma gondii* acquired during pregnancy can result in congenital toxoplasmosis (chorioretinitis, recurrent seizures, hydrocephalus, intracranial calcifications) present at birth or appearing later. A woman can be affected only once, so a woman who is immune prior to pregnancy (for example approximately 25% in London), is not at risk of transmitting the organism to her infant. Infection may be associated with malaise, fever, fatigue, and lymphadenopathy, but is usually asymptomatic. Diagnosis is by finding a high antibody level to *T.gondii* in the serum and routine screening for this is conducted in some countries (France, Belgium) but not in others (UK, Netherlands).

The risk of transmission from mother to baby is higher in the third trimester (65%) than in the first trimester (17%) but infection in the first trimester results in more severe disease with 14% of fetuses affected after first-trimester transmission and none affected with third-trimester transmission. Some advocate termination of pregnancy if infection occurs in the first trimester as an alternative to the current treatment which is the antiprotozoan drug spiromycin (Wang and Smaill 1989).

Human Immunodeficiency Virus

Pregnancy does not usually result in progression of HIV-related infection and pregnant women do not have an enhanced risk of miscarriage. The risk of transmission from mother to baby varies throughout the world; in Europe it is approximately 15%. Women transmitting infection during one pregnancy may not necessarily do so in a subsequent one. The baby may also be infected during birth. Treatment of HIV-infected mothers with zidovudine reduced transmission by two thirds, but the long-term effects have yet to be studied. Delivery by Caesarean section may halve the rate of viral transmission. Breastfeeding confers an additional risk of approximately 14% over and above the risk of intrauterine and intrapartum infection in women who were infected prenatally, therefore women for whom bottle-feeding is a safe alternative should be advised against breastfeeding (Wang and Smaill 1989).

Syphilis

Despite the relatively low incidence of maternal syphilis in the UK, there is still a benefit on cost grounds in continuing a screening programme. Congenital syphilis can largely be prevented by treatment of the mother and as most women are asymptomatic, they can only be identified by serological testing. The accepted procedure is to perform a venereal disease research laboratory (VDRL) test at the beginning of pregnancy, followed by treponemal serology if the test is positive. Women considered to be at increased risk of acquiring the infection may need this repeated later in the pregnancy. Treatment of infected mothers should be with antibiotics, preferably penicillin. Infants and sexual partners should also be checked, and treated if infected (Wang and Smaill 1989).

Gonorrhoea

Infection with *Neisseria gonorrhoeae* in pregnancy can be asymptomatic, but pregnancy appears to increase the likelihood of both arthritis and systemic disease. Pregnant women may also present with the same symptoms as the non-pregnant. Ascending infection may result in pelvic inflammatory disease, including septic abortion after the 12th week of gestation. Where local patterns of infection make screening worthwhile, cervical swabs for culture can be obtained at the first antenatal visit, and repeated if the woman is thought to be at particular risk. Treatment with penicillin or, where penicillin resistance is high, a third-generation cephalosporin is recommended (Wang and Smaill 1989).

Herpes simplex

Herpes simplex infection of the newborn is a potentially serious but fortunately rare condition (Chapter 16). Although there is a wide range of opinion concerning the management of recurrent genital herpes in pregnancy, some recommendations have been made aimed at limiting the number of women requiring Caesarian section which is one method used for preventing neonatal infection (Brocklehurst *et al.* 1995). The recommendations are:

- A history of recurrent genital herpes should be specifically requested from all women at their first antenatal visit.

- Women with a history of recurrent genital herpes infection should be alerted early in pregnancy to the importance of a recurrence at the time of labour. They should be encouraged to record the frequency of their recurrence during their pregnancy.

- In women who are anxious or who have frequent recurrences, weekly examination of the genitalia toward the end of pregnancy may be useful, although there is no merit in taking viral cultures unless the diagnosis is in doubt.

- Women should be encouraged to present early in labour if they have an active recurrence and should present immediately when the membranes rupture.

- If there is clinical evidence of herpetic lesions at the time of delivery, Caesarean section should be recommended in order to bypass the infected birth canal. If there is no evidence of recurrent disease then vaginal delivery can be permitted.

- In the neonatal period, any evidence suggesting neonatal infection should be managed promptly with acyclovir to minimize mortality and morbidity.

Obstetric cholestasis

Obstetric cholestasis affects one per 1000 pregnant women during the third trimester. It presents as pruritis, and jaundice can develop later. The perinatal mortality rate is increased by up to five times so referral to an obstetrician is mandatory (Department of Health 1994).

Haemoglobinopathies

Sickle-cell disorder primarily affects the Afro-Caribbean population whereas thalassaemia is mainly found in individuals from the Mediterranean and from the Indian subcontinent. It is important to screen for these specific defects before conception or early in pregnancy. The clinical effects may complicate obstetric management and appropriate precautions can be taken. It is now possible to offer prenatal diagnosis to those women carrying a fetus at risk of a serious defective haemoglobin synthesis or structure at a time when termination of pregnancy is feasible (Standing Medical Advisory Committee 1993).

Substance misuse

This is an increasing problem for us. It is considered in detail in Chapter 12.

Conclusion

We try to be expert in dealing with the common discomfitures and illnesses of pregnancy despite any strong evidence base for much of what we do. Community-based research is badly needed. Good teamwork is important as well as being enjoyable. Sound relationships with secondary care facilitates the treatment of the rarer conditions which it is our job to detect.

References

Banatvala, J. E. (1996). Viral infections in pregnancy In: *Oxford textbook of medicine Vol. 2* (3rd edn) (ed. D. J. Weatherall, J. G. G. Ledingham, and D. A. Warrell). Oxford University Press, Oxford.

Brocklehurst, P., Carney, O., Ross, E., and Mindel, A. (1995). The management of recurrent genital herpes infection in pregnancy: a postal survey of obstetric practice. *British Journal of Obstetrics and Gynaecology*, **102**, 791–7.

Davison, J. and Bayliss, C. (1995). Renal disease. In: *Medical disorders in obstetric practice* (ed. M. de Swiet). Blackwell Science, Oxford.

Department of Health (1992a). *Management and prevention of listeriosis and other food-borne infections in pregnancy.* PL/CMO (92) 19. HMSO, London.

Department of Health (1992b). *Folic acid and the prevention of neural tube defects.* HMSO, London.

Department of Health (1994). *Obstetric cholestasis.* CMOs update 4. HMSO, London.

Department of Health (1995). *Health information for overseas travel.* HMSO, London.

Department of Health (1996a). *While you are pregnant: how to avoid infection from food and from contact with animals.* HMSO, London.

Department of Health (1996b). *Report on confidential enquiries into maternal deaths in the United Kingdom 1991–1993.* HMSO, London.

Department of Health (1996c). *Immunization against infectious disease.* HMSO, London.

Department of Health and Social Security (1990). *Vitamin A and pregnancy.* PL/CMO (90)11. DHSS, London.

Enders, G., Miller, E., Craddock-Watson, J., Bolley, I., and Ruehalgh, M. (1994). Consequences of varicella and herpes infection in pregnancy: prospective study of 1739 cases. *Lancet*, **343**, 1548–51.

Enkin, M., Keirse, M. J. N. C., Renfrew, M. J., and Neilson, J. (1995). *A guide to effective care in pregnancy and childbirth* (2nd edn). Oxford University Press, Oxford.

Everett, C., Ashurst, H., and Chalmers, I. (1987). Reported management of threatened miscarriage by general practitioners in Wessex. *British Medical Journal*, **295**, 998.

Forbes, K. (1995). Management of first-trimester spontaneous abortions. *British Medical Journal*, **310**, 1426.

Halliday, H. L., McCreid, M., and McClane, G. (1982). Results of heavy drinking in pregnancy. *British Journal of Obstetrics and Gynaecology*, **89**, 829.

Health Education Authority (1996). *New pregnancy book*. HEA, London.

Hill, L. V. H., Luther, E. R., Young, D., Pereira, L., and Embil, J. A. (1988). Prevalence of lower genital tract infections in pregnancy. *Sexually Transmitted Diseases*, **15**, 5–10.

Lumley, J. (1994). *Behaviour strategies for reducing smoking in pregnancy*. Review no. 03397. The Cochrane Pregnancy and Childbirth Database.

Lumley, J. and Astbury, J. (1989). Advice for pregnancy. In: *Effective care in pregnancy and childbirth* (ed. I. Chalmers, M. Enkin, and M. J. N. C. Keirse). Oxford University Press, Oxford.

Marsh, G. N. (1985*a*). *Modern obstetrics in general practice* (edited.) Oxford University Press. Oxford.

Marsh, G. N. (1985*b*). New programme of antenatal care in general practice. *British Medical Journal*, **291**, 646.

Marsh, G. N. and Channing, D. M. (1989). Audit of 26 years of obstetrics in general practice. *British Medical Journal*, **298**, 1077.

Royal College of Radiologists and Royal College of Obstetricians and Gynaecologists (1995). *Ultrasound procedures for early pregnancy*. RCR and RCOG, London.

Smaill, F. (1994*a*). *Single dose vs four–seven day antibiotic for bacteriuria*. Review no. 03171. The Cochrane Pregnancy and Childbirth Database.

Smaill, F. (1994*b*). *Broad-spectrum penicillin vs cephalosporin for bacteriuria in pregnancy*. Review no. 03172. The Cochrane Pregnancy and Childbirth Database.

Smaill, F. (1994*c*). *Single dose vs seven-day course of antibiotics for bacteriuria*. Review no. 03176. The Cochrane Pregnancy and Childbirth Database.

Smaill, F. (1994*d*). *Oral vs intravenous antibiotics for acute pyelonephritis*. Review no. 07204. The Cochrane Pregnancy and Childbirth Database.

Smaill, F. (1994*e*). *Nitrofuantoin vs surveillance after pyelonephritis*. Review no. 03166. The Cochrane Pregnancy and Childbirth Database.

Smaill, F. (1994*f*). *Intrapartum antibiotics for Group B streptococcal colonization*. Review no. 003006. The Cochrane Pregnancy and Childbirth Database.

Smaill, F. (1994*g*). *Antepartum antibiotics for Group B streptococcal colonization*. Review no. 003005. The Cochrane Pregnancy and Childbirth Database.

Standing Medical Advisory Committee (1993). *Report of a working party of the Standing Medical Advisory Committee on Sickle Cell, Thalassaemia, and Other Haemoglobinopathies*. HMSO, London.

van Royen (1993). *Vaginal discharge and bacterial vaginosis in family practice.* PhD thesis. Antwerpen.

Venkatesan, P. (1996). *Chickenpox in pregnancy: how dangerous? Practitioner,* **240**, 256–9.

Wang, E. and Smaill, F. (1989). Infection in pregnancy. In: *Effective care in pregnancy and childbirth* (ed. I. Chalmers, M. Enkin, and M. J. N. C. Keirse). Oxford University Press, Oxford.

Wise, R. (1995). Antibiotics. In: *Prescribing in pregnancy* (ed. P. Rubin). BMJ Publications, London.

Young, G. L. (1994*a*). *Clotrimazole for vaginitis in pregnancy.* Review no. 06810. The Cochrane Pregnancy and Childbirth Database.

Young, G. L. (1994*b*). *Imidazoles vs nystatin for vaginal candidiasis.* Review no. 06810. The Cochrane Pregnancy and Childbirth Database.

Young, G. L. (1994*c*). *Four day vs seven-day treatment for vaginal candidiasis.* Review no. 03151. The Cochrane Pregnancy and Childbirth Database.

Young, G. L. (1994*d*). *Seven day vs fourteen-day treatment for vaginal candidiasis.* Review no. 076811. The Cochrane Pregnancy and Childbirth Database.

CHAPTER TWENTY-ONE

Care in labour

Rosemary Mander

The term 'normal' is difficult to define (Downe 1996). For clarity, therefore, this chapter covers care of the woman with an uncomplicated labour and birth where medical/high-tech intervention is not required. The environment for labour and birth is discussed first, followed by support in labour and the control of pain. These three factors are fundamental and closely interrelated in the care of women in labour. Routines in care are then examined, the evidence base and its quality are described, and the extent to which that evidence informs present practice.

There is no reason why care in uncomplicated labour should differ from setting to setting, and so it is described irrespective of the place of birth.

The environment for labour and birth

Place of birth is discussed in Chapter 2 and will not be dealt with in detail here. In summary, care-givers should discuss the woman's wishes with her early in pregnancy, and every effort should be made to help her to give birth in an environment where she feels comfortable and safe. This may be in her own home, in a GP or midwife-led unit, or in a hospital. Whatever the setting, and whoever the care-givers are, she should have her views listened to and respected, and should be able to have the companions she chooses, whether partner, family member, or friend.

Support in labour and at birth

There is good evidence that support of women during labour, either by professionals or by lay women, is beneficial not only in improving women's feelings about labour and delivery but also by decreasing interventions and adverse clinical outcomes (Hodnett 1997; Chapter 13). Support may be offered by the woman's formal care providers, such as the midwife, as well as her companions or informal carers, such as her partner.

The presence of another person is crucial for a woman in labour (Keirse *et al.* 1989), although it is less clear which elements of support are most effective.

Praise and encouragement were offered by the lay care-givers in some of the studies reviewed by Hodnett (1997). Other elements of support were examined in a Canadian study which found that 'physical comfort measures', 'emotional support', 'information/instruction', and 'advocacy' were all important (Hodnett and Osborn 1989). Other forms of support include physical contact such as hand-holding, making conversation, and an empathetic attitude. It is possible that the strength of the active management practised by O'Driscoll and colleagues (O'Driscoll and Meagher 1980) is that in addition to clinical management, it also spells out the support to be offered to the mother, including close physical proximity and eye contact (Thornton and Lilford 1994).

Care is needed, therefore, to make support in labour as effective as possible, and for that support to continue throughout labour and birth.

Control of pain

One of the features of labour that women are most anxious about is pain and their reaction to it. Control of pain should not simply be seen as the use of pharmacological measures, but should also include support (see above), mobility and posture, and supportive measures including non-pharmacological pain relief. The perception of pain is, of course, heightened by fear and anxiety. Providing good support and encouraging women to have control over their own movement and choice of pain-relief measures is likely to increase their feelings of control thus lessening their fear and anxiety.

Mobility and posture

Restricting women's mobility to a recumbent position in labour increases interventions and the use of pharmacological analgesia. It may also lengthen labour (Mendez-Bauer *et al.* 1975; Flynn *et al.* 1978; McManus and Calder 1978; Golay *et al.* 1993), although the quality of evidence is not high. Women should be free to move around and to adopt the most comfortable positions they can find; they may need advice and suggestions for alternatives. Extra pillows and bean bags will help to support women in some postures.

Supportive measures

General supportive measures include relaxation, touch, and education, as well as specific interventions such as hypnotherapy and immersion in water. The quality of evidence in this field is not good but relevant studies are summarized here.

Relaxation, which usually includes breathing exercises, is the method of pain control most frequently used in the UK (Steer 1993). Together with education, it is a traditional cornerstone of prepared childbirth. Research to demonstrate the effectiveness of relaxation in childbirth *per se* has, however, been confounded by the many different sources of information and advice given to women during pregnancy. In one study, however, Enkin *et al.* (1972) examined 'psychoprophylactic preparation classes'. They found that the trained group used significantly less pharmacological analgesia than either of the control groups, even after controlling for self-selection bias.

Hypnotherapy (Booth 1993) requires more intense training than relaxation. Following their review of three randomized controlled trials (RCTs), Spanos *et al.* (1994) concluded that hypnotherapy does not reduce labour pain. Some women, however, may find it helpful.

Biofeedback involves teaching to control autonomic responses such as pain. The two studies of this technique have conflicting results (St James-Roberts *et al.* 1982; Duchene 1989), and there is no strong evidence to support its use. If it is used, it is likely to require relatively intense training prior to labour.

Transcutaneous electronic nerve stimulation (TENS) has not been well evaluated. Hardy's RCT (1991) could not be completed. She found that women using TENS were more likely to use no additional analgesia, but larger numbers are needed.

In recent years, women have been offered the opportunity to use birthing pools in labour in addition to using traditional baths and showers. Although it appears to reduce pain and the use of pharmacological pain relief, and women report feelings of relaxation, more information is needed before immersion in water should be offered without careful monitoring and audit (McCandlish and Renfrew 1993; Alderdice *et al.* 1995). This is especially the case if women stay in water for the second stage and the birth where questions need to be addressed about perineal outcome and the well-being of the baby (Garland and Jones 1994; Alderdice *et al.* 1995; Hawkins 1995).

Other methods of non-pharmacological pain control include massage, therapeutic touch, acupressure, and acupuncture; they have been subjected to little research.

Pharmacological pain relief

Nitrous oxide and oxygen (Entonox) is the analgesic most frequently used in labour in the UK; 60% of women were reported as using it in the survey by Chamberlain *et al.* (1993). Evidence about its effectiveness is limited. Studies suggest that women experience good pain relief (Bonica and McDonald 1990), although this may be a result of distraction and the role it can play in assisting with relaxation and breathing exercises (Wraight 1993).

Opioid drugs act by raising the woman's pain threshold (Way and Way 1992), but their side-effects involve depressant and excitatory effects on various receptors throughout the body. Thus, opioids in labour carry serious implications; Apgar scores and breastfeeding, for example, may be adversely affected (Freeborn *et al.* 1980; Matthews 1989). Progress in labour has traditionally been assumed to be facilitated by opioids (De Voe *et al.* 1969), but one study serendipitously showed longer first and second stages of labour as the amount of opioid (pethidine) increased (Thomson and Hillier 1994). Evidence is limited, and because of potential side-effects they should be used with caution.

Epidural analgesia is unquestionably the most effective pain control method. Some epidural blocks are ineffective, however, although it is not clear what proportion (Howell and Chalmers 1992). Epidural analgesia has a number of drawbacks; it can only be used in a hospital with an anaesthetic service and it results in a 'medicalization' of labour and birth, with an increased number of obstetric interventions being used (Williams *et al.* 1985). Epidurals slow labour, especially the second stage (Williams *et al.* 1985, Chestnut *et al.* 1987). The instrumental delivery rate is higher (Morton *et al.* 1994; Ramin *et al.* 1995; Scott and Tunstall 1995), although later epidurals (after 5 cm dilatation) may reduce the likelihood of an operative birth (Chestnut *et al.* 1994). The limited data on women's perceptions of the costs and benefits of epidurals (Howell and Chalmers 1992; Mander 1994) suggests that their views require more detailed study.

Complications recorded range from immobility to maternal hypotension; approximately 2% of women who have epidural analgesia require ephedrine (Pursey 1994; Ramin *et al.* 1995). Bladder sensation may also be reduced resulting in bladder distension (Williams *et al.* 1985). There are a small number of reports of long-term effects of epidural in labour, such as headache and backache, but no prospective studies. MacArthur *et al.* (1991) found that nearly 19% of the mothers in their retrospective survey who had an epidural reported new backache compared with 10.5% in other mothers. Knowledge of neonatal effects is also limited (Howell and Chalmers 1992). Maternal pyrexia associated with epidural analgesia is likely to lead to fetal tachycardia after eight hours of labour. This can be diagnosed as fetal distress resulting in intrapartum and neonatal interventions (Fusi *et al.* 1989).

It has been suggested that variations in anaesthetic technique, such as the combination spinal/epidural (Morgan and Kadim 1994), will resolve the problems. There is no evidence, as yet, that this is the case (Morey *et al.* 1994).

In summary; it is striking that in spite of the clear need for safe, effective pain relief in labour, strong evidence on which to base practice is lacking. Such evidence as does exist is not always communicated to women to inform their choice.

Routines in care

The development of agreed policies, including the use of routine practices which have been shown to be beneficial, can prevent wide variations in the implementation of care (Chalmers *et al.* 1989). Such policies can be part of quality assurance, and can protect both staff and clients from care which is not evidence based. Routine practices can, however, promote the unquestioning continuation of traditional and outdated care. There is a danger that unresponsiveness to new knowledge can be inherent in a system where there are large numbers of staff, and this can delay or even prevent the implementation of change and the regular updating of policies. If not examined regularly and updated to incorporate new evidence, policies can become a straightjacket (Mander 1995), especially if they do not allow for the views of the individual woman and her family.

Neilson (Chapter 13) states that practices and interventions in labour should have evidence to support their use before they are used routinely. In the next section, the evidence for routine practices is reviewed.

Routines in the first stage of labour

Admission procedures

For women who plan to give birth at home, entry into a strange environment is a challenge they will hope to avoid. For women who labour and give birth in a maternity unit, however, admission in labour will be a part of a transition to hospital care. For many, it will be their first adult 'in-patient' experience, and therefore issues such as autonomy and control will be important.

Garcia and Garforth (1989) identified the social and clinical significance of admission and initial assessment when they observed admission procedures from the viewpoints of the woman, midwife, and manager. Concern was voiced about 'routine preparation procedures' including enema and shaving, about the partner being excluded during admission, and about poor individualization of care. Although some routine procedures, such as pubic shaving, are much less likely to occur now, it is possible that the routinized, or ritualized, character of admission and preparation procedures persist. Alternatives might now include routine admission cardiotocography, vaginal examination, and discussion of the birth plan. Some routines may be beneficial but they should be subject to regular review.

Eating and drinking in labour

Not allowing women to eat and drink in labour is a response to fear of maternal acid aspiration (Mendelson's syndrome) if the woman needs a general anaesthetic. There is wide variation in policies relating to this practice, with some units routinely allowing food or fluid in labour while many others routinely forbid it (Garcia and Garforth 1989; Michael *et al.* 1991). The effects of such restrictions are not known, partly because the nutritional demands of labour are unclear. In one study in the USA, however, the temporary introduction of a nil-by-mouth policy was associated with a fivefold increase in augmentation of labour, a 36% increase in operative births, and a 69% increase in neonatal unit admissions (Ludka 1987). It is also not clear what proportion of women are likely to become distressed by such regimes; many women do not wish to eat, especially in the later phases of labour. Some women experience hunger and thirst, and the routine withholding of food and drink should be questioned.

Women at risk are those who ultimately need a general anaesthetic. The original *raison d'être* for the policy has declined, therefore, because the use of epidural analgesia has decreased the likelihood of general anaesthesia. Anaesthetic deaths due to aspiration of gastric contents continue (Clinical Resource and Audit Group 1996; Department of Health 1996). The quality of anaesthetic technique is an important factor and physical and chemical prophylaxis can be used to protect against this complication. Physical prophylaxis comprises cricoid pressure combined with a cuffed endotracheal tube (Sellick 1961). The original manoeuvre has been modified to a two-handed technique because it not only protects the airway but also maintains head extension and neck flexion (Crowley and Giesecke 1990). These techniques require that skilled personnel assist the anaesthetist. Trained anaesthetic assistants are generally available in maternity units (Cook and McCrirrick 1994), but although cricoid pressure was found always to be used in this survey, the two-handed technique was used in a small minority of units. These authors question the value of recommendations which do not change practice.

Chemical prophylaxis employed to reduce the acidity of the stomach contents and lessen the risk of pulmonary damage involves the administration of particulate antacids, such as aluminium hydroxide. These prophylactic drugs have largely been replaced (Gibbs *et al.* 1981). A survey of obstetric anaesthetic departments showed that 93% now use ranitidine (Greiff *et al.* 1994).

Routine observations

Observations are used routinely in labour to monitor progress. Whether monitoring is seen as a tool to identify potentially pathological deviations (Crowther *et al.* 1989) or to ensure physiological progress depends on the orientation of the observer. Routine four-hourly vaginal examination in labour is a good example of a maternal observation which should be questioned because of its inherent unpleasantness, women's limited control over it (Bergstrom *et al.* 1992), and the potential for long-term psychological sequelae (Menage 1996). One survey showed that only 9% of women in labour were examined less than four-hourly, whereas 71% were examined more frequently (Clinical Standards Advisory Group 1995). There is no indication of the proportion of examinations which constituted 'checks' on other staff's observation. Twenty per cent of women were examined five times more than recommended.

The problem of over-examination is aggravated by questionable accuracy of the examination itself. A study of midwifery sisters' and obstetricians' examinations (n = 60) showed that obstetricians tended to underestimate cervical dilatation whereas midwives overestimated it; marked intra-observer inconsistency featured in both groups (Tuffnell *et al.* 1989). Among students (n = 14) and qualified staff (n = 38), qualification and experience bore no relation to accuracy of vaginal examination (Robson 1992). Although the researchers recognized the subjective nature of this intervention, they asked only for better education rather than reflecting on its benefits to care.

Health care providers have been criticized for assuming that an intervention which benefits a small client group with a specific problem will inevitably benefit the larger, healthier population. This principle has resulted in the unproven assumption underpinning the routine use of electronic fetal monitoring (EFM) that more information inevitably improves perinatal outcomes. Fetal heart rate monitoring may be by intermittent auscultation using a Pinard stethoscope or Doppler, continuous EFM using an abdominal transducer or fetal scalp electrode, or a combination of methods and frequency. Monitoring may be supported by fetal blood sampling (Chapter 13).

The evidence does not support the routine use of electronic fetal monitoring, and 'in a normal labour auscultation using a Pinard stethoscope or hand-held Doppler ultrasound device could not be regarded as inadequate or negligent assessment' (Neilson 1994). This evidence is of major importance to those practising midwifery away from hi-tech centres.

Active management

The active management of labour was developed in a large maternity hospital in Dublin (O'Driscoll and Meagher 1980), and its alleged advantages widely disseminated before evaluation was carried out. Active management aims to identify delay in labour and to remedy this. This first requires a definition of the 'normal' duration of labour. But diagnosing the onset of labour is easier with hindsight. The duration of 'normal' labour, currently defined as 12 hours, is derived from a small and inadequately detailed study (Friedman 1955). Crowther and colleagues (1989) discussed the value of the retrospective diagnosis of normal labour and the role of the 'partogram'. The diagnosis of prolonged labour or 'failure to progress' (Olah and Neilson 1994) which is thus facilitated does not necessarily benefit the woman: 'augmentation [shortens] the labour and commitment of her care-givers' (Keirse 1989). The benefits to the system, rather than the woman, become apparent in Keirse's description of active management as a 'framework in which thousands of women needed to be delivered within the confines and infrastructure of what a single institution in a relatively poor country (Ireland) could offer' (Keirse 1993).

Active management in the first stage incorporates precise diagnosis of onset of labour, early amniotomy and oxytocin, and continuous professional support (Thornton and Lilford 1994). In their systematic review of RCTs, Thornton and Lilford regret that research focuses on components of the process rather than the total package. Amniotomy has been examined, for example, but not in conjunction with continuous professional support, which may in fact be the most important element (see above). One RCT which examined a number of the components of the package together involved 306 women, of whom 152 received active management (Cammu and van Eeckhout 1996), and showed that the first stage was only shortened by 30 minutes (254 minutes vs 283 minutes, p = 0.087). Additionally, the Caesarean section rate was higher following active management and spontaneous births lower.

Thornton and Lilford (1994) reported similar findings – trials of amniotomy and oxytocin which they identified showed no reduction in operative births. Although both groups of authors deny advantages in routine active management, early amniotomy alone has been found by a systematic review of eight RCTs to reduce the duration of labour by between 7% and 40% (Fraser *et al.* 1996).

The partograph, fundamental to active management, has been recommended for worldwide use (World Health Organization 1994). The basis of this recommendation is a flawed study which serves to reflect little more than the 'unnecessarily high' rates of intervention in some Third World countries (Rosser 1994). Concerns arise that inadequately researched interventions may be exported to settings where they are even less appropriate.

Care in the second stage of labour

Diagnosis of full dilatation

Care in the second stage presents many challenges and diagnosis is the first of these. Cervical assessment is not a precise art and, even if it were, it would be difficult to ascertain the exact moment when full dilatation is reached. Diagnosis of the second stage may therefore be made either when no cervix is palpable or when the head appears at the vulva (Thomson 1988).

Interventions to shorten the second stage are often recommended in spite of the problems of diagnosing full dilatation (Downe 1996). There is little evidence, however, to support such intervention simply on the basis of time. Although, traditionally, the serious risk in prolonged second stage has been perceived to be its harm for the fetus/neonate due to placental compromise (Thomson 1988), work by Saunders and colleagues (1992) suggests that this is not so. These researchers analysed retrospectively the records of 25 069 women experiencing uncomplicated term labour. They found that duration of the second stage and neonatal morbidity were unrelated and they concluded that a second stage of up to three hours carries no undue fetal/neonatal risks. It is possible that fetal compromise, traditionally attributed to prolonged second stage, may be due to haemodynamic changes associated with supine posture. This, in combination with the other mainstay of conventional second stage care – directed pushing – may be responsible for the long-recognized deterioration in fetal condition. Such problems may therefore be iatrogenic.

Posture in second stage

The position of the woman during second stage may affect the feto–maternal haemodynamics, uterine activity, risk of perineal damage, and effectiveness of pushing (Thomson 1988). The latter is known to be influenced by gravity and by pelvic dimensions (Paciornik 1990). Borell and Fernestron (1960) used radiographic techniques to show that the anteroposterior diameter of the pelvic outlet could increase by 1–2 cm if the sacroiliac joints were 'freed' by the change to a non-recumbent posture. Squatting was shown, using anthropological studies, to facilitate this freeing-up (Paciornik 1990).

One RCT of squatting using a supportive cushion in the second stage (Gardosi *et al.* 1989) found fewer instrumental births (9% vs 16%) and shorter second stages (mean length 31 minutes vs 45) in women in the squatting group compared with the semi-recumbent group. Perineal tears were less likely in the squatting group, but not labial damage. The fetal/neonatal condition, blood loss, and vulval oedema showed no difference. Maintaining a vertical posture may be difficult at the end of labour, but 82% of the squatting group remained upright.

However, most of the RCTs on non-recumbent positions in the second stage involved the woman sitting on a bed or birthing chair/stool. Hofmeyr and Nikodem's systematic review of such studies (1996) shows that the advantages include less perineal/vaginal trauma, less operative intervention, easier expulsive efforts, shorter non-augmented second stage, and less minor/severe pain. The disadvantages include more labial lacerations and larger measured blood loss when chairs and stools are used.

Some women are reluctant to adopt a 'non-traditional' position and research is needed to identify the factors which would support them in assuming more effective postures.

Pushing

Directed pushing, a mainstay of traditional second-stage care, has been compared to a 'rugby scrum' (Thomson 1988) where all present encourage the woman to push harder using the Valsalva (closed glottis) manoeuvre. To assess the effectiveness of this regime, 100 primigravidae were encouraged to push intuitively and comparisons were made with 393 using directed pushing (Beynon 1957). There was no difference in the duration of the second stage between the two groups but in the intuitive group instrumental birth or perineal repair were less likely, lending little support to the 'rugby scrum' regime.

Episiotomy

Episiotomy is another intervention used to shorten the second stage (Banta and Thacker 1982). An RCT undertaken to ascertain its short- and long-term effects compared a more liberal and a more restrictive use of episiotomy (Sleep 1984). No significant differences were found in terms of the perineal pain experienced at 10 days or at three months. However, the women in the restrictive group resumed sexual intercourse significantly earlier. A more restrictive approach to episiotomy was therefore associated with more women giving birth without perineal damage. A follow-up study three years later (Sleep and Grant 1987) found no clear differences between the two groups. Other trials have subsequently confirmed the results of this study. There are no grounds for performing episiotomy routinely (Enkin *et al.* 1995).

Perineal management

The techniques used to supposedly protect the perineum from damage during the second stage are legion. They range from the more 'hands-on' approaches such as perineal massage and 'ironing' the perineum, through 'guarding' the perineum, to the 'hands-off' approaches (Kitzinger 1990). There is, however, little or no evidence to guide us in which approach is best in preventing perineal trauma and pain, although there is a large, ongoing trial which will report in 1997–98. In principle, the midwife continues to observe the well-being of the mother and fetus at this time, as well as more specific observations of the progress of labour, and making preparations for the birth. The birth of the baby's head should be gentle and unhurried, as should the birth of the rest of the baby's body. The mother can, if she wishes, complete the delivery herself by lifting the baby up into her arms (Enkin *et al.* 1995).

Care in the third stage of labour

The third stage of labour offers a number of challenges and paradoxes; for example, women have limited interest in this stage but there is the potential for dire pathology (Prendiville and Elbourne 1989). Third-stage care aims to deliver the placenta and minimize haemorrhage, so this section focuses on these.

Active management of the third stage has prevailed in various forms in the UK since the mid-twentieth century (Prendiville and Elbourne 1989), but the research basis for this approach is unclear. This is partly because, like active management of labour, it comprises a package which may be implemented and researched in its entirety *or* piecemeal (Gyte 1994). The essential components of active management are oxytocic administration, cord clamping, and controlled cord traction. They allow considerable scope for variation in the route, timing, and nature of the oxytocic, the timing of cord clamping, maternal posture, and the use of nipple stimulation. Each of these elements and the results of a series of systematic reviews have been summarized (Enkin *et al.* 1995). In brief, trials suggest that active management results in less blood loss, fewer blood transfusions, shorter third stages, therapeutic oxytocic medication, and women are more likely to vomit. These findings have provoked extensive debate (Gyte 1994).

Midwives' unfamiliarity with physiological management may make it difficult for them to cooperate confidently in these trials (Gyte 1994). Additionally, women may resent the extra time taken by a physiological third stage. These difficulties may be resolved by two ongoing trials where midwives and women are accustomed to expectant management (Rogers *et al.* in Simms *et al.* 1994; Herschdorfer, personal communication).

Studies have compared the use of oxytocin versus an oxytocin/ergometrine combination widely used in the UK. McDonald and colleagues (1993), in a large RCT, found that PPH rates were not significantly different between groups of women given oxytocin or an oxytocin/ergometrine combination. The combined preparation was also more likely to cause nausea, vomiting, and hypertension. Another study also found a similar blood loss in both groups, and gastric problems, mean rise in blood pressure, and headache were less in the oxytocin-only group (Khan *et al.* 1995). Unlike the previous studies, Yuen and colleagues (1995) did identify significant differences between the two groups in terms of blood loss and likelihood of post-partum haemorrhage (PPH). These researchers found that oxytocin/ergometrine was associated with a 40% reduction in the risk of PPH. They also identified a significantly higher incidence of retained placenta with the combined preparation and found that gastric upsets, headache, and hypertension were 'uncommon'. The differences between the latter and the two former studies is hard to understand, although the setting of care – the trials were carried out on three different continents – may have had an effect.

Care of the baby at birth

Routine neonatal care involving standard components for all babies is all too easily provided in an institution but may not always be in the baby's best interests. Such routines are less likely to occur in the community. It may be that such routines benefit the institution or individual staff members (Thomson and Westreich 1989), and these benefits may only be enhanced by the common perception of the maternity unit as staff rather than women's territory. It is necessary, therefore, to examine practices which commonly occur within hours of the baby's birth.

Contact between mother and baby

Mother–baby interaction immediately after birth aroused much interest following the early work of Kennell and Klaus (Kennell *et al.* 1974). Their studies were carried out at a time and in circumstances where contact between mothers and their babies was very restricted after birth, and were influential in supporting changes in attitudes and in practice.

There are no grounds for placing any restrictions on the close and intimate contact between mother and baby after birth (Enkin *et al.* 1995).

The actual extent of initial skin-to-skin contact was observed by Garcia and Garforth (1990) in their study of maternity routines in the UK. They noted that in only 45% of births which they observed was the baby delivered on to the mother's body. They also observed the separation of the mother and baby for transfer from the labour room, which happened in half of the study births. The circumstances of this separation varied in terms of requests, explanations, and rationale.

First examination of the baby

The first examination of the baby being undertaken in the birthing room is welcomed by some mothers (Garcia and Garforth 1990). Little is known, however, about the value of this examination in diagnosing real or potential health problems or whether this is a valid use of midwifery time in view of the subsequent examinations which the baby routinely receives (Chapter 23).

Early breastfeeding

Early breastfeeding is important to both mother and baby (Chapter 24). In summary, every opportunity should be made to support the mother in breastfeeding her baby soon after birth. There is no 'critical period' for the establishment of breastfeeding, however, and women who cannot or do not wish to breastfeed in the first hour or so after birth should neither be discouraged from trying when they are ready nor made to think that they will have problems if they delay (Renfrew and Lang 1994).

Vitamin K

Routine prophylactic vitamin K has long been recommended for intramuscular administration to prevent haemorrhagic disease of the newborn (American Academy of Pediatrics 1961; Chapter 23).

Care of the mother after birth

The care of the woman in the minutes and hours after the birth has attracted limited research interest. The length of time which the woman spends in the one-to-one care of the midwife and/or in the birthing room, and the events which happen during this time, are traditionally prescribed. They include a wash or a shower, quiet time with partner and baby, routine observations of pulse, temperature, blood pressure, fundus, bladder, and blood loss, and the offer of a cup of tea. This time also offers an opportunity to share a time with the mother, her partner, and the baby when they are exploring and finding out about their baby. It may be, therefore, that it is a unique opportunity to answer their questions and to talk with them about the care of their baby.

Conclusion

The extent to which relevant research exists and is used is very variable in this area. For some topics, such as posture in labour and immediate care after birth, more information is needed. Existing research is not always used, however, as is apparent in the frequent use of electronic fetal monitoring and in the frequent administration of opioid medication. Further, practice may be based on tradition or other priorities, as is evident in the widespread use of routines such as vaginal examination. Research on a number of topics related to care in labour is seriously overdue, and this should include ways of changing practice where strong and relevant information exists.

References

Alderdice, F., Renfrew, M., Marchant, S., Ashurst, H., Hughes, P., Berridge, G., *et al.* (1995). Labour and birth in water in England and Wales: survey report. *British Journal of Midwifery*, 3(7), 375–82.

American Academy of Pediatrics Committee on Nutrition (1961). Vitamin K compounds and the water-soluble analogues – use in therapy and prophylaxis in pediatrics. *Pediatrics*, 28, 501–7.

Andrews, C. M. and Chrzanowski, M. (1990). Maternal position, labour, and comfort. *Applied Nursing Research*, 3 Jan/Feb, 7.

Banta, D. and Thacker, S. B. (1982). Benefits and risks of episiotomy. *Birth*, 9(1), 25–30.

Beech, B. L. (1995). Water labour water birth. *AIMS Journal*, 7(1), 1–3.

Begley, C. M. (1990). A comparison of 'active' and 'physiological' management of the third stage of labour. *Midwifery*, 6(1), 3–17.

Bergstrom, L., Roberts, J., Skillman, L., and Seidel, J. (1992). 'You'll feel me touching you, sweetie'. *Birth*, 19(1), 10–18.

Beynon, C. (1957). The normal second stage of labour: a plea for the reform of its conduct. *Journal of Obstetrics and Gynaecology of the British Empire*, 64, 815–20.

Bonica, J. J. and McDonald, J. S. (1990). The pain of childbirth. In: *The management of pain* (ed. J. J. Bonica), pp1313. Lea and Febiger, Philadelphia.

Booth, B. (1993). Hypnotherapy. *Nursing Times*, 89(40), 42–5.

Borell, U. and Fernestron, I. (1960). The movement of the sacroiliac joints and their importance to change in the pelvic dimensions during parturition trial. *Acta Obstetrica et Gynaecologica Scandinavica*.

Cammu, H. and van Eeckhout, E. (1996). A randomized controlled trial of early versus delayed use of amniotomy and oxytocin infision in nulliparous labour. *British Journal of Obstetrics and Gynaecology*, 103(4), 313–18.

Chalmers, I., Garcia, J., and Post, S. (1989). Hospital policies for labour and delivery. In: *Effective care in pregnancy and childbirth Vol. II* (ed. I. Chalmers, M. Enkin, and M. J. N. C. Keirse), pp.815–19. Oxford University Press, Oxford.

Chamberlain, G., Wraight, A., and Steer, P. (1993). Findings and recommendations of the NBT survey. In: *Pain and its relief in childbirth: the results of a national survey conducted by the National Birthday Trust* (ed. G. Chamberlain, A. Wraight, and P. Steer), pp.115–17. Churchill Livingstone, Edinburgh.

Chestnut, D. H., Vandewalker, G. E., Owen, O. L., Bates, J. N., and Choi, W. W. (1987). The influence of continuous epidural bupivicaine analgesia on the second stage of labour and method of delivery on the nulliparous woman. *Anesthesiology*, 66, 774–80.

Chestnut, D. H., McGrath, J. M., Vincent, R. D., Penning, D. H., Choi, W. W., Bayes, J. N., *et al.* (1994). Does early administration of epidural analgesia affect obstetric outcome in nulliparous women who are in spontaneous labour? *Anaesthesiology*, 80, 1201–8.

Clinical Standards Advisory Group (1995). *Women in normal labour*. HMSO, London.

Cook, T. M. and McCrirrick, A. (1994). A survey of airway management during induction of general anaesthesia in obstetrics. *International Journal of Obstetric Anaesthesia*, 3, 143–5.

Clinical Resource and Audit Group (1996). *Report on pain relief in labour*. CRAG working group on maternity services, Edinburgh Scottish Office.

Crowley, D. S. and Giesecke, A. H. (1990). Bimanual cricoid pressure. *Anaesthesia*, 45, 588–9.

Crowther, C., Enkin, M., Keirse, M. J. N. C., and Brown, I. (1989). Monitoring the progress of labour. In: *Effective care in pregnancy and childbirth Vol II* (ed. I. Chalmers, M. Enkin, and M. J. N. C. Keirse), pp.833–45. Oxford University Press, Oxford.

Davies, J. and Young, G. (1995). ACBMC Northern Region Home Birth Survey. *Association of Community-based Maternity Care Newsletter,* 11, 6.

Department of Health (1996). Report on Confidential Enquiries into Maternal Deaths in the UK 1991–93. HMSO, London.

De Voe, S., De Voe Jr, K., Rigsby, W. V. C., and McDaniels, B. A. (1969). Effect of meperidine on uterine contractility. *American Journal of Obstetrics and Gynecology,* 105, 1004–7.

Downe, S. (1996). Concepts of normality in maternity services: applications and consequences. In: *Ethics and midwifery: issues in contemporary practice* (ed. L. Frith), pp.86–103. Butterworth Heinemann, Oxford.

Duchene, P. (1989). Effects of biofeedback on childbirth pain. *Journal of Pain and Symptom Management,* 4, 117–23.

Duigan, N. M., Studd, J. W. W., and Hughes, A. O. (1977). Characteristic of normal labour in different racial groups *British Journal of Obstetrics and Gynaecology,* 82(8), 593–601.

Ekelund, H., Finnstrom, O., and Gunnarskog, J. (1993). Administration of vitamin K to newborn infants and childhood cancer. *British Medical Journal,* 307, 89–91.

Elbourne, D. R. (1996). Care in the third stage of labour In: *Midwives, research, and childbirth Vol.* 4(ed. S. Robinson and A. M. Thomson), pp.192–207. Chapman and Hall, London.

Enkin, M. (1989). Commentary: why do the Caesarean section rates differ? *Birth,* 16(4), 207–8.

Enkin, M., Keirse, M. J. N. C., Renfrew, M. J., and Neilson, J. (1995). *A guide to effective care in pregnancy and childbirth.* Oxford University Press, Oxford.

Enkin, M. W., Smith, S. L., Dermer, S. W., and Emmett, J. O. (1972). An adequately controlled study of the effectiveness of PPM training. In: *Psychosomatic medicine in obstetrics and gynaecology* (ed. N. Morris). Karger, Basel.

Flynn, A. M., Kelly, J., and Hollins-Lynch, P. F. (1978). Ambulation in labour. *British Medical Journal,* 2, 591–3.

Fraser, W. D., Krauss, I., Brisson-Carrol, G., Thornton, J., and Breart, G. (1996). Amniotomy to shorten spontaneous labour In: Cochrane Database (see below).

Freeborn, S. F., Calvert, R. T., and Black, P. (1980). Saliva and blood pethidine concentrations in the mother and newborn baby. *British Journal of Obstetrics and Gynaecology,* 87, 966–9.

Friedman, E. A. (1955). Primigravid labour – a graphicostatistical analysis. *American Journal of Obstetrics and Gynecology,* 6, 567–89.

Fusi, L., Maresh, J. A., and Steer, P. J. (1989). Maternal pyrexia associated with the use of epidural analgesia in labour. *Lancet,* i, 1250–2.

Garcia, J. and Garforth, S. (1989). Labour and delivery routines in English consultant maternity units. *Midwifery,* 5(4), 155–63.

Garcia, J. and Garforth, S. (1990). Parents and newborn babies in the labour ward. In: *The politics of maternity care* (ed. J. Garcia, R. Kilpatrick, and M. Richards), p.175. Clarendon, Oxford.

Gardosi, J., Hutson, N., and Lynch, B. C. (1989). Randomized controlled trial of squatting in the second stage of labour. *Lancet*, **Jul 8**, 74–7.

Garforth, S. and Garcia, J. (1987). Admitting – a weakness or a strength? Routine admission of a woman in labour. *Midwifery*, **3**(1), 10–24.

Garland, D. and Jones, K. (1994). Waterbirth: first stage immersion or non-immersion? *British Journal of Midwifery*, **2**(3), 113–20.

Gibbs, C. P., Sophr, L., and Schmidt, D. (1981). *In vitro* and *in vivo* evaluation of sodium citrate as an antacid. *Anaesthesiology*, **55**, A31.

Golay, J., Vedam, S., and Sorger, L. (1993). The squatting position for the second stage of labour. *Birth*, **20**(2), 73–8.

Golding, J., Greenwood, R., and Birmingham, K. (1992). Childhood cancer, intramuscular vitamin K, and pethidine given during labour. *British Medical Journal*, **305**, 341–6.

Greiff, J. M. C., Tordoff, S. G., Griffiths, R., and May, A. E. (1994). Acid aspiration prophylaxis in 202 obstetric anaesthetic units in the UK. *International Journal of Obstetric Anaesthesia*, **4**, 137–42.

Gyte, G. M. L. (1994). Evaluation of the meta-analyses on the effects, on both mother and baby, of the various components of 'active' management of the third stage of labour *Midwifery*, **10**(4), 183–99.

Hardy, J. (1991). *A randomized controlled trial into the use of TENS in labour*. Research and the Midwife Conference Proceedings 1990, Manchester.

Harris, M. (1992). The impact of research findings on current practice in relieving post-partum perineal pain in a large district general hospital. *Midwifery*, **8**(3), 125–31.

Hawkins, S. (1995). Water vs conventional births: infection rates compared. *Nursing Times*, **91**(11), 38–40.

Hodnett, E. D. (1994). Support from care-givers during childbirth. In: Cochrane Database (see below under Neilson *et al.*).

Hodnett, E. and Osborn, R. (1989). A randomized trial of the effects of monitrice support during labour: mothers' views two to four weeks post-partum. *Birth*, **16**(4), 177–83.

Hofmeyr, G. J. and Nikodem, V. C. (1996). Achieving mother and baby friendliness: the evidence for labour companions. In: *Baby friendly mother friendly* (ed. S. F. Murray). Mosby, London.

Howell, C. J. and Chalmers, I. (1992). A review of prospectively controlled comparisons of epidural with non-epidural forms of pain relief during labour. *International Journal of Obstetric Anesthesia*, **1**, 93–110.

Hunt, J. M. (1981). Indicators for nursing practice: the use of research findings. *Journal of Advanced Nursing*, **6**(3), 189–94.

Keirse, M. J. N. C. (1989). Augmentation of labour. In: *Effective care in pregnancy and childbirth Vol. II* (ed. I. Chalmers, M. Enkin, and M. J. N. C. Keirse). Oxford University Press, Oxford.

Keirse, M. J. N. C. (1993). A final comment managing the uterus, the woman, or whom? *Birth*, **20**(3), 159–61.

Keirse, M. J. N. C. and Chalmers, I. (1989). Methods for inducing labour. In: *Effective care in pregnancy and childbirth Vol. II* (ed. I. Chalmers, M. Enkin, and M. J. N. C. Keirse). Oxford University Press, Oxford.

Keirse, M. J. N. C., Enkin, M., and Lumley, J. (1989). Social and professional support during labour. In: *Effective care in pregnancy and childbirth Vol. II* (ed. I. Chalmers, M. Enkin, and M. J. N. C. Keirse). Oxford University Press, Oxford.

Kennell, J., Klaus, M., McGrath, S.,Robertson, S., and Hinkley, C. (1991). Continuous emotional support during labour in a US hospital: a randomized controlled trial. *Journal of the American Medical Association*, **265**(17), 197–201.

Kennell, J. H., Jerauld, R., Wolfe, H., Chester, D., Kreger, N., Macalpine, W., *et al.* (1974). Maternal behaviour one year after early and extended post-partum contact. *Developmental Medicine and Child Neurology*, **16**, 172–9.

Kennell, J. H., Klaus, M., McGrath, S., Robertson, S., and Hinkley, C. (1988). Medical intervention: the effect of social support *Paediatric Research*, **23**, 211A.

Khan, G. Q., John, I. S., Chan, T., Wani, S., Hughes, A.,O. and Stirrat, G. M. (1995). Abu Dhabi third-stage trial: oxytocin versus syntometrine in the active management of the third stage of labour *European Journal of Obstetrics and Gynaecology and Reproductive Biology*, 58(2), 147–51.

Kitzinger, S. (1990). Pelvic floor awareness. In: *Episiotomy and the second stage of labour* (2nd edn) (ed. S. Kitzinger and P. Simkin). Pennypress, Seattle.

Klaus, M. H., Kennell, J. H., Robertson, S. S., and Sosa, R. (1986). Effects of social support during parturition on maternal and infant morbidity. *British Medical Journal*, **293**(6), 585–7.

Klebanoff, M. A., Read, J. S., Mills, J. L., and Shiono, P. H. (1993). The risk of childhood cancer after neonatal exposure to vitamin K. *The New England Journal of Medicine*, **329**(13), 905–8.

Lenstrup, C., Schantz, A., Berget Afeder, E., Roseno, H., and Hertel, J. (1987). Warm tub bath during delivery. *Acta Obstetrica et Gynaecologica Scandinavica*, **66**(8), 709–12.

Ludka, L. (1987). *Fasting during labour.* Paper presented at the International Confederation of Midwives 21st Congress in the Hague, August 1987.

MacArthur, C., Lewis, M., and Knox, E. G. (1991). *Health after childbirth.* HMSO, London.

McCandlish, R. and Renfrew, M. (1993). Immersion in water during labour and birth: the need for evaluation. *Birth*, **20**(2), 79–85.

McDonald, S. J., Prendiville, W. J., and Blair, E. (1993). Randomized controlled trial of oxytocin alone versus oxytocin and ergometrine in active management of third stage of labour. *British Medical Journal*, **307**, 1167–71.

Macleod, J., Macintyre, C., and McClure, J. H. (1995). Backache and epidural analgesia: a retrospective survey of mothers one year after childbirth. *International Journal of Obstetric Anaesthesia*, 4(1), 21–5.

McManus, T. J. and Calder, A. A.. (1978). Upright posture and the efficiency of labour. *Lancet*, **1**, 72–4.

Mander, R. (1994). Epidural analgesia. 2: research basis. *British Journal of Midwifery*, 2(1), 2–16.

Mander, R. (1995). The care of the mother grieving a baby relinquished for adoption. Avebury, Aldershot.

Matthews, M. K. (1989). The relationship between maternal labour analgesia and delay in the initiation of breastfeeding in healthy neonates in the early neonatal period. *Midwifery*, 5(1), 3–10.

Meah, S., Luker, K. A., and Cullum, N. A. (1996). An exploration of midwives' attitudes to research and perceived barriers to research utilization. *Midwifery*, 12(2), 73–84.

Menage, J. (1996). Post traumatic stress disorder following obstetric/gynaecological procedures. *British Journal of Midwifery*, 4(10), 532–3.

Mendez-Bauer, C., Arroyo, J., Garcia-Ramos, C., Mendendez, A., Lavilla, M., Isquierdo, F., *et al.* (1975) Effects of standing position on spontaneous uterine contractility and other aspects of labour. *Journal of Perinatal Medicine*, 3, 89–100.

Michael, S., Reilly, C. S., and Caunt, J. A. (1991). Policies for oral intake during labour: a survey of maternity units in England and Wales. *Anaesthesia*, 46(12), 1071–3.

Morey, R. J., Macdonald, R., Fisk, N. M., *et al.* (1994). Patient control of combined spinal epidural anaesthesia. *Lancet*, **344**, 1238.

Morgan, B. M. and Kadim, M. Y. (1994). Mobile regional analgesia in labour. *British Journal of Obstetrics and Gynaecology*, **101**(10), 839–41.

Morton, S. C., Williams, M. S., Keeler, E. B., Gambone, J. C., and Kahn, K. L. (1994). Effect of epidural anesthesia for labor on the Cesarean delivery rate. *Obstetrics and Gynecology*, **6**, 1045–52.

Neilson, J. P. (1994). Electronic fetal heart rate monitoring during labour: information from randomized trials. *Birth*, **21**(2), 101–4.

Neilson, J. P., Crowther, C. A., Hodnett, E. D., Hofmeyer, G. J., Keirse, M. J. N. C., and Renfrew, M. J. (eds.) Cochrane Database of systematic reviews (Updated April 1997). Cochrane Library, Oxford.

O'Driscoll, K. and Meagher, D. (1980). *Active management of labour.* W. B. Saunders, London.

Olah, K. S. J. and Neilson, J. P. (1994). Failure to progress in the management of labour. *British Journal of Obstetrics and Gynaecology*, **101**(1), 1–3.

Paciornik, M. (1990). Arguments against episiotomy and in favour of squatting for birth *Birth*, **17**(2), 104–5.

Prendiville, W. J., Elbourne, D. R., and Chalmers, I. (1988a). The effects of routine oxytocic administration in the management of the third stage of labour. *British Journal of Obstetrics and Gynaecology*, 95, 3–16.

Prendiville, W. J., Harding, J. E., Elbourne, D. R., and Stirrat, G. M. (1988b). The Bristol third stage trial: active versus physiological management of the third stage of labour. *British Medical Journal*, 297, 1295–300.

Prendiville, W. and Elbourne, D. (1989). Care during the third stage of labour. In: *Effective care in pregnancy and childbirth Vol. II* (ed. I. Chalmers, M. Enkin, and M. J. N. C. Keirse), pp.1145–69. Oxford University Press, Oxford.

Pursey, M. (1994). Mobile epidural – the only analgesia without anaesthesia. *Paediatric Post*, **Spring/Summer**, 3.

Ramin, S. M., Gambling, D. R., and Lucas, M. J. (1995). Randomized trial of epidural versus intravenous analgesia during labour. *Lancet*, 345, 1413–16.

Renfrew, M. J. and Lang, S. (1994). Early initiation of breastfeeding and its effect on duration. In: Cochrane Database (see below).

Robson, S. (1992). Variation of cervical dilatation estimation by midwives, doctors, student midwives, and medical students – a small study using cervical simulation methods. In: *Research and the Midwife Conference Proceedings 1991*. University of Manchester.

Rosser, J. (1994). World Health Organization partograph in management of labour. *MIDIRS Midwifery Digest*, 4()4), 436–7.

Salariya, E. M., Easton, P. M., and Cater, J. I. (1978). Duration of breastfeeding after early initiation and frequent feeding. *Lancet*, 2, 1141–3.

Saunders, N. S. G., Paterson, C. M., and Wadsworth, J. (1992). Neonatal and maternal morbidity in relation to the duration of the second stage of labour. *British Journal of Obstetrics and Gynaecology*, 99(5), 381–5.

Scott, D. B. and Tunstall, M. E. (1995). Serious complications associated with epidural/spinal blockade in obstetrics: a two-year prospective study. *International Journal of Obstetric Anaesthesia*, 4, 133–9.

Scottish Home and Health Department (1985). *Obstetric anaesthesia and analgesia in Scotland*. National Medical Consultative Committee, Scottish Home and Health Department, Edinburgh.

Sellick, B. A. (1961). Cricoid pressure to control regurgitation of stomach contents. *Lancet*, 2, 404–6.

Simms, C., McHaffie, H., Renfrew, M., and Ashurst, H. (1994). *The midwifery research database: MIRIAD*. Hale, Haigh, and Hochland, Cheshire.

Sleep, J. (1984). The West Berkshire Episiotomy Trial. In: *Research and the Midwife Conference Proceedings 1983* (ed. A. Thomson and S. Robinson). University of Manchester.

Sleep, J. and Grant, A. (1987). West Berkshire Perineal Management Trial: three years follow-up. *British Medical Journal*, 295, 749–51.

Sosa, R., Kennell, J. H., Klaus, M., Robertson, S., and Urrutia, J. (1980). The effect of a supportive companion on perinatal problems, length of labor, and mother–infant interaction. *New England Journal of Medicine*, 303, 597–600.

Spanos, N. P., Carmanico, S. J., and Ellis, J. A. (1994). Hypnotic analgesia. In: *Textbook of pain* (3rd edn) (ed. P. D. Wall and R. Melzack), pp.1349–66. Churchill Livingstone, Edinburgh.

Steer, P. (1993). The methods of pain relief used. In: *Pain and its relief in childbirth* (ed. G. Chamberlain, A. Wraight, and P. Steer). Churchill Livingstone, Edinburgh.

St James-Roberts, I., Hutchinson, C., Haran, F., and Chamberlain, G. (1982). Biofeedback as an aid to childbirth. *British Journal of Obstetrics and Gynaecology*, 90, 56–60.

Thilaganathan, B., Cutner, A., Latimer, J., and Beard, R. (1993). Management of the third stage of labour in women at low risk of post-partum haemorrhage *European Journal of Obstetrics and Gynaecology and Reproductive Biology*, 48(1), 19–22.

Thomson, A. M. (1988). Management of the woman in the normal second stage of labour: a review. *Midwifery*, 4(2), 77–85.

Thomson, A. M. and Hillier, V. F. (1994). A re-evaluation of the effect of pethidine on the length of labour. *Journal of Advanced Nursing*, 19(3), 448–56.

Thomson, M. and Westreich, R. (1989). Restriction of mother–infant contact in the immediate postnatal period. In: *Effective care in pregnancy and childbirth Vol. II* (ed. I. Chalmers, M. Enkin, and M. J. N. C. Keirse), pp.1322–32. Oxford University Press, Oxford.

Thornton, J. G. and Lilford, R. J. (1994). Active management of labour: current knowledge and research issues. *British Medical Journal*, 309, 366–9.

Tuffnell, D. J., Bryce, F., Johnson, N., and Lilford, R. J. (1989). Simulation of cervical changes in labour: reproducibility of expert assessment. *Lancet*, ii, 1089–90.

Way, W. L. and Way, E. L. (1992). Opioid analgesics and antagonists. In: *Basic clinical pharmacology* (5th edn) (ed. B. G. Katzung), pp.420–36. Lange, East Norwalk.

Widstrom, A.-M., Ransjo-Arvidson, A. B., Christensson, K., Matiesen, A.-S., Winberg, J., and Uvnas-Moberg, K. (1987). Gastric suction in healthy newborn infants: effects on circulation and developing feeding behaviour. *Acta Paediatrica Scandinavica*, 76, 566–72.

Williams, S., Hepburn, M., and McIlwaine, G. (1985). Consumer view of epidural anaesthesia. *Midwifery*, 1(1), 32–6.

Woodcock, H. C., Read, A. W., Bower, C., Stanley, F. J., and Moore, D. J. (1994). A matched cohort study of planned home and hospital births in Western Australia 1981–1987. *Midwifery*, 10(3), 125–35.

World Health Organization (1994). World Health Organization partograph reduces complications of labour and childbirth. Press release, 7th June.

Wraight, A. (1993). Coping with pain. In: *Pain and its relief in childbirth* (ed. G. Chamberlain, A. Wraight, and P. Steer). Churchill Livingstone, Edinburgh.

Yuen, P. M., Chan, N. S., Yim, S. F., and Chang, A. M. (1995). A randomized double-blind controlled trial of syntometrine and syntocinon. *British Journal of Obstetrics and Gynaecology*, 102(5), 377–80.

CHAPTER TWENTY-TWO

Care of the mother after birth

Jo Garcia and Sally Marchant

'Having a baby really changes your life. I feel that you get lots of help and attention in the first few weeks but after that you are on your own. My husband now seems to think "Well, that's all over so we should be back to normal" . . . I'm not too worried as I know everything will straighten itself out; the baby will sleep more, my husband will pay more attention to him as he gets older, my daughter will realize baby is no threat to her and Mummy doesn't love her any less, and I will, *eventually*, get my body back!!'

This comment, from a mother who took part in a study of postnatal care (Garcia and Marchant 1992), was chosen to illustrate two things: first, that care is given in the wider context of family support and the woman's varied responsibilities; and second, that women's physical health and mental well-being are closely related. The first section of this chapter describes current patterns of postnatal care in this country. Next is a section about women's health in the period after a birth. We then explore what the purposes of postnatal care might be and look at evidence about interventions in the postnatal period.

The present pattern of postnatal care

After the birth women are attended by various health professionals with the aim of providing care, advice, and support for the new mother and her baby. Care is given in hospital and at home by midwives, specialists, GPs, and health visitors. Midwives are the main care-givers in the immediate puerperium. If the birth takes place in hospital the stay is very variable in length, ranging from a few hours to several days, depending on the health of mother and baby, the family's wishes, and local policies. National data for average lengths of stay have recently been published (Department of Health 1997) and these show a steady decline in lengths of stay since the 1970s. In a national sample survey of women who had given birth in 1995, 22% stayed in hospital for less than 24 hours, a further 31% stayed for one or two days, and the remaining 47% stayed for three days or longer (Garcia *et al.* 1998).

Once women return home they are visited routinely by midwives.

Midwives have a statutory obligation to provide care for women after the birth (Garcia and Marchant 1996). These visits usually take place every day in the first few postnatal days and then at varying intervals up to the 10th day. After that, women in most districts may be visited by a midwife up to the 28th day if there seems to be a need or if local policy sets out routine days for such a visit. Visiting patterns are sometimes guided by explicit policies which say, for example, that visits can be omitted on days seven and nine if all is well. Other places have policies which offer a flexible pattern, allowing the midwife to plan visits with the individual mother (Garcia *et al.* 1994).

The 1995 data collected by the Audit Commission show that 29% of women were visited every day and 32% on every day but one, up to 10 days after the birth. Most studies show that very few women get *no* home visits from a midwife after the birth (around 1% in the Audit Commission survey) and these women are more likely to have stayed in hospital for longer than average, or to have had a baby who needed a longer stay in hospital (Garcia *et al.* 1998).

At some point around 14 days after the birth the woman will be contacted by a health visitor whose role is to provide advice and support for mother and baby and to assess the health and development of babies and children. Women are also encouraged to take their babies to local child health clinics for advice on milk feeding, weaning, child development, minor illnesses, safety, and family health. Computerized systems are used to remind parents to take their children to the clinic for routine screening and immunization. Health visitors can also continue to visit at home. In the Audit Commission survey, 98% of women had been visited at home by a health visitor since the birth of their baby.

GPs are involved routinely in the postnatal period mainly through the postnatal check which is carried out at around six weeks after the birth. In the survey carried out for the Audit Commission, 93% of women reported that they had had a postnatal check and nine tenths of these were done in the GPs surgery, almost always by the GP (Garcia *et al.* 1998).

In addition, some GPs aim to visit all new mothers in the immediate postnatal period. In a survey of GPs carried out by the Audit Commission (Audit Commission 1997), three quarters of GPs said that they did this. Two thirds of respondents to the survey of mothers said that they had had at least one visit from a GP in the period after the birth to 'check on you and your baby's progress'. In addition, many mothers and babies receive home visits from GPs because of sickness. There is probably quite a lot of practice to practice variation in the extent of GP involvement over and above the postnatal check. In a smaller survey carried out in 1992 and 1993 in two hospitals in the former North East Thames Region, none of the women who had given birth in an inner-city hospital reported home visits by a GP in the diaries they filled in on days four, eight, or 12 after the birth. In contrast, a fifth of those who had given birth in a town outside London reported that the GP visited on day four and the same proportion reported a visit on day eight (Garcia *et al.*, unpublished data).

Women's health in the postnatal period

Information from research about postnatal health and health care is accumulating (MacArthur *et al.* 1991; Glazener *et al.* 1993; Glazener 1997). Women often have substantial health problems in the postnatal period, some of which may be long lasting. For example, in the immediate puerperium, perineal trauma resulting from episiotomies, tears, or bruising may affect the mother's ability to sit or walk comfortably and care for her baby. In the longer term, poorly healed perineal tissue may affect the sexual relations between a couple for months after the birth (Sleep 1991). A study which looked at the longer-term health of women following childbirth found that 47% of women developed at least one health problem lasting more than six weeks within the first three months after delivery of the baby (MacArthur *et al.* 1991). Research about postnatal care in one region in Scotland showed that 87% of postnatal women had at least one health problem once they were at home, 46% of these being major problems which included bleeding or high blood pressure, and 78% relatively 'minor' problems such as tiredness, backache, constipation, piles, or headache (Glazener *et al.* 1995).

Problems with mental health are also common (Romito 1989; Brown *et al.* 1994; Glazener 1997). Transient sadness affects as many as four fifths of women in the first few days. In the study of women who had given birth in two English maternity units, the self-reported mood of the women taking part showed a marked dip at day four after the birth (Garcia *et al.*, unpublished data). Figures for the proportion of women who are depressed after the birth vary between studies, ranging from 10–20%. Much of this depression is long lasting (Glazener 1997) and it may well have an adverse effect on the relationship with the baby and his or her development (Murray 1992; Chapter 18). Some other mental health issues are also important in addition to depression. Some women find that their experiences of childbirth leave them feeling distressed and frightened; they may be reluctant to consider another pregnancy and may suffer from nightmares (Menage 1993; Smith and Mitchell 1996). Experiences in the postnatal period may lead to long-term anxieties for parents even when the baby has been judged to be well by caregivers (Kemper *et al.* 1990). A large proportion of these illnesses are taken to GPs for advice and continuing care: the volume of work is considerable.

A high proportion of breastfeeding mothers suffer morbidity from poor positioning at the breast and resultant sore nipples, and a small number develop infection in the breast (White *et al.* 1992, Renfrew *et al.*, in press; Chapter 24). Bottle-feeding mothers also have some problems of pain and engorgement but these tend to be of shorter duration. Postnatal care is crucial because it has the potential to alleviate some of the burden of physical and psychological ill health for mothers (Glazener *et al.* 1993). It can also be seen as a positive source of support for parents and a way of helping them to develop good relationships with their children and to make appropriate use of the health services. Postnatal care also has the advantage that it reaches almost all child-bearing women (e.g. Murphy-Black 1989; Audit Commission 1997).

What is postnatal care for?

What information do we have about the effectiveness of postnatal interventions and how useful is the present pattern of care likely to be in addressing the main types of morbidity? We would suggest that postnatal care has three main purposes as far as the new mother is concerned: to safeguard her health; to enable her to develop a good relationship with the new baby; and to provide her and her family with support and advice. The immediate care and longer-term health of the baby are also of concern to the three main care-givers in the postnatal period (Chapter 23). In common with many other areas of health care, research evidence is very limited about the effectiveness of the clinical components of postnatal care. In addition, the postnatal health of the mother and baby is affected by the events and in some cases the care given in pregnancy and at the birth, as well as care given after the birth (Green *et al.* 1990; Hodnett 1997). It is easier to access information about the effects of intrapartum care than of subsequent care because of the focus of research up to now.

In addition to uncertainty about the clinical aspects of care, there are also doubts about the most effective ways to organize the service. For example, one key issue for postnatal care is whether it should be a universal service with a large component of routine care or whether, in contrast, care should be aimed mainly at women with specific needs. This debate is relevant to both the clinical and the social aspects of care. At present, the service probably has a large component of routine care with some selective elements. We know little, though, about the actual balance between these two in current practice nor the impact of different approaches on the welfare of mothers and families. There are many other specific issues about the organization of postnatal care that are being discussed and researched at present: the pattern of postnatal home visiting (Twaddle *et al.* 1993; Garcia *et al.* 1994); the postnatal check (Bick and MacArthur 1994); length of postnatal hospital stay (Norr and Nacion 1987; Brown *et al.* 1995); and the offer of 'debriefing' for women who have had a difficult birth (Smith and Mitchell 1996). The next sections highlight some of the evidence that we do have about effective care.

Safeguarding maternal health

Although this chapter focuses on postnatal care, it is worth noting that intrapartum care is likely to affect women's physical health after the birth. A reduction in operative and instrumental births, were it desirable on balance, would be likely to reduce maternal perineal and abdominal pain and infection (Glazener *et al.* 1993). Assisted delivery by vacuum extractor leads to less maternal trauma than the use of forceps (Johanson 1995*a*). On the basis of the trials so far we can estimate that antibiotic prophylaxis at Caesarean section reduces the rate of post-partum infection from around 10% to 4%

(Smaill 1995). Active management of the third stage of labour, including the use of oxytocic drugs, reduces post-partum haemorrhage, though its impact on longer-term vaginal loss and iron status is not yet known (Prendeville *et al.* 1997). Types of suturing materials, and techniques for repair have an impact on maternal pain and other outcomes in the shorter and longer term (Johanson 1995*b*).

Many of the clinical components of postnatal care have not been adequately studied. In some cases, such as vaginal bleeding in the puerperium, there is not even a clear idea of what would count as illness (Marchant and Garcia 1995). However, some clinical interventions have been evaluated and help inform clinicians about effectiveness. In a recent review about perineal care (Sleep 1995), the author concluded that paracetamol was the best first choice for pain relief; the local application of 5% lignocaine spray or gel reduces discomfort; topical steroids should be avoided for perineal care because they seem to impair healing; and so far there is no evidence that pulsed electromagnetic energy (used by physiotherapists) is effective in reducing pain or initiating earlier healing. Where a perineal wound breaks down, there is evidence from one small trial (Monberg and Hammen 1987) that primary resuturing and prescribing antibiotics is more effective than waiting.

Although morbidity from urinary and faecal incontinence is quite substantial following a birth, so far effective treatments have not been demonstrated. Some studies are in progress and a Cochrane Review Group has been formed to bring together all those interested in evidence about effective treatments for incontinence (Glazener 1997).

What type of service is likely to contribute to reducing maternal morbidity? In this country, care in the postnatal period is largely based on a framework of routine observations and tests directed towards the detection of disease and screening for pathological problems such as secondary post-partum haemorrhage or virulent infection. These problems were important at a time when maternal mortality was high and this contributed to setting up and codifying formal maternity care in this country. For example, before the introduction of antibiotics earlier this century, the presence of uterine sepsis accounted for a very high proportion of maternal deaths (Loudon 1986). Although similar conditions are still major causes of maternal mortality and morbidity in the developing world, they would appear to have less importance for the majority of mothers in the developed world.

The underlying health of mothers has changed in the last 70 years, and the care provided should reflect this. Re-evaluation of the routine aspects of postnatal care might look more towards reducing the occurrence of the most common types of morbidity which affect both the ability of the mother to return to reasonable health and to care for the new baby rather than screening everyone for serious conditions which affect only a few. We need to be cautious, though, and evaluate any changes to practice – both those which are innovations and those where current care based on tradition is discarded. Research studies which both describe the extent of any morbidity and then the usefulness of current routine practices to assess this morbidity are one way forward (Alexander *et al.* 1997). There are currently studies in progress to look at the benefits and disadvantages of different ways of providing clinical care in the puerperium.

Supporting the relationship between mother and baby

Care in pregnancy, at the birth, and after may affect the way that the mother relates to her baby later, as judged by the results of randomized controlled trials. For example, mothers cared for by a small team of midwives were more confident about their babies at six weeks after the birth when compared with mothers getting usual care (Flint 1991). Women provided with supportive visits from a research midwife during pregnancy were less likely to be worried about their babies at six weeks after the birth (Oakley 1992). Many studies, though, do not follow up for long enough, or do not cover the relationship between mother and baby. In addition, few of the interventions that are designed to improve parents' understanding of the new baby or offer support with problems have been evaluated. Infant feeding is one area where there has been a considerable amount of research, though there are still gaps in key areas of knowledge (Chapter 24).

Providing support and advice for the woman and family

The benefits of social and psychological support have been demonstrated for some aspects of maternity care, such as care in labour (Hodnett 1997) and postnatal depression (Holden *et al.* 1989; Holden 1990). Care-givers need to look at these aspects of their work in the light of the evidence, and map out what they hope to achieve with the support they offer. Research may be needed to demonstrate the value of other aspects of their care (health promotion, general support, contact with parent networks, etc.) and the best ways of providing care that have been shown to work. For example, the Edinburgh Postnatal Depression Scale (EPDS) has been used in research for some years (Cox *et al.* 1987). It is a self-administered scale which provides a reasonable detection of depression in women following a birth. Recently it has begun to be used in community-based interventions, usually by health visitors (McClarey and Stokoe 1995; Painter 1995). In these two examples protocols for its use were drawn up, suggesting what care to offer to women who scored above a certain number on the scale, and how to liaise with other care-givers. However, one small study indicated that some health visitors were using the EPDS without being confident about how to do so (Almond 1996). Although some small audits have been carried out, we are not aware of a methodologically rigorous evaluation of the use of the EPDS as a routine part of care. There is research in progress, though, about other aspects of support in the postnatal period, including an Australian trial of the offer of 'debriefing' after a Caesarean section.

The conventional view is that despite education in the antenatal period for postnatal events, many parents feel ill-equipped to care for the newly born infant. The roles of the midwife and health visitor have shifted more towards increasing parents' confidence in their abilities to cope when they need to on their own. These staff have an important role to play in supporting women who choose to breastfeed and have not had experience of breastfeeding before (Chapter 24). They have a responsibility to see that social conditions are suitable for both the mother and the new baby and this may involve liaison with social services. Health education information is appropriate at this time both to help to avoid ill health in the baby and to raise mothers' awareness about their own health. There is evidence that many women do not seek professional help for health problems in the postnatal period (MacArthur *et al.* 1991). If they did so, common physical and psychological problems could be raised and issues such as cervical smears and adequate contraception could be discussed. Although some of these areas may be covered by giving out leaflets and booklets, the work of the midwife and health visitor in visiting the mother at home provides a more immediate access to health services and involves one-to-one interactions alongside practical demonstrations of infant care, and being available to parents who seek reassurance about their own competence can be invaluable.

Although the midwife is the primary care-giver in the early stages, she is supported by the general practitioner and later transfers care to the health visitor. The lines of responsibility between care-givers in the postnatal period can become confused as the midwife may visit for up to 28 days after the birth. In the absence of any complications it is usual for the health visitor to assume care for the mother shortly after the 10th postnatal day and for women to be followed up through community or GP clinics. In the past, screening for physical problems was central to the purpose of the midwife's visit and provided a clear purpose for the midwife in the postnatal period in both the hospital and the mothers' own home. With increasing awareness of the need for psychological and social support and parent and health education, the roles of midwife and health visitor are becoming blurred.

Conclusions

The increased interest in the well-being of women following a birth is encouraging. In the past, those who wrote about postnatal mental health, for example, rarely read journals where articles about breastfeeding were published. There is now more writing and research that bridges the gap between physical and mental health and between mother and baby (Brown *et al.* 1994). On the other hand, changes in maternity care, and in health care more widely, are likely to have intended and unintended effects on the care that is offered to women and families. It is far from clear how the complex changes in NHS management and the promotion of commissioning groups will affect the type of service that is provided.

More specifically, many aspects of the organization of postnatal care are currently under debate. For example, changes in the organization of midwifery care may be exacerbating problems that women experience in postnatal care in hospital. If women are supposed to be cared for by a team midwife they may not be able to get help with, say, breastfeeding when they need it. How should this be resolved? Should fewer women stay in hospital after the birth, or even give birth in hospital? Or should care in the wards be mainly carried out by midwives based there and not 'following' women? There are also questions about the pattern of postnatal home visiting, the content of care, and the content and value of the postnatal check. The appropriate type of staff to provide the different aspects of care has been raised. Some of these issues are being explored in research projects that are now in progress. It is to be hoped that the results will allow more rational care in the future.

References

Alexander, J., Garcia, J., and Marchant, S. (1997). *The BLiPP Study: blood loss in the postnatal period. Final Report.* National Perinatal Epidemiology Unit, Oxford.

Almond, P. (1996). How health visitors assess the health of postnatal women. *Health Visitor*, **69**, 495–8.

Audit Commission (1997). *First class delivery: improving maternity services in England and Wales.* Audit Commission, London.

Bick, D. E. and MacArthur, C. (1994). Identifying morbidity in post-partum women. *Modern Midwife.*

Brown, S., Lumley, J., Small, R., and Astbury, J. (1994). *Missing voices: the experience of motherhood.* Oxford University Press, Oxford.

Brown, S., Lumley, J., and Small, R. (1995). *Reasons to stay – reasons to go: Victorian women talk about early discharge.* Centre for the Study of Mothers' and Children's Health, Melbourne.

Cox, J. L., Holden, J. M., and Sagovsky, R. (1987). Detection of postnatal depression: development of the 10-item Edinburgh Postnatal Depression Scale. *British Journal of Psychiatry*, **150**, 782–6.

Department of Health (1997). *NHS Maternity Statistics, England, 1989–90 to 1994–5.* Statistical Bulletin 1997/28. Department of Health, London.

Flint, C. (1991). Continuity of care provided by a team of midwives – the Know Your Midwife scheme. In: *Midwives, research and childbirth Vol. II* (ed. S. Robinson and A. M. Thomson). Chapman and Hall., London.

Garcia, J. and Marchant, S. (1992). The NPEU Postnatal Care Project. *Research and the Midwife Conference Proceedings.* University of Manchester.

Garcia, J., Renfrew, M., and Marchant, S. (1994). Postnatal home visiting by midwives. *Midwifery* **10**(1), 40–3.

Garcia, J. and Marchant, S. (1996). The potential of postnatal care. In: *Midwifery care for the future: meeting the challenge* (ed. D. Kroll). Balliere Tindall, London.

Garcia, J., Redshaw, M., Fitzsimons, B., and Keene, J. (1998). *First class delivery: a national survey of women's views of maternity care.* Audit Commission, London.

Glazener, C. (1997). Postnatal morbidity. In: *Royal College of Obstetricians and Gynaecologists' Yearbook* (ed. P. M. S. O'Brien).

Glazener, C., MacArthur, C., and Garcia, J. (1993). Postnatal care: time for a change. *Contemporary Reviews in Obstetrics and Gynaecology*, **5**, 130–6.

Glazener, C., Abdalla, M., Stroud, P., Naji, S., Templeton, A., and Russell, I. (1995). Postnatal maternal morbidity: extent, causes, prevention, and treatment. *British Journal of Obstetrics and Gynaecology*, **102**, 282–7.

Green, J. M. (1990). *Calming or harming? A critical review of psychological effects of fetal diagnosis in pregnant women.* Galton Institute occasional paper no.2.

Hodnett, E. D. (1997). Support from care-givers during childbirth. In: Pregnancy and Childbirth Module of the Cochrane Database of Systematic Reviews (ed. J. P. Neilson, C. A. Crowther, E. D. Hodnett, G. J. Hoffmeyer, and M. J. N. C. Keirse). The Cochrane Collaboration. Issue 2. Update Software, Oxford.

Holden, J. M. (1990). Emotional problems associated with childbirth. In: *Postnatal care – a research-based approach* (ed. A. Alexander, V. Levy, and S. Roch). Macmillan, London.

Holden, J. M., Sagovsky, R., and Cox, L. J. (1989). Counselling in a general practice setting: a controlled study of health visitor intervention in the treatment of postnatal depression. *British Medical Journal*, **298**, 223–6.

Johanson, R. B. (1995*a*). Vacuum extraction versus forceps delivery. In: Pregnancy and Childbirth Module of the Cochrane Database of Systematic Reviews (ed. M. J. N. C. Keirse, M. J. Renfrew, J. P. Neilson, and C. Crowther). The Cochrane Collaboration. Issue 2. Update Software, Oxford.

Johanson, R.B. (1995*b*). Continuous vs interrupted sutures for perineal repair. In: Pregnancy and Childbirth Module of the Cochrane Database of Systematic Reviews (ed. M. W. Enkin, M. J. N. C. Keirse, M. J. Renfrew, and J. P. Neilson). The Cochrane Collaboration. Update Software, Oxford.

Kemper, K. J., Forsyth, B. W., and McCarthy, P. L. (1990). Persistent perceptions of vulnerability following neonatal jaundice. *Americal Journal of Diseases in Childhood*, **144**(2), 238–41.

Loudon, I. (1986). Obstetric care, social class, and maternal mortality. *British Medical Journal*, **293**, 606–8.

MacArthur, C., Lewis, M., and Knox, E. G. (1991). *Health after childbirth.* HMSO, London.

McClarey, M. and Stokoe, B. (1995). A multidisciplinary approach to postnatal depression. *Health Visitor*, **68**, 141–3.

Marchant, S. and Garcia, J. (1995). Routine clinical care in the immediate postnatal period. In: *Aspects of midwifery practice: a research-based spproach* (ed. J. Alexander, V. Levy, and S. Roch). Macmillan, Basingstoke.

Menage, J. (1993). Post-traumatic stress disorder in women who have undergone obstetric and/or gynaecological procedures. *Journal of Reproductive and Infant Psychology*, **11**, 221–8.

Monberg, J. and Hammen, S. (1987). Ruptured episiotomia resutured primarily. *Acta Obstetrica et Gynaecologica Scandinavica*, **66**, 163–4.

Murphy-Black, T. (1989). *Postnatal care at home: a descriptive study of mothers' needs and the maternity services.* A report of the Scottish Home and Health Department Nursing Research Unit, University of Edinburgh.

Murray, L. (1992). The impact of postnatal depression on infant development. *Journal of Child Psychology and Psychiatry*, **33**, 543–61.

Norr, K. and Nacion, K. (1987). Outcomes of post-partum early discharge 1960–1986. *Birth*, **14**(3), 135–41.

Oakley, A. (1992). *Social support and motherhood.* Blackwell, Oxford.

Painter, A. (1995). Health visitor identification of postnatal depression. *Health Visitor*, **68**, 138–40.

Prendeville, W. J., Elbourne, D. E., McDonald, S. (1997). Active versus expectant management of the third stage of labour. In: Pregnancy and Childbirth Module of the Cochrane Database of Systematic Reviews (ed. J. P. Neilson, C. A. Crowther, E. D. Hodnett, G. J. Hoffmeyer, and M. J. N. C. Keirse). The Cochrane Collaboration. Issue 2. Update Software, Oxford.

Renfrew, M. J., Ross McGill, H., and Woolridge, M. W. (1996). Enabling women to breastfeed: interventions which support or inhibit breastfeeding. A structured review of the evidence. HMSO, London.

Romito, P. (1989). Unhappiness after childbirth. In: *Effective care in pregnancy and childbirth* (ed. I. Chalmers, M. Enkin, and M. J. N. C. Keirse). Oxford University Press, Oxford.

Sleep, J. (1991). Perineal care: a series of five randomized controlled trials. In: *Midwives, research and childbirth* vol. II (ed. S. Robinson and A. Thomson). Chapman and Hall, London.

Sleep, J. (1995). Postnatal perineal care revisited. In: *Aspects of midwifery practice: a research-based approach* (ed. J. Alexander, V. Levy, and S. Roch). Macmillan, Basingstoke.

Smaill, F. (1995). Prophylactic antibiotics for elective Caesarean section. In: Pregnancy and Childbirth Module of the Cochrane Database of Systematic Reviews (ed. M. J. N. C. Keirse, M. J. Renfrew, J. P. Neilson, and C. Crowther). The Cochrane Collaboration. Issue 2. Update Software, Oxford.

Smith, J. A. and Mitchell, S. (1996). Debriefing after childbirth: a tool for effective risk management. *British Journal of Midwifery*, **4**, 581–6.

St Mary's Maternity Information System (1992). *North West Thames Region annual maternity figures.* St Mary's Hospital Medical School, London.

Twaddle, S., Liao, X., and Fyvie, H. (1993). An evaluation of postnatal care individualized to the needs of the woman. *Midwifery*, **9**, 154–60.

White, A,, Freeth, S., and O'Brien, M. (1992). *Infant feeding 1990.* Social Survey Division, Office of Population Censuses and Surveys, London.

CHAPTER TWENTY-THREE

Newborn babies and how to treat them

Sara Watkin and Cath Henson

Ninety-three per cent of newborn babies are born at term and of these between 95% and 99% are in good condition. They require no resuscitation and have no abnormalities on routine baby check and biochemical screening. Caring for the newborn demands the skills and expertise of working in partnership with parents. It is very easy to 'tell' rather than to teach but such interactions only lead to short-term remedies where the parent has to return repeatedly for further advice. Acknowledging a family's right to participate in decision-making and to respect their knowledge about their baby is important. Working in this manner enables the family to make health choices that result in them 'owning' their baby's health.

Definitions and statistics

In 1994, 7% of all infants born in England and Wales were of low birthweight (i.e. < 2500 g) and 1.1% of very low birthweight (i.e. < 1500 g). Data on mortality are available from the Office of National Statistics (ONS). Mortality following pregnancy is defined in several ways (Table 23.1). On 1 October 1992 the definition of a stillbirth was changed from an infant born after 28 weeks to an infant born after 24 weeks. OPCS data for 1992 did not report stillbirths of < 28 weeks' gestation. This change in definition has resulted in an apparent increase in both the stillbirth and perinatal mortality rates.

The major contributor to the stillbirth rate was antepartum stillbirth (79%) followed by congenital abnormalities (9%) (Table 23.1).

Seventy-eight per cent of neonatal deaths were due to either congenital abnormalities or conditions related to immaturity. All indices of mortality increase with fall in social class; see, for example, the data on PNMR in Table 23.2.

Information regarding long-term morbidity has not been collected in a standardized or comparable way either within or between countries. Published studies mainly assess morbidity in relation to low birthweight or prematurity and are mainly cohort rather than population based. Where whole populations have been studied the major cause of severe isolated

Table 23.1 *Definitions of mortality and rates for England and Wales, 1994*

	Definition	**Rate**
Stillbirth rate (SBR)	No. of infants born after 24th week of gestation who do not breath or show any other sign of life per 1000 total births	5.7
Perinatal mortality rate (PNMR)	No. of still births + no. of deaths at 0–6 days following live birth per 1000 total births	8.9
Neonatal mortality rate (NMR)	No. of deaths at 0–27 days after a live birth per 1000 live births	4.1
Infant mortality rate	No. of deaths under 1 year after live birth per 1000 live births	6.1

Source: OPCS (1995).

Table 23.2 *Relationship between social class on perinatal mortality rate in 1994. (Data based on infants born within marriage and on father's occupation at death registration)*

Social class	**Perinatal mortality rate**
I	6.7
II	7.4
III (non-manual)	8.1
III (manual)	8.1
IV	9.6
V	10.7
Other*	10.3

*Other includes the armed forces, persons with inadequately described occupations, the permanently sick, etc.
Source: OPCS (1995).

mental handicap has been found to be genetic in origin – for example, Down's syndrome – or due to congenital malformation – for example, neural tube defect. Contrary to popular opinion, only 8% of cases of cerebral palsy are associated with (and even then not necessarily caused by) birth asphyxia (Blair and Stanley 1988). Obstetric interventions have not been shown to reduce the incidence of cerebral palsy (Niswander *et al.* 1984; MacDonald *et al.* 1985; Chapter 13). The incidence of cerebral palsy increases with falling gestation and birthweight (Powell *et al.* 1986).

Resuscitation of the newborn

Over 99% of babies born in Sweden at more than 32 weeks' gestation following an uncomplicated normal vaginal delivery required no resuscitation except simple stimulation or facial oxygen (Palme-Kilander 1992). These babies could be handed happily to their mothers at or soon after delivery. Only 0.8% of babies weighing over 2500 g required mask ventilation and only 0.2% required endotracheal intubation both with or without external cardiac massage. More recently, Arya *et al.* (1996) have shown retrospectively that 5.2% of low-risk pregnancies delivered by normal vaginal delivery in North Staffordshire require assisted ventilation with 0.4% requiring intubation. The vast majority of term babies therefore need no resuscitation and those that do can be resuscitated by professionals trained in mask ventilation occasionally with external cardiac massage. However, because these resuscitation skills are needed so infrequently it is extremely important that they are assessed and updated frequently, preferably annually.

Tracheal intubation should only be performed by trained individuals who have sufficient practice to maintain this skill. Parents requesting home birth must therefore be aware of the limitations – albeit tiny – of neonatal resuscitation within the home.

All personnel must familiarize themselves with the resuscitation equipment available in their area and how further help can be summoned. Not all areas with home deliveries have a neonatal flying squad. If further advanced resuscitation of a neonate is required, it may be preferable to immediately transport the baby to hospital via an emergency ambulance. Training of paramedics in neonatal intubation may help facilitate this. Written procedures for the unexpected resuscitation and transfer of infants born at home are available in all districts.

Further information can be found in *Neonatal resuscitation: a report of a British Paediatric Association working party* (BPA 1993).

Relevant physiology

In response to the physiological and normal asphyxia which occurs around the time that the umbilical cord is clamped, a healthy, term baby usually takes its first breath within 60 seconds. Respiratory efforts are further provoked by physical stimuli, such as release of the chest wall, as it is delivered. The first spontaneous breath generates a negative pressure of -40 to -100 cm H_2O. This is required to overcome lung surface tension, the viscosity of the fluid filling the airways and the elastic recoil and resistance of the chest walls, lungs, and airways. Once the lungs are opened, subsequent breaths are not so forceful. Surfactant lines the alveoli, reducing surface tension and preventing alveolar collapse at the end of expiration. Its production is reduced by hypothermia, hypoxia, and acidosis.

Following acute asphyxia a baby will stop making breathing movements (primary apnoea). Primary apnoea is of variable duration. If asphyxia continues, deep gasping respirations every 10–20 seconds develop. Finally, gasping stops and the baby becomes apnoeic once more (terminal apnoea). Without intervention death follows (Dawes *et al.* 1963).

Practical aspects of resuscitation

The delivery room should be warmed (25°C), the obstetric history confirmed, equipment checked, hands washed and gloved. The equipment available will depend on the place of delivery. In hospital this is likely to be a purpose-built and equipped resuscitaire. Within the home ensure adequate heating, an appropriate padded surface at table height, prewarmed towels, an oxygen supply with facilities to regulate both the pressure and the flow rate, suction equipment, and an appropriate-sized bag (500 ml) and face masks (00 to 2).

At delivery of the baby the exact time should be noted. Frequently the mother requests for the baby to be delivered onto her bare abdomen. This direct skin contact is an ideal way of maintaining the baby's temperature. Immediately assess the baby's colour, breathing, and heart rate (see below) and decide if any intervention is required. If the baby does not start to breath or is apnoeic, he/she should be transferred to the resuscitation surface, dried off, and any wet towels removed. The baby should be rewrapped in dry towels. Resuscitation should then follow a logical sequence of airway, breathing, and circulation (ABC).

Breathing or crying, heart rate > 100 beats per minute (bpm), and centrally pink (approximately 83% of term babies (Arya et al. *1996))*

Maintain skin-to-skin contact if possible. Encourage the mother to put her baby to the breast if she wishes. If the mother does not wish skin contact, wrap the baby to prevent heat loss.

Blue, apnoeic/gasping respirations but heart rate > 100 bpm (approximately 12–16% of term babies (Arya et al. *1996))*

Stimulate the baby; for example rub with a towel, gently tap feet, perform gentle oral suction, or blow cold oxygen onto the face. If there is no response by one minute of age (approximately 5% of babies) then mask ventilation should be commenced. If the mother has received opiate analgesia and the baby pinks up and has a good heart rate but no spontaneous respirations with the onset of mask ventilation then naloxone (10 micrograms/kg intramuscularly) may be given. Naloxone must not be used as a substitute for adequate resuscitation. If, despite adequate mask ventilation (i.e. there is a patent airway and equal bilateral air entry), the heart rate continues to fall then the infant requires tracheal intubation and help must be sought. This is an extremely rare occurrence in normal, term babies.

Breathing inadequate after stimulation or heart rate < 100 bpm or pale (approximately 1–5% of term babies (Arya et al. *1996))*

Mask ventilation should be commenced immediately. If there is no response in heart rate within two minutes then intubation should be undertaken. If the heart rate falls to < 60 bpm, external cardiac massage (ECM) must be commenced. The commonest cause for the heart rate to fail to improve is inadequate lung ventilation. It is very rare for the heart rate not to respond if adequate mask ventilation is being performed. This should always be checked prior to commencing ECM.

Apnoeic, white, heart rate < 60 bpm (a rare event in normal, term babies)

Full cardiopulmonary resuscitation is required. Remember to get someone to call for help immediately. This baby is going to require intubation and probably venous access and cardiac drugs such as adrenaline.

Meconium-stained liquor

The oropharynx and then the nares should be suctioned prior to the delivery of the baby to prevent postnatal aspiration of meconium (Carson *et al.* 1976). Whether this reduces the risk of meconium aspiration syndrome is unknown and a controlled trial is unlikely. The baby's chest wall should not be held in an attempt to prevent inspiration as the baby is only likely to struggle vigorously and potentially aspirate further. This advice has developed as a result of retrospective reviews or cohort studies and not clinical trials (Gregory *et al.* 1974; Ting and Brady 1975). It is not necessary to suction the trachea where the liquor has only been lightly stained with meconium. If the liquor is heavily stained with particulate matter then a professional experienced in endotracheal intubation should ideally be present at the delivery; if at all possible the mother should be transferred to a maternity unit where such skills are available. If at delivery the baby is pink, vigorous attempted intubation may cause later complications (Linder *et al.* 1988). Suction of the oropharynx followed by the nostrils is therefore sufficient. If the baby is not active then suction of the oropharynx under direct laryngoscopy is required. If meconium is present at the cords the baby requires intubation and direct suction applied to the endotracheal tube. This should be repeated until all meconium is withdrawn unless the heart rate falls to < 60 bpm. At this stage ventilation should be commenced.

If transfer of the mother to a maternity unit is not possible, for example if the birth of the baby is imminent, then as much meconium as possible should be removed from the oropharynx using the mucus extractor or suction apparatus available. It must be accepted that this baby may aspirate meconium and if there is any respiratory distress or the baby requires oxygen he/she must be transferred to a neonatal intensive care unit.

Principles of resuscitation techniques

Airway opening techniques

The baby should be positioned on a flat surface with the head in a neutral position and the chin lifted forward (Figure 23.1). The mouth and then the nostrils should be gently suctioned using a size 10 G suction catheter at a pressure not exceeding 4" or 100 mmHg. If a suction unit is not available, a suction bulb should be used in preference to an oral mucus extractor which may put the user at risk of infection.

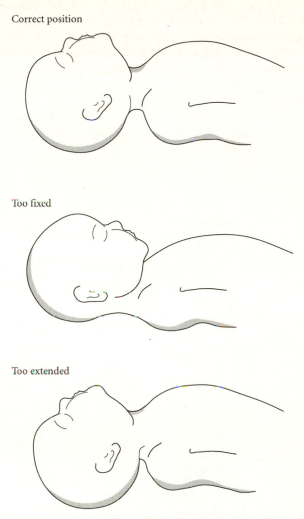

Correct position

Too fixed

Too extended

Figure 23.1 Correct positioning of the head for resuscitation. (Reproduced with permission from the Royal College of Paediatrics and Child Health and the Royal College of Obstetricians and Gynaecologists (1997).)

Mask ventilation

Face masks ranging from size 00 to 2 are usually available to the primary care-giver. One big enough to cover the face from the bridge of the nose to below the mouth should be chosen. A good seal must be obtained. A 500 ml resuscitation bag with a 40 cm H_2O cut-off valve and a reservoir bag is usually available. It should be used with an oxygen flow rate of 4–6 litres per minute. The first five breaths should be given slowly with the fingertips trying to maintain inflation times of 1–2 seconds. Ventilation should then occur at a rate of 30 breaths per minute. The chest wall should be observed for equal movement. Auscultation of both lung fields and the stomach should be performed. Once the chest wall is moving, pressures can be reduced by decreasing the amount of squeezing. If the baby's heart rate does not increase with bag and mask ventilation, review the head position, resuction the airway, and confirm that sufficient pressure is being used.

External cardiac massage

There are two techniques (Figure 23.2), the first of which is more effective but can be less convenient if there is only a single resuscitator (David 1988; Menegazzi *et al.* 1993):

(a)

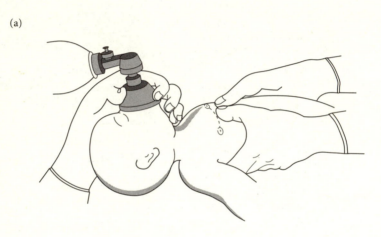

(b)

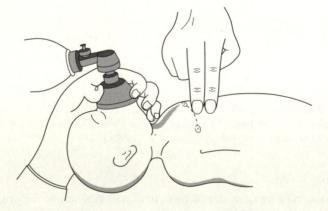

Figure 23.2 (a) Two thumb and (b) two finger techniques for cardiac massage. (Reproduced with permission from the Royal College of Paediatrics and Child Health and the Royal College of Obstetricians and Gynaecologists (1997).)

(1) the chest is encircled with both hands so that the fingers lie behind the baby and the thumbs are opposed over the mid-sternum

(2) two fingers are used over the mid-sternum.

The thumbs or fingers should be positioned 1 cm below the inter-nipple line. They should be compressed to a depth of 1.5–2 cm at a rate of 100–120 bpm. A ratio of 3:1 compressions to lung inflations should be used.

Common perinatal trauma

Fortunately, most birth trauma, although initially distressing to parents, resolves without treatment and parents can be reassured that there will be no long-term sequelae.

Many babies have superficial injuries, e.g. traumatic cyanosis, forceps or ventouse marks (chignon). Where there has been significant bruising the baby should be observed for subsequent jaundice. Oedema caused by pressure over the presenting part (caput succaedaneum) usually subsides in two to three days.

Cephalohaematoma, which are localized subperiosteal collections of blood, are seen in approximately 1% of newborn babies. They often present after a few days, usually over one or both parietal bones. The extent of the bleed is limited by the suture lines. Over a few days a hard ridge develops around the periphery of the cephalohaematoma. This may be suspected to be a fracture by the inexperienced. Cephalohaemotoma can take up to three months to disappear. They require no treatment.

Subconjunctival haemorrhages are common and resolve in a few weeks. Facial nerve palsy may occur after both forceps and normal delivery. It is detected when the infant cries. The eye on the affected side does not close and the mouth is pulled across to the opposite side. Facial palsy does not interfere with feeding and recovers within a few weeks.

Erb's palsy is most commonly seen following shoulder dystocia. Contusion of the upper trunks of the brachial plexus results in injury of the fifth and sixth cervical nerve roots and a characteristic waiter's tip posture with an immobile extended and pronated arm. Function should begin to return within one month. If it does not then the chance of recovery is still good but likely to take up to 18 months. The child should be treated with passive physiotherapy to maintain movement and prevent contractures.

Shoulder dystocia may also result in fracture of the clavicle or humerus. Fractures in the newborn have the great capacity to fully reheal within two to three weeks. They do not require accurate reduction or immobilization except to provide relief from pain.

Examination of the newborn

Newborn infants are examined on several occasions during the first few days of life. Traditionally, this has been by the midwife present at delivery, by a paediatrician or GP in the second 24 hours of life, and by the midwife daily until at least 10 days of age. Care of the baby is likely to be improved if it is carried out by a minimum number of professionals all giving the same information.

Following delivery of a baby, an external check should be undertaken by the midwife to determine sex, exclude major congenital abnormality, and to exclude illness needing active treatment such as respiratory distress. If there was polyhydramnios, a wide-bore nasogastric tube should be passed and acid aspirated to confirm that the baby does not have oesophageal atresia. The detailed baby check should not be undertaken at this stage for several reasons:

- the infant is usually covered in blood and /or vernix, making finer details difficult and often impossible to assess

- detailed examination takes 10–15 minutes. This is a time when the newborn baby is bright, alert, and often keen to suckle. The parents should be given time with their baby to get to know and welcome him/her into the world

- routine hip examination soon after birth possibly increases the risk of instability

- cardiac murmurs are frequently detected. Many of these represent normal changes in cardiac haemodynamics following delivery. Their detection causes unnecessary parental concern.

Doctors or midwives fully trained in examination of the newborn should examine the baby in detail within the second 24 hours of life (Figure 23.3). The two most important things this examination detects are cardiovascular and hip problems. No additional major abnormalities will be detected by repeating this detailed examination again during the first few days of life. Many excellent reviews of newborn examination are available (Gandy 1992; Roberton 1996). Experience of the vast range of normal variation will only come from examining as many babies as possible. If doubt exists over a particular feature then someone more experienced must be asked to review the baby.

The newborn examination should always be done in the mother's presence. It provides an opportunity for her to ask any questions regarding her baby and for the professional to offer reassurance and advice. Always check the maternal medical, obstetric, and social history prior to examining the baby. If the mother is not previously known to you, ask her about: the pregnancy and delivery; how is her baby feeding and is it going well; has her baby passed urine and opened its bowels; has she any worries about her baby; and, if in hospital, when does she plan to go home?

The newborn examination should proceed in a logical order. Look at the baby's size, proportions, maturity, colour, facies, breathing pattern, posture, and movement. Often the baby will start to cry on being undressed, therefore examine the anterior fontanelle, cardiovascular system, and eyes for bilateral red retinal reflexes before doing this. Once the baby is undressed, work from

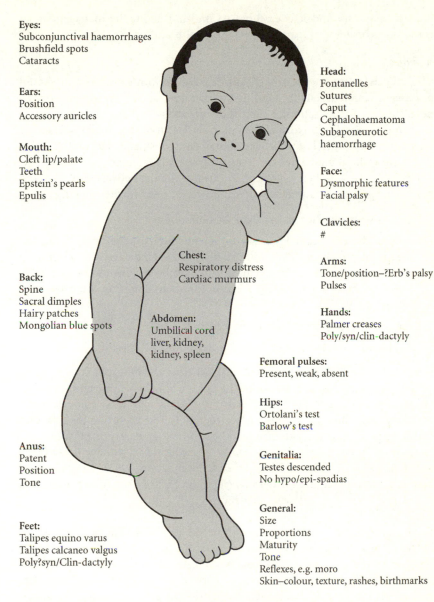

Eyes:
Subconjunctival haemorrhages
Brushfield spots
Cataracts

Ears:
Position
Accessory auricles

Mouth:
Cleft lip/palate
Teeth
Epstein's pearls
Epulis

Back:
Spine
Sacral dimples
Hairy patches
Mongolian blue spots

Anus:
Patent
Position
Tone

Feet:
Talipes equino varus
Talipes calcaneo valgus
Poly?syn/Clin-dactyly

Head:
Fontanelles
Sutures
Caput
Cephalohaematoma
Subaponeurotic
haemorrhage

Face:
Dysmorphic features
Facial palsy

Clavicles:
#

Arms:
Tone/position–?Erb's palsy
Pulses

Hands:
Palmer creases
Poly/syn/clin-dactyly

Chest:
Respiratory distress
Cardiac murmurs

Abdomen:
Umbilical cord
liver, kidney,
kidney, spleen

Femoral pulses:
Present, weak, absent

Hips:
Ortolani's test
Barlow's test

Genitalia:
Testes descended
No hypo/epi-spadias

General:
Size
Proportions
Maturity
Tone
Reflexes, e.g. moro
Skin–colour, texture, rashes, birthmarks

Figure 23.3 Scheme for examination of the newborn.

head to toe. It is essential to have a check-list to prevent potential problems being overlooked (Figure 23.3). Remember that minor external abnormalities may give clues to major internal ones (Smith 1977).

Common problems detected during routine newborn examination

Some common problems and their management are described either below or in the section on minor illness presenting in the first few weeks of life. Local practice may vary and it is essential to find out about the management of common neonatal problems within your health authority.

Jaundice

Clinically assessing the severity of jaundice comes with experience. It should be observed in natural light, standing by a window, and by pressing the baby's nose gently. Facial jaundice becomes detectable when bilirubin is 85 micromoles per litre. Normal bilirubin levels and the levels warranting treatment vary with both the gestational and postnatal age of the baby. Reference to local guidelines for treatment levels is required.

Physiological jaundice is present in 30% of infants between day two and four. Four groups of jaundiced babies, however, need further investigation:

(1) babies with jaundice at less than 24 hours of age

(2) babies whose bilirubin levels are sufficiently high to require phototherapy (see local guidelines). This will usually include all babies with a bilirubin > 260 micromoles per litre. This group have been shown to be extremely likely to have a pathological cause for their jaundice (Matthew and Wharton 1981)

(3) babies who are unwell and jaundiced

(4) babies who remain or become jaundiced after 14 days of age.

For babies in the final group, establish whether the bilirubin is conjugated or unconjugated. Ask parents about the colour of baby's urine and stools. In conjugated jaundice the urine is persistently yellow and never colourless and the stools are white due to absent bile pigment. Test the urine for bilirubin (positive in conjugated jaundice) and perform a split serum bilirubin. All conjugated jaundice must be referred to a paediatrician without delay (Hull and Kelly 1991; Children's Liver Disease Foundation 1993). Unconjugated jaundice may also require further investigation, e.g. for urinary tract infection.

Erythema toxicum

Erythema toxicum is common in term babies (20–50%) but rare in preterm babies. The aetiology is unknown (Berg and Solomon 1987). It may be a reaction to the infusion of maternal white cells during labour (Stern 1992). The rash usually appears within the first three days of life but can occur as late as two weeks. It is characterized by white papules 1–3 mm in diameter surrounded by a variable area of erythema. If the spots are atypical, vesicular or pustular, or are present at birth, then other causes must be considered. The rash is asymptomatic, regresses spontaneously, and requires no treatment. A useful review of neonatal skin conditions can be found by Walker and Champion (1992).

Birth marks

It is important that these are well documented. Mongolian blue spots are commoner in babies with dark skin and are usually found in the sacral region or over the buttocks. They may be suspected in later childhood as having been caused by non-accidental injury. The blue discolouration is, however, permanent and, unlike a bruise, it does not fade. Strawberry birth marks (cavernous haemangiomas) are rarely present at birth. They begin as a small, bright red mark which increases in size over the first year of life. The lesion then slowly regresses over the next four to six years, leaving either no visible skin change or an area of slight pallor. They should not be treated unless they involve an area which puts the baby at risk of medical sequelae, for example blindness if they cover the eye.

Port-wine stains (capillary haemangiomas) are flat, reddish-purple lesions. They do not fade and can be treated with pulsed dye laser (Reyes and Geronemus 1990). There are no long-term controlled trials of this and the optimal age of treatment is unknown. To allay any parental anxiety, children should be referred within the first year of life to a dermatologist.

Conjunctivitis

Conjunctivitis affects up to 12% of neonates. It varies from mild crusting along the lid to a copious purulent discharge. The frequency of responsible organisms varies widely but include *Staphylococcus aureus, Haemophilus* species, *Streptococcus viridans, Chlamydia,* and gonococcus. Mild conjunctivitis can be treated by regular cleaning with sterile saline every four to six hours for two to three days. Treat with antibiotics if cultures are positive, if it persists longer than 48 hours, or there is conjunctiva or lid oedema. Use drops rather than ointment as they irrigate the eye. A profuse purulent discharge within the first 24 hours of life suggests gonococcal infection. A swab must be sent to the microbiology laboratory for gram stain and culture. Without treatment, gonococcus rapidly destroys the cornea, resulting in blindness. Chlamydial conjunctivitis is important as some babies will develop chlamydial pneumonia. The conjunctivitis presents between five and 12 days of age. Culture necessitates immunoassay or immunofluorescence of corneal scrapings. Treatment is with erythromycin for two weeks. This prevents later pneumonia (Heggie *et al.* 1985; Rettig 1986). Late-onset and recurrent conjunctivitis is commoner if there is a blocked lacrimal duct. In most cases the duct will clear spontaneously, but occasionally probing is required in later infancy.

Cataracts

Examine for cataracts using a +10 dioptre lens held six to eight inches from the eye. If a red retinal reflex is present then the lens is clear.

Tongue tie

This is due to a short frenulum. It rarely needs treatment unless it appears to be interfering with breastfeeding – it can make feeding painful for the mother – or later with pronunciation.

Heart murmurs, femoral pulses, and congenital heart disease

A low-amplitude ejection systolic murmur is audible in up to 60% of normal newborn babies either over the mid-precordium or in the pulmonary area. Eighty to ninety per cent of these will disappear within the first year, most within the first three months. Eight per 1000 of all newborn babies, however, will have congenital heart disease and one to two per thousand will present with life-threatening symptoms during the neonatal period.

Murmurs are more difficult to interpret in the neonatal period than at other times (Wilkinson and Cooke 1992). Because of rapid postnatal changes in the circulation, cardiac signs can vary from examination to examination. When a murmur is discovered the child should be examined carefully for other signs of congenital heart disease, such as respiratory distress, cyanosis, impalpable or poor volume pulses, shock, or hepatomegaly. The presence of any of these, or a loud murmer or a diastolic component, requires urgent referral to a paediatrician.

The majority of babies with a murmur at the newborn examination will be asymptomatic. Parents are always greatly distressed when told of the murmur and a great deal of support and reassurance may be required. Explain that murmurs can be heard in approximately half of all infants at some stage and that they rarely signify an abnormality. Their baby will be reviewed at six weeks. By then the murmur may well have gone. If it is still present their baby will need referral to a paediatrician. The baby will then be reviewed either until the murmur has gone or until the paediatrician is completely happy that all is normal. Parents should be given both verbal and written information regarding the cardiac symptoms they should look for, such as sweating with feeds, and the action they should take.

Absent femoral pulses even without other cardiac symptoms suggests coarctation of the aorta, requiring urgent referral. If there is any doubt about the presence of femoral pulses, always request an immediate second opinion.

Undescended testicles

An undescended testis is one which does not reside spontaneously in the scrotum and which cannot be manipulated to the bottom of the scrotum without undue tension on the spermatic cord. A retractile testis is one which is descended, but the cremasteric reflex is active and causes it to retract out of the scrotum. This cremasteric reflex is either weak or absent at birth, making this the ideal time to examine the testis.

In 1.3% of male babies one or both testes will be undescended in the newborn period. Impalpable or undescended testicles on a second check at six weeks require referral to a paediatric surgeon. The optimal age for orchidopexy is 9–12 months. A descended testis which shows marked retractibility should be followed up regularly by a paediatric surgeon as a proportion will 'ascend' (Atwell 1985).

Hydrocoeles

These are common, harmless, and almost always resolve spontaneously. Persistence beyond one year necessitates referral to a paediatric surgeon.

Unstable hips

One in 1000 unscreened babies will eventually require surgery for complete or partial dislocation of the hip (Leck in press). A detailed description of screening newborns, adapted from Ortolani (1948) and Barlow (1962), is available (Department of Health and Social Security 1986). Hip screening, however, should always be taught by an individual experienced in its use as, incorrectly performed, it may induce hip instability (Moore 1989). Despite meticulous examination at birth some infants will later be found to have dislocation of the hip. Repeat hip screening should therefore be performed at the 6–8 week, 8–9 month, and 18–24 month checks (Hall 1989).

Newborn babies with hip instability require referral for further assessment and possible splinting. It has been suggested that only babies with definite ultrasound changes at two weeks of age require splinting (Clarke 1994). A multicentre trial is ongoing.

Predisposing factors include a family history, breech presentation, oligohydramnios, and neuromuscular disorders. Many units now undertake routine ultrasound screening at approximately two weeks of age in this group.

Hairy patches, sacral pits

Sacral dimples or sinuses are found in about 3% of neonates (French 1985). Sacral pits above S2 (very rare) should always be investigated as they are likely to communicate with the spinal tract. Cutaneous abnormalities over the spine, such as hypertrichosis, raise the possibility of occult spinal dysraphism. Investigation of the spine in babies with sacral pits or cutaneous abnormalities is best done by ultrasonography in the first few weeks of life. If this is delayed then MRI scanning is required.

Talipes

Talipes calcaneovalgus is usually due to positioning *in utero*. It will correct with or without simple manipulation. If the foot is in an equinovarus position, try to correct it by abduction and dorsiflexion so that the little toe touches the outside of the leg. If this is successful only gentle physiotherapy is required; if not then get an urgent orthopaedic referral.

Syndactyly and polydactyly

Syndactyly (i.e. fused digits) and polydactyly (i.e. extra digits) are often familial and a check must be made for other dysmorphic features. Polydactyly should be treated surgically rather than by ligating with a suture (Hensinger and Jones 1992). Syndactyly of the second and third toe does not require treating.

Preventative medicine

Vitamin K deficiency bleeding/haemorrhagic disease of the newborn (HDN)

All newborn babies are deficient in Vitamin K. Untreated, this results in classical (early) haemorrhagic disease of the newborn in 0.4–1.7% of babies in the first week of life (Merenstein *et al.* 1993). Late haemorrhagic disease is much rarer (4.4–10.5 per 100 000 births) and associated with a higher mortality and morbidity. It presents almost exclusively in breastfed babies of two to 12 weeks of age who did not receive intramuscular vitamin K at birth or who received only a single oral dose. Breastfed babies are more susceptible since human milk has less vitamin K than formula (Canfield *et al.* 1991).

In 1992, owing to concern that neonatal vitamin K prophylaxis might cause childhood cancer (Golding *et al.* 1990; 1992), parental vitamin K prophylaxis for all newborn babies was abandoned in the UK and replaced largely with an oral vitamin K policy whereby the intramuscular preparation was given by the oral route (British Paediatric Association 1992). A licensed oral preparation of vitamin K has recently been introduced.

The present recommended practice (British Paediatric Association 1992) is as follows:

- all babies should receive vitamin K (preferably orally) on the day of birth

- if oral prophylaxis is used, a single dose of 0.5 mg is adequate for formula-fed babies; breastfed babies need further doses at 7–10 days, 4–6 weeks, and perhaps monthly thereafter while solely breastfed. Since the compliance rates are poor (Croucher and Azzopardi 1994), any minor bleeding manifestation requires urgent investigation.

Recent studies confirm that HDN can be completely eradicated using intramuscular vitamin K without the threat of leukaemia or childhood cancer (Klebanoff *et al.* 1993; Olsen *et al.* 1994; Ansell *et al.* 1996; von Kries *et al.* 1996), so this route can be reconsidered (Zipurski 1996).

Umbilical cord care

Good cord care significantly reduces the incidence of infection in the newborn baby (Cushing 1985). Several research studies compare one antibiotic application against another (Barrett *et al.* 1979; Elias-Jones 1986; Gladstone *et al.* 1988). Other studies have shown that colonization of the cord, usually by *Staphylococcus aureus*, can be traced to the hospital environment (Verber and Pagan 1993). If babies room in with, and are cared for by, their mothers this is significantly reduced (Rush 1990), as is probably the case for babies born at home. Advising mothers to keep the cord clean and dry and explaining that separation should occur within 10 days is all that is necessary (Barr1984; O'Kane 1995). They should report any peri-umbilical flare or discharge. Prompt treatement of infection prevents it becoming generalized. Granulomas may be treated by the judicious use of silver nitrate.

Biochemical screening

National biochemical screening is undertaken in the UK for phenylketonuria (PKU) and hypothyroidism. Other screening tests, for example for cystic fibrosis and the haemoglobinopathies, are performed on a regional basis. All parents should receive both verbal and written information on neonatal screening. In PKU (incidence one in 10 000 babies), phenylalanine accumulates in the blood, resulting in severe mental retardation. This can be prevented by a diet low in phenylalanine. Surveys of infants with congenital hypothyroidism (one in 4000) have shown that early thyroxine prevents brain injury (Klein *et al.* 1972).

Hypothyroidism and PKU are tested for on-heel capillary blood obtained on day six of life. The diagnosis of PKU is dependent on an adequate milk intake for at least 48 hours. If this has not been achieved the test must still be performed to screen for hypothyroidism, and repeated 48 hours later to test for PKU. In PKU, phenylalanine levels will be high by 14 days regardless of feed and screening must not be delayed beyond this stage.

Immunization in the first week of life

BCG immunization should be offered to all newborn babies of immigrants from countries with a high prevalence of tuberculosis or any newborn baby with a family history of active tuberculosis. Relative and absolute contra-indications have been published (Department of Health 1996).

It is important to be aware of parental concerns regarding immunization. Parents should be given both verbal and written information in their own language to enable them to make an informed choice.

Reducing the risk of Sudden Infant Death Syndrome (SIDS)

This condition is defined as: the sudden death of any baby and young child, which is unexpected by history, and in which a thorough post-mortem examination fails to demonstrate an adequate cause of death (Bergman *et al.* 1970).

Confidential Enquiry into Sudden Deaths in Infancy (CESDI 1994) showed that SIDS was more common in babies of younger mothers and less often affects the first child. Other factors included low birthweight, low gestational age at birth, and an excess of deaths in boys. The previously recognized association between SIDS and socio-economic deprivation now seems more marked. The association between SIDS and parental smoking is still clearly present with a suggestion that the greater the exposure to tobacco smoke, the greater the risk.

Health professionals have a duty to ensure that all parents are fully aware of the CESDI report's key recommendations that babies should be put on their backs to sleep, sleep in a smoke-free zone, sleep in a way that their head does not become covered, and that they should not become too hot. Prompt medical help should be sought for babies that become unwell. The report also recommends that babies sleep in their cots, but before telling parents not to sleep with their babies in their bed, it should be remembered that there are strong confounding factors of sleeping position and exposure to parents' smoking.

These and the known risk factors must be explained to parents in a way that is practical and supportive and not hostile and guilt inducing.

Minor illness and abnormalities

Most mothers visit the baby clinic for advice and reassurance. They often attend weekly until the time of the first immunization and then less frequently as they become confident in their own abilities and decisions. Some issues seem to cause concern to the majority of parents and in this section we touch briefly on the most common.

Colic

The causes of infantile colic are unclear. Mothers may have tried several remedies and hope that the health professional can produce a miracle cure. No one product is completely effective so health professionals should be able to offer a range of remedies, including empathizing with the problem, drug treatment, and massage.

There are many proprietary medicines available to treat the irritability caused by colic and wind (gripe mixtures, colic drops). In very severe cases, an underlying cause should be sought. There is some evidence that allergy to cows' milk protein may cause abdominal pain in some babies from formula milk or when the mother drinks lots of cows' milk (Jacobsson and Linberg 1983).

Posseting and vomiting

It is common for babies to bring back milk during 'winding' or movement after a feed. Inform the mother of the size of the baby's stomach relative to the volume of feed. Small, frequent feeds may help.

Congenital pyloric stenosis must be excluded. This commonly presents between four and six weeks. It is characterized by a projectile vomit immediately after or during a feed. Peristaltic waves are observed and the pyloric tumour can be felt, by experienced doctors, on palpation during a feed.

Bowel movements

Differing feeding methods will influence the appearance of the stool. Inform the parent what a normal stool may look like. In constipation, the stool is hard and infrequent. If truly constipated, obtain a picture of the feeding regime. Simple adjustments to the mother's feeding practice will frequently solve the problem. Should further choices be offered, the practitioner should be fully aware of the implications – for example, dilution of feeds results in undernourishment. Written guidance is helpful.

Diarrhoea can be serious in babies due to their susceptibility to dehydration and weight loss. It is increasingly common in formula-fed babies. Poverty, resulting in lack of basic cleaning and storage equipment, compounds the problem. Tailor information to fit the parents' home situation, offering realistic choices. The incidence of diarrhoea in breastfed babies is considerably lower (Howie *et al.* 1990). There are no storage problems and the milk has antibacterial properties and other factors which will aid recovery.

Treat formula-fed babies promptly with an oral rehydration solution for 24 hours. Breastfed babies should continue to be breastfed and offered extra oral rehydration fluid for 24 hours. Offering diluted feeds over several days is not necessary and results in inadequate nutrition. After the 24 hours of rehydration fluid the baby should be recommenced on its regular milk feeds. If a baby is dehydrated, hospital admission may be necessary depending upon the degree of dehydration, the mother's capabilities and confidence, and the social circumstances.

Viral gastroenteritis can damage the lining of the small intestine, impairing its ability to absorb nutrients. This may lead to temporary lactose intolerance and secondary diarrhoea lasting several weeks. It is treated by giving the baby a lactose-free milk formula until the symptoms settle.

Snuffles

Snuffles can be caused by changes in atmospheric pressure and humidity. If the condition cannot be alleviated by simply clearing the nose with a wisp of cotton wool, suggest that the parent keeps the bedroom well ventilated but not cold or draughty. There are no proprietary medicines suitable for babies under three months. If symptoms persist and interfere with feeding, nasal decongestant drops should be prescribed.

Raised temperature

A raised temperature is a frequent symptom in infancy. There are two causes: pyrexia and overheating (Rutter 1994).

Pyrexia

It is now known that febrile responses assist in the immune response so it is not recommended that every fever be treated (Carmicheal 1992). It is reasonable to advise anti-pyrexials, such as paracetamol at an age-related dose, if the temperature remains over 38.5°C. Tepid sponging is no longer recommended (Working Party of the Royal College of Physicians 1991).

Overheating

The newborn baby has been used to a constant uterine temperature of 37° C. The normal newborn axillary temperature is 36.5–37.2° C. After birth a baby has to adjust to a lower and changing environmental temperature. Before six months of age the heat-regulating mechanism is not fully matured and the environmental temperature has an effect (Johnson 1992). Although it is important to prevent a baby becoming cold, becoming too hot is also a danger. Room heating is not required at night except in very cold weather. Babies' bedrooms should be at a temperature overnight which is comfortable for a lightly clothed adult (16–20°C).

Minor skin problems

Nappy rash

Peri-anal rashes during the first few days of life are thought to be due to irritation by faeces rather than urine. Ammonical dermatitis is commoner after the first month. Erythema, ulceration, and blisters which spare the flexures appear over the thighs, lower abdomen, and perineum. The rash usually resolves following frequent nappy changes, exposure, or the use of barrier creams. Secondary *Candida* infection should be treated. Occasionally, topical steroids are required.

Candida nappy rash involves the flexures. Superficial desquamation of the skin occurs and there are characteristic satellite lesions. A topical anti-fungal agent should be used two to three times per day only.

Hernias

Umbilical hernias (commoner in Afro-Caribbean babies) usually resolve by two years. Those that persist can be repaired. Inguinal hernias are uncommon in term infants but become increasingly common with decreasing gestation. Term infants should be promptly referred for surgery to reduce the risk of incarceration and strangulation. Parents should be advised that, while awaiting surgery, any obvious distress or inability to reduce the hernia necessitates an urgent medical opinion. Hernias in preterm babies should be repaired prior to discharge from hospital.

Major illness

This section describes briefly the signs and symptoms of major illness arising in the first few days of life which require prompt action. Parents are warned in the child health record (the 'red book') that an ill baby may be unusually sleepy, hard to wake up, unusually quiet, refuse food, have difficulty breathing, cry as if in pain, dirty nappies frequently, vomit frequently, and go blue all over. Other parents may use the 'baby check' system (Thornton *et al.* 1990). Such symptoms cause parents to request the advice of their midwife or GP.

Midwives presented with a clearly ill baby should get immediate medical advice via a GP. 'Collapsed babies' should go direct to accident and emergency or the paediatric or neonatal unit, depending on local policies. An emergency ambulance should always be summoned.

Respiratory distress

Signs of respiratory distress, including tachypnoea (i.e. rate > 60), recession, grunting, and cyanosis in the first four to six hours of life suggest respiratory distress syndrome, transient tachypnoea of the newborn, congenital pneumonia, or other rarer respiratory disorders. Any baby who is deteriorating or whose respiratory distress has not settled by four hours needs admission to a neonatal unit. Respiratory distress presenting after six hours will be due to either pneumonia or congestive cardiac failure. Admission to hospital is mandatory.

Quiet, listless, floppy (baby 'not right')

This baby needs urgent assessment by a doctor – usually the GP. The differential diagnosis includes sepsis and inborn errors of metabolism. The signs of sepsis in the newborn are very non-specific. Because of a relative immune deficiency the newborn baby is both at risk of infection and of rapid dissemination.

Cyanosis

Central cyanosis must be differentiated from peripheral, peri-oral, or traumatic cyanosis. This is best done by observing the colour of the tongue. Central cyanosis may be due to both respiratory and cardiovascular problems. Both require further, urgent investigation.

Gastroenteritis

This should be recognized promptly to prevent dehydration (see above). Bile-stained vomiting requires urgent surgical referral.

Care of preterm babies

Preterm or low birthweight babies commonly require admission to a neonatal unit. Many do not receive neonatal care in their local maternity hospital, having been transferred to the most appropriate care provider. Tertiary neonatal units care for the smallest, sickest babies and admit more babies with suspected abnormalities (Redshaw *et al.* 1993). Some maternity units offer transitional care, allowing babies with feeding problems, hypoglycaemia, and jaundice to stay with their mothers on the postnatal wards. Most babies in neonatal care will require some form of assistance with feeding. Breast milk is the food of choice for premature babies.

Parents are often faced with enormous practical and financial problems with travel and child care. Facilitating contact and involving parents in their baby's care is a potentially valuable approach to overcoming the emotional problems that can arise in the short term, and of avoiding some of the longer-term consequences of separation. Participating in and taking over the care of the baby are important to both parents, especially true when progress is slow and babies stay in hospital for a long time (Redshaw *et al.* 1993).

Effective communications between hospital and community are essential. The practicalities of having a baby on a neonatal unit may make it very difficult for family doctors and community midwives to keep in regular contact with the new family at a most vulnerable time.

The teaching necessary before discharge actually begins on admission with the identification of parental learning need. Babies with ongoing special needs will need a continuing care plan after discharge (Department of Health 1989). A meeting of all involved professionals and the parents, prior to discharge, often ensures a smooth transition from hospital to home. Before discharge, family doctors may be invited to examine the baby in the presence of the paediatrician. Any changes in the post-discharge period can then be quickly identified. When a baby is discharged or dies it is vital that the information reaches the community professionals as rapidly as possible.

Premature babies should be discharged home when their parents feel competent and confident to care for them. The age and weight criteria of the past have been largely abandoned.

As small and vulnerable babies are discharged more quickly into the community, the evidence for the need for specialist support is becoming increasingly apparent. What that support consists of differs throughout the country, but most providers of neonatal care offer some system of community support. It is important for families to receive care from professionals who they have met while their baby is in hospital, therefore hospital-based community visitors are ideally placed to offer this specialized service.

Discharged babies fall into two categories: those who are well and need a short-term follow-up to provide nutritional support, growth monitoring, and parental reassurance by neonatal community teams; and those who need long-term specialist follow-up by paediatric community teams. Each baby should receive a planned programme of home visiting targeted to his or her needs that will ensure both a smooth transition from hospital to home and adequate care for the baby within the community.

References

Ansell, P., Bull, D., and Roman, E. (1996). Childhood leukaemia and intramuscular vitamin K: findings from a case–control study. *British Medical Journal*, 313, 204–5.

Arya, R., Pethen, T., Johanson, R. B., and Spencer, S. A. (1996). Outcome in low-risk pregnancies. *Archives of Disease in Childhood*, 75, 97–101.

Atwell, J. D. (1985). Ascent of the testis: fact or fiction. *British Journal of Urology*, 57, 473–7.

Barlow, T. G. (1962). Early diagnosis and treatment of congenital dislocation of the hip joint. *Journal of Bone and Joint Surgery*, 44B, 292–310.

Barr, J. (1984). The umbilical cord: to treat or not to treat. *Midwives Chronicle*, July, 224–6.

Barrett, F. F., Mason, F. O., and Flemming, D. (1979). The effect of three cord care regimens on bacterial colonization of normal newborn infants. *Journal of Pediatrics*, 94, 769–99.

Barton, J. S., Tripp, J. H., and McNinch, A. W. (1995). Neonatal vitamin K prophylaxis in the British Isles: current practice and trends. *British Medical Journal*, 310, 632–3.

Berg, F. J. and Solomon, L. M. (1987). Erythema neonatorum toxicum. *Archives of Disease in Childhood*, **62**, 327–8.

Bergman, A. B., Beckwith, J. B., and Ray, C. C. (1970). *Sudden Infant Death Syndrome*. University of Washington Press, Seattle.

Blair, E. and Stanley, F. J. (1988). Intrapartum asphyxia: a rare cause of cerebral palsy. *Journal of Pediatrics*, **112**, 515–19.

British Paediatric Association (1992). Vitamin K prophylaxis in infancy: report of an expert committee funded by the department of child health. BPA, London.

British Paediatric Association (1993). Neonatal resuscitation: a report of a British Paediatric Association working party. BPA, London.

Canfield, L. M., Hopkinson, J. M., Lima, A. F. Silver, B., and Garza, C. (1991). Vitamin K in colostrum and mature human milk over the lactation period – a cross-sectional study. *American Journal of Clinical Nutrition*, **53**, 730–5.

Carmicheal, A. (1992). Common disorders in infancy and childhood. In: *Baby and family health in Australia: a textbook for community health workers* (ed. A. Clements), pp.307. Churchill Livingstone, London.

Carson, B., Losey, R., Bowes, W., and Simmons, M. (1976). Combined obstetric and pediatric approach to prevent meconium aspiration syndrome. *American Journal of Obstetrics and Gynecology*, **126**, 712–15.

Children's Liver Disease Foundation (1993). *Early identification of liver disease in infants*. W. S. & G. Advertising and Sales Promotion Agency, Guildford.

Clarke, N. M. P. (1994). Role of ultrasound in congenital hip dysplasia. *Archives of Disease in Childhood*, **70**, 362–3.

Confidential Enquiry into Stillbirths and Deaths in Infancy (1994). *Third Annual Report Executive Summary and Recommendations*. DoH, London.

Croucher, C. and Azzopardi, D. Compliance with recommendations for giving vitamin K to newborn infants. *British Medical Journal*, **308**, 894–5.

Cushing, A. H. (1985). Omphalitis: a review. *Paediatric Infectious Disease*, **4**, 282–5.

David, R. (1988). Closed-chest cardiac massage in the newborn infant. *Pediatrics*, **81**, 552–4.

Dawes, G. S., Jacobson, H. N., Mott, J. C., Shelley, H. J., and Stafford, A. (1963). The treatment of asphyxiated, mature fetal lambs and rhesus monkeys with intravenous glucose and sodium carbonate. *Journal of Physiology*, **169**, 167–84.

Department of Health (1989). Discharge of patients from hospital. *Health Circular*, **5**.

Department of Health and Social Security (1986). *Screening for congenital dislocation of the hip*. HMSO, London.

Department of Health, Welsh Office, Scottish Office Department of Health, DHSS Northern Ireland (1996). *Immunization against infectious disease*. HMSO, London.

Elias -Jones, A. C. (1986). Triple antibiotic spray application to umbilical cords. *Early Human Development*, **13**, 299–302.

Foundation for the Study of Infant Deaths (FSID) (1996). *Reduce the risk of cot death*. DoH leaflet.

French, B. N. (1985). Midline fusion defects and defects of formation. In: *The tethered spinal cord* (ed. R. N. N. Holtzman and B. M. Stein), pp.3–13. Thieme- Stratton, New York.

Gandy, G. M. (1992). Examination of the neonate including gestational age assessment. In: *Textbook of neonatology* (2nd edn) (ed. N. R. C. Roberton), pp.199–216. Churchill Livingstone, Edinburgh.

Gladstone,I. M., Clapper, I., Thorpe, J. W., and Wright, D. I. (1988). Randomized study of six cord care regimes. *Clinical Paediatrics*, 27, 127–29.

Golding, J., Paterson, M., Kinlen, L. J. (1990). Factors associated with childhood cancer in a national cohort study. British Journal of Cancer, 62, 304–8.

Golding, J., Greenwood, R., Birmingham, K., and Mott, M. (1992). Childhood cancer, intramuscular vitamin K, and pethidine given in labour. *British Medical Journal*, 305, 341–6.

Gregory, G. A., Gooding, C. A., Phibbs, R. H., and Tooley, W. H. (1974). Meconium aspiration in infants – a prospective study. *Journal of Pediatrics*, 85, 848–52.

Hall, D. M. B. (1989). *Health for all children* (1st edn), pp.20–3. Oxford Medical Publications, Oxford.

Heggie, A. D., Jaffe, A. C., Stuart, L. A., Thombre, P. S., and Sorensen, R. U. (1985). Topical sulphacetamide vs oral erythromycin for neonatal chlamydial conjunctivitis. *American Journal of Diseases in Children*, 139, 564–6.

Hensinger, R. N. and Jones, E. T. (1992). Orthopaedic problems in the newborn. In: *Textbook of neonatology* (2nd edn) (ed. N. R. C. Roberton), pp. 904. Churchill Livingstone, Edinburgh.

Howie, P. W., Forsyth, J. S., Ogston, S. A., Clark, A.du V., and Florey, C. (1990). Protective effects of breastfeeding against infections. *British Medical Journal*, 300, 11–16.

Hull, J. and Kelly, D. A. (1991). Investigation of prolonged neonatal jaundice. *Current Paediatrics*, 1, 228–30.

Jacobsson, I. and Linberg, T. (1983). Cows' milk as a cause of infantile colic in breastfed babies: a double-blind crossover study. *Paediatrics*, 71, 268–71.

Johnson, A. (1992). Examination of infants and young children. In: *Baby and family health in Australia: a textbook for community health workers* (ed. A. Clements), pp.98. Churchill Livingstone, London.

Klebanoff, M. A., Read, J. S., Mills, J. L., and Shiono, P. H. (1993). The risk of childhood cancer after neonatal exposure to vitamin K. *New England Journal of Medicine*, 329, 905–8.

Klein, A. H. Meltzer, S., and Kenny, F. M. (1972). Improved prognosis in congenital hypothyroidism treated before age 3 months. *Journal of Pediatrics*, 81, 912–15.

von Kries, R., Gobel, U., Machmeister, A., Kaletsch, U., and Michaelis, J. (1996). Vitamin K and childhood cancer: a population based case-control study in Lower Saxony, Germany. *British Medical Journal*, 313, 199–203.

Leck, I. (In press). Congenital dislocation of the hip. In: *Antenatal and neonatal screening* (2nd edn) (ed. N. J. Wald). Oxford Univerity Press, Oxford.

Linder, N., Aranda, J. V., Tsur, M., Matoth, I., Yatsiv, I., Mandelberg, H., *et al.* (1988).

Need for endotracheal intubation and suction in meconium-stained neonates. *Journal of Pediatrics*, 112, 613–15.

MacDonald, D., Grant, A., Sheridan-Pereira, M., Boylan, P., and Chalmers, I. (1985). The Dublin randomized controlled trial of intrapartum fetal heart rate monitoring. *American Journal of Obstetrrics and Gynecology*, 152, 524–39.

Matthew, P. M. and Wharton, B. A. (1981). Investigation and management of neonatal jaundice. A problem-orientated case record. *Archives of Disease in Childhood*, 56, 949–53.

Menegazzi, J. J., Auble T. E., Nicklas, K. A., Hosack, G. M., Rack, L., and Goode, J. S. (1993). Two-thumb versus two-finger chest compressions during CPR in a swine infant model of cardiac arrest. *Annals of Emergency Medicine*, 22, 235–9.

Merenstein, K., Hathaway, W. E., Miller, R. W., Paulson, J. A., and Rowley, D. L. (1993). Controversies concerning vitamin K and the newborn. *Pediatrics*, 91, 1001–2.

Moore, F. H. (1989). Examining infants' hips: can it do harm? *Journal of Joint and Bone Surgery*, 71B, 4–5.

Niswander, K., Henson, G., Elbourne, D., Chalmers, I., Redman, C., Macfarlane, A., *et al.* (1984). Adverse outcome of pregnancy and the quality of obstetric care. *Lancet*, ii, 827–31.

Office of Population Censuses and Surveys (1995). OPCS Monitor DH3 95/3. HMSO, London.

O'Kane, M. (1995). Evaluating cord care. *Nursing Times*, 91, 57–8.

Olsen, J. H., Hertz, H., Blinkengerg, K., and Verder, H. (1994). Vitamin K regimens and incidence of childhood cancer in Denmark. *British Medical Journal*, 308, 895–6.

Ortolani, M. (1948). *La lussazione dell' onca*. Capelli, Bologna.

Palme-Kilander, C. (1992). Methods of resuscitation in low-Apgar-score newborn infants – a national survey. *Acta Paediatrica*, 81, 739–44.

Powell, T. G., Pharoah, P. O. D., and Cooke, R. W. I. (1986). Survival and morbidity in a geographically defined population of low birthweight infants. *Lancet*, i, 539–43.

Redshaw, M. E., Harris, A., and Ingram, J. C. (1993). *The neonatal unit as a working environment: a survey of neonatal nursing*. Institute of Child Health, University of Bristol.

Rettig, P. J. (1986). Chlamydial infection in pediatrics: diagnostic and therapeutic considerations. *Pediatric Infectious Disease Journal*, 5, 158–61.

Reyes, B. and Geronemus, R. (1990). Treatment of port-wine stains during childhood with the flashlamp-pumped pulsed dye laser. *Journal of American Academy of Dermatology*, 23,1142–8.

Roberton, N. R. C. (1996). *A manual of normal neonatal care* (2nd edn), pp.87–113. Arnold, London.

Royal College of Paediatrics and Child Health and the Royal College of Obstetricians and Gynaecologists (1997). *Resuscitation of babies at birth*. BMJ Publishing Group, London.

Rush, J. (1990). Care of the umbilical cord. In: *Postnatal care: a research-based approach* (ed. J. Alexander, V. Levy, and S. Roch), pp.84–97. Macmillan Education, Basingstoke.

Rutter, N. (1994). Temperature control and its disorders. In: *Textbook of neonatology* (ed. N. R. C. Roberton), pp.211–31. Churchill Livingstone, Edinburgh.

Smith, D. W. (1977). *Recognizable patterns of human malformation.* W. B. Saunders, Philadelphia.

Stern, C. M. (1992). Neonatal infection. In: *Textbook of neonatology* (2nd edn) (ed. N. R. C. Roberton), pp.934. Churchill Livingstone, Edinburgh.

Thornton, A., Morley, C., and Kohner, N. (1990). *Baby check.* BluePrint, Cambridge.

Ting, P. and Brady, J. (1975). Tracheal suction in meconium aspiration. *American Journal of Obstetrics and Gynecology,* **122**, 767–71.

Verber, I. G. and Pagan, F. S. (1993). What cord care – if any? *Archives of Disease in Childhood,* 68, 594–6.

Walker, N. P. J. and Champion, R. H. (1992). Neonatal dermatology. In: *Textbook of neonatology* (2nd edn) (ed. N. R. C. Roberton), pp.865–77. Churchill Livingstone, Edinburgh.

Wilkinson, J. L. and Cooke, R. W. I. (1992). Cardiovascular disorder. In: *Textbook of neonatology* (2nd edn) (ed. N. R. C. Roberton), pp. 559–604. Churchill Livingstone, Edinburgh.

Working Party of the Royal College of Physicians (1991). Guidelines for the management of convulsions with fever. *British Medical Journal,* **303**, 934–6.

Zipurski, A. (1996). Vitamin K at birth. *British Medical Journal,* **313**, 179–80.

Further reading

Beasley, S. W. (1994). Assessment of the undescended testis. *Current Paediatrics,* **4**, 174–7.

British Paediatric Association (1993). *Neonatal resuscitation: a report of a British Paediatric Association working party.* BPA, London.

Gandy, G. M. (1992). Examination of the neonate including gestational age assessment. In: *Textbook of neonatology* (2nd edn) (ed. N. R. C. Roberton), pp.199–216. Churchill Livingstone, Edinburgh.

Johnston, P. G. B. (1994). *Vullliamy's the newborn child* (7th edn), pp.113–24. Churchill Livingston, Edinburgh.

Passmore, S. J. and McNinch, A. W. (1995). Vitamin K in infancy. *Current Paediatrics,* **5**, 36–8.

Redington, A. N. (1991). Clinical assessment of the neonate and infant with suspected congenital heart disease: how to avoid some of the pitfalls. *Current Paediatrics,* **1**, 65–72.

Roberton, N. R. C. (1996). *A manual of normal neonatal care* (2nd edn), pp.87–113. Arnold, London.

CHAPTER TWENTY-FOUR

Breastfeeding

Sally Inch and Chloe Fisher

Breastfeeding rates in Great Britain

Since 1975 the Office of Population Censuses and Surveys (now the Office of National Statistics) has carried out national infant feeding surveys at five-yearly intervals. The 1995 survey found that 67% of all women who gave birth started breastfeeding. By the end of the first week only 57% of women were breastfeeding, by the end of the second week 53%, and by the end of the sixth week only 43%. By four months only 28% of babies were receiving any breast milk (White *et al.* 1992; Foster *et al.* 1997).

Initiation of breastfeeding

Ninety-three per cent of women have decided on their method of feeding before their baby is born (White *et al.* 1992). Those who choose to bottle-feed may well be aware that 'breast is best', but may also feel that the differences between breast milk and substitutes are so small that they can allow social and cultural factors to influence the decision (Ross *et al.* 1983). Regrettably, many health professionals are similarly misinformed (Inch 1991). Since 1994, scientific data on some of the differences in composition between breast milk and breast milk substitutes have been readily available (see Further reading, below).

A leaflet for women entitled *Feeding your baby – breast or bottle?* has been produced by the Midwives Information and Resource Service (MIDIRS) and the NHS Centre for Reviews and Dissemination. In it, the real differences between breast and bottle are spelled out; for example, bottle-fed babies are five times more likely to be admitted to hospital with diarrhoea or to suffer from urinary infections; twice as likely to be admitted with a chest infection; and twice as likely to suffer from eczema, wheeze, diabetes, or a middle-ear infection. This leaflet should be given to every pregnant woman.

Duration of breastfeeding

From birth to hospital discharge

In 1990, 12% of mothers who started to breastfeed had given up before they left hospital (at a time when most mothers spent three to five days there). This figure was unchanged in 1995 even though the hospital stay was shorter. An OPCS survey in 1990 showed a strong association between certain hospital practices and the success or failure of breastfeeding:

- delaying the first breastfeed (20% of breastfed babies were more than four hours old before they first went to the breast. In 1995, 18% of babies were more than four hours old)

- giving artificial feeds to breastfed babies (45% of breastfed babies received formula in hospital. In 1995 this had dropped to 36%)

- reduced contact between mother and baby (37% of healthy, breastfed babies were separated from their mothers some of the time. In 1995 this had dropped to 26%)

- restrictions of feed frequency and duration (11% of breastfed babies were not fed 'on demand').

In addition, 30% of mothers developed sore or damaged nipples in hospital and 31% had difficulty attaching the baby to the breast themselves. Lack of knowledge and, more recently, the loss of skills seem to underpin the current situation.

Box 24.1 *Ten steps to successful breastfeeding*

Every facility providing maternity services and care for newborn infants should:

(1) have a written breastfeeding policy that is routinely communicated to all health care staff
(2) train all health care staff in skills necessary to implement the breastfeeding policy
(3) inform all pregnant women about the benefits and management of breastfeeding
(4) help mothers initiate breastfeeding within half an hour of birth
(5) show mothers how to breastfeed and how to maintain lactation even if they are separated from their infants
(6) give newborn infants no food or drink other than breast milk, unless medically indicated
(7) practise rooming-in, allowing mothers and infants to remain together 24 hours a day
(8) encourage breastfeeding on demand
(9) give no artificial teats or pacifiers (also called dummies or soothers) to breastfeeding infants
(10) foster the establishment of breastfeeding support groups and refer mothers to them on discharge from hospital or clinic.

These, and other practices, are currently being rigorously reassessed by hospitals who want to achieve the prestigious UNICEF UK Baby Friendly Hospital Award. This requires that facilities providing maternity services fully implement the '10 steps' to successful breastfeeding (Box 24.1) and that at least 50% of mothers are breastfeeding on discharge from hospital.

The background to the current situation

Medical involvement in feed management started early this century. In the beginning these doctors were mainly concerned with artificial feeding, which at the time was very unsafe, but which they also believed would be the feeding method of choice for the future. Desire for control over artificial feeding then spread to breastfeeding. Their ignorance did not deter them.

'Now, it is clear that we cannot have the same control over the chemical constitution of maternal milk that we possess in the case of cows' milk . . . in what respects can we so adapt the food . . . as to render this method of feeding one that is scientific and exact? . . . Although we must leave to nature the qualitative modification of milk, we can on the other hand control the quantity' (Pritchard 1904).

Vincent (1904) began to advocate restricting the duration of the early feeds:

'. . . the infant should be put to the breast and allowed to suck for two or three minutes'.

Within a few years this was also being advocated as a means of preventing sore nipples:

'. . . sucking at each breast at first for under two minutes, the second day for three minutes, and so on. Prolonged sucking, at first, is apt to cause tenderness and cracking of the nipples' (King 1913).

This unresearched advice was continuously enshrined in print from 1973 to 1992: the *Textbook of paediatrics* contained the instruction to restrict the early feeds to 3, 5, and 7 minutes per breast for the first three days (Arneil and Stroud 1984). The fact that this advice is of no value (sore nipples are frequently the result of poor attachment (Woolridge 1986)) would be of less concern if it did no harm. However, restricting the duration of feeds causes breast engorgement (Moon and Humenick 1989), a restricted milk intake, and inadequate vitamin K for the baby (von Kries *et al.* 1987).

Further breastfeeding control was effected by restricting frequency (Sarjeant 1905; Chavasse 1906; Pritchard 1907; Vincent 1913; Langmead 1916; Liddiard 1924–1958) and, ultimately, their duration (King 1913; King 1934; Myles 1956). As a result, babies who would, if left to themselves, have fed more often, were underfed. Liddiard, an advocate of four-hourly feeding, noted that many breastfed babies took six months to double their birthweight. In their first nine editions, Patterson and Smith (1926–1955) also expected that most babies would take six months to double their birthweight.

With good attachment and unrestricted feeding, a baby can easily double his birthweight by four months (Ahn and MacLean 1980; Hitchcock *et al.* 1981).

Evidence-based modern management can be found in Inch (1989), Inch and Garforth (1989), Inch and Renfrew (1989), Enkin *et al.* (1995), and the Cochrane Database. These have been used in the preparation of texts for health care professionals (e.g. *Successful breastfeeding* – see Further reading, below).

At the beginning of the century, when these unhelpful 'rules' were being introduced, many midwives were still skilled at helping women attach their babies to the breast correctly. However, as breastfeeding rates dropped, experienced midwives retired and these skills were eroded. Staffing shortages have compounded the problem as even those midwives who have the necessary skills may be unable to spend enough time with an individual mother and baby.

The provision of at least one skilled, specialist practitioner in a district health authority would help to alleviate the situation until the skills training programme required by hospitals seeking to become Baby Friendly has reskilled more midwives.

Hospital discharge to six weeks

In 1990, 26% of women who left hospital breastfeeding had stopped by the time their baby was six weeks old; although this figure was slightly improved in 1995, the situation remains broadly the same. Eight per cent of this drop occurred at the time when midwifery care in the community was at its most intensive (up to the end of the second week). Eighteen per cent of the drop occurred whilst the health visitor and the GP were likely to be seeing the mother most intensively. Sore nipples and an apparently insufficient milk supply were the two most common reasons.

Nipple soreness is almost always due to incorrect attachment. The solution is not nipple shields, creams, sprays, or lotions but referral to a midwife who can watch and improve the woman's feeding technique. The exception to this is nipple thrush (see p. 444).

A mother may feel that she has insufficient milk if her baby feeds frequently or for prolonged periods and yet seldom seems satisfied. The baby may or may not be gaining weight adequately. Since very few women are physiologically unable to produce sufficient milk for their infants (Chetley 1986), it is likely that the baby is simply not effectively obtaining the milk that is in the breast.

Again, the solution is to improve the attachment, not to give complementary or supplementary feeds. Unfortunately, artificial feeds are seen as a panacea for breastfeeding problems, and have been since 1900!

Women who want to breastfeed actually *want* to breastfeed – they are not merely trying to do what is best. Many mothers feel that they form a particularly special bond with their breastfed baby. The emotional and psychological consequences of feeling that they 'failed' to breastfeed may stay with them for the rest of their lives.

Six weeks to four months

In 1990, 23% of women who were breastfeeding at six weeks had stopped by four months. For 91% this was earlier than planned. Poor breastfeeding technique was still likely to have been the underlying cause despite the reasons women gave (insufficient milk, baby refusing the breast, feeds taking too long). Although women who were breastfeeding were less likely than those who were bottle-feeding to have introduced solids by three months, 94% of babies were having solids by four months.

Giving solids to a breastfed baby who is under four months old does not increase the total calorie intake. All that happens is that milk intake is reduced. If the original problem is 'insufficient milk', the early introduction of solids will compound it (Cohen *et al.* 1994; Borresen 1995). Solids should not be introduced before four months (and could be delayed until six months) (Department of Health 1994).

The proportion of women who gave up breastfeeding because they were going back to work increased considerably between 1985 and 1990: an 8% increase at two to three months and a 17% increase at three to four months. In 1995, 33% of those who gave up at three to four months did so because they were returning to work; a further 10% rise from the 1990 figure. Some of these women may have been unaware that it is possible to combine working and breastfeeding as the two are not mutually exclusive (see Breastfeeding and working).

Advantages of breastfeeding

The advantages to a baby of being breastfed rather than receiving an artificial substitute are overwhelming (Figures 24.1 and 24.2).

These advantages to the baby will have a knock-on effect for general practitioners:

- fewer GP consultations

- fewer paediatric admissions

- fewer night calls

- ultimately, fewer ongoing chronic conditions, such as diabetes, asthma, and eczema.

In *Breastfeeding: good practice guidance to the NHS* (Department of Health 1995), it is estimated that savings in reduced hospital admissions for gastroenteritis alone, if all babies were breastfed, would be '£35 million for the country as a whole and £300 000 for the average district'. Realistically, a 1% increase in breastfeeding would save £4000 per district; £500 000 in England and Wales. The impact in monetary terms on the reduced incidence of gastroenteritis, insulin-dependent diabetes mellitus, necrotizing enterocolitis (NEC), and pre-menopausal breast cancer of even a 1% increase in breastfeeding might be as high as £3 million for the health districts in England and Wales.

Breastfeeding shown to be associated with:

Reduced risk of infant mortality

Neonatal necrotizing enterocolitis (NNEC) in preterm infants:
Lucas & Cole, Lancet, 1990, 336: 1519-23

Sudden Infant Death
Ford et al, Intl J Epidemiol, 1993, 22: 885-9*
(Frederikson et al, Amer J Dis Child, 147: 460 Abstract)
Klonoff-Cohen et al, JAMA, 1995, 273: 795-8 (Non-smokers)
*see also Gilbert et al, BMJ, 1995, 310: 88-90

Reduced infant morbidity from infection

Gastrointestinal infections
Howie et al, BMJ, 1990, 300: 11-16

Respiratory infections
Victora et al, Intl J Epidemiol, 1989, 18: 918-25
Wright et al, BMJ, 1989, 299: 946-9

Urinary tract infections
Marild et al, Lancet, 1990, 339: 942
Pisacane et al, J Pediatrics, 1992, 120: 87-90
(Coppa et al, Lancet, 1990, 335: 569-71 - Oligosacch. & bact.
adhesion)

Otitis media
Duncan et al, Pediatrics, 1993, 91: 867-72
Aniansson et al, Pediatr Infect Dis J, 1994, 13: 183-8
Paradise et al, Pediatrics, 1994, 94: 853-60 (Cleft palate)

Enhanced immunity

Pabst & Spady, Lancet, 1990, 336: 269-71

Reduced atopic disease (where family history of atopy)

Eczema
Lucas et al, BMJ, 1990, 300: 837-840
Saarinen & Kajosaari, Lancet, 1995, 346: 1065-9 (at age 17 yrs)

Respiratory wheeze
Burr et al, J Epidemiol Commun Health, 1989, 43: 125-32
Wright et al, Arch Pediatr Adolesc Med, 1995, 149: 758-63
Saarinen & Kajosaari, Lancet, 1995, 346: 1065-9 (at age 17 yrs)

Increased intelligence (cognitive development) in:

Term babies
(Rogan & Gladen, Early Human Development, 1993, 31: 181-93)
Pollock, Develop Med Child Neurol, 1994, 36: 429-40

Preterm babies
Lucas et al, Lancet, 1992, 339: 261-4*
*but see also Morley et al, Arch Dis Childhd, 63: 1382-5

Reduced risk of auto-immune disease

Diabetes
Mayer et al, Diabetes, 1988, 37: 1625-32
Karjalainen J et al, New Eng J Med, 1992, 327: 302-7

Reduced risks to mother of:

Breast cancer
Layde et al, J Clin Epidemiol, 1989, 42: 963-73
Chilvers - UKNCCSG, Brit Med J, 1993, 307: 17-20
Newcomb et al, New Eng J Med, 1994, 330: 81-87
c.f. Michels et al, Lancet, 1996, 347: 431-6

Ovarian cancer
Gwinn et al, J Clin Epidemiol, 1990, 43: 559-68
Rosenblatt et al, Intl J Epidemiol, 1993, 22: 192-7

Hip fractures (in elderly)
Cumming & Klineberg, Intl J Epidemiol, 1993, 22: 684-91

Additional benefits (requiring further substantiation) to infant:

• Dental malocclusion
  Labbok & Hendershot, Amer J Prev Med, 3: 227-32
• Childhood lymphoma
  Davis et al, Lancet, 1988, ii, 356-8
  (Golding et al, Br J Cancer, 1990, 62: 304-8)
• Inflammatory bowel disease
  Calkins & Mendeloff, Epidem Rev, 1986, 8: 60-9
• Coronary heart disease
  Barker et al, Arch Dis Childhd, 1988, 63: 867-9
• Autoimmune thyroid disease
  Fort et al, J Am Coll Nurs, 1986, 5: 439-41
• Crohn's disease
  Koletzko et al, Brit Med J, 1989, 1617-8
• Coeliac disease (delay in)
  Kelly et al, Arch Dis Childhd, 1989, 64: 1157-60
• Neonatal tetany
  Specker et al, Amer J Dis Child, 1991, 145: 941-5
• Multiple sclerosis
  Pisacane et al, Brit Med J, 1994, 308: 1411-2
• Appendicitis
  Pisacane et al, Brit Med J, 1995, 310: 836-7

to mother:

• Rheumatoid Arthritis (death)
  Brun et al, Brit J Rheumatol, 1995, 34: 542-6

Further sources:

Cunningham et al, 'Breastfeeding, Growth & Illness', 1992, UNICEF.
Standing Committee on Nutrition of the British Paediatric.
Association. 'Is breastfeeding beneficial in the UK?' Arch Dis
Chldhd, 71: 376-80

Compiled by M Woolridge for the UNICEF UK Baby Friendly Initiative,
April 1996.

Figure 24.1 *UNICEF/UK Baby Friendly Initiative list of advantages. (Reproduced with kind permission.)*

Breast milk also plays a major role in the prevention of NEC, an often fatal condition associated with prematurity. The mothers of preterm infants are often unable to provide their babies with their own milk initially, and the provision of banked human milk can make the difference between life or death. Thirteen districts operate a human milk bank, and breastfeeding mothers could be encouraged to donate excess milk. Screening tests similar to those required of blood donors are mandatory (British Paediatric Association 1994).

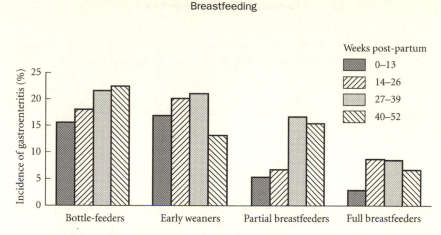

Figure 24.2 *The incidence of gastroenteritis by feeding method over time. (Source: Howie et al. (1990).)*

Drugs in breast milk

There are relatively few conditions for which it is not possible to find a form of therapy that is compatible with breastfeeding and authoritative reference books, such as the *British National Formulary* or *MIMMS*, and local or regional drug information services give advice on request.

The technique of breastfeeding

In 1995, in Great Britain, almost three-quarters of all babies were bottle-fed by the time they were four months old. This figure has persisted for 20 years. As a corollary, the art of breastfeeding has largely been lost. The myth has emerged that women can breastfeed 'naturally'. This overlooks the crucial fact that breastfeeding has to be learned. Most women have only seen bottle-feeding and probably try and use their breast in the same way. For example, they may well try to push their nipple into the baby's mouth instead of putting the baby to the breast.

Holding and putting the baby to the breast

Finding the right position on the breast often takes time and practice for mothers and babies alike. Importantly, the mother should be sitting comfortably with her back straight and her lap almost flat. Wrapping the baby's hands out of the way is useful and the mother can then concentrate on the mouth/breast relationship.

The way a mother holds her baby is most important. The baby's shoulders and chest should be turned towards the mother, with the nose opposite the nipple. The mother should then bring the *baby* up to the *breast*, supporting her baby across the shoulders, thus allowing the head to extend slightly so that the chin will make the first contact with the breast. She may find it helpful to support her breast from the base, not close to the nipple. The stimulation of moving the baby gently against the breast causes the baby to gape, that is, open his mouth wide whilst darting the tongue down and forward.

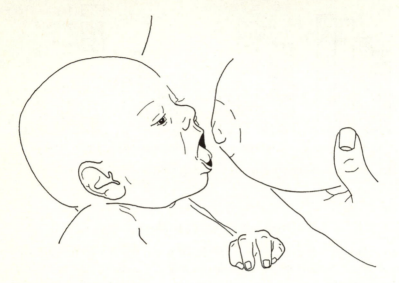

Figure 24.3 *A baby gaping.*

Once the baby gapes, the mother brings him quickly but gently to the breast, aiming the bottom lip as far away from the nipple as she can. This enables him to scoop in as much breast as possible, creating a teat from which to feed effectively.

Once the baby is well attached, he should be allowed to finish the feed in his own time and relinquish the breast spontaneously. The exception to this is if the baby needs to come off to bring up wind after a minute or two of feeding, after which he should return to the same breast until finished on that side. This is the only way the mother has of ensuring that her baby has taken all he needs from the first breast. The baby can then be offered the second breast which he will take, or not, according to his appetite.

A well-attached baby feeds with a wide mouth and an active tongue, and this will be evident from the rhythm of the feed. After an initial burst of short sucks the baby will switch into long, deep sucks. Occasional pauses will become more frequent as the feed progresses. His body will be relaxed as he feeds and he will have no difficulty breathing. Throughout, the feed will be comfortable and pain free for the mother.

Prevention and treatment of breastfeeding problems

'One of the characteristics of health care that attracts a lot of attention is the time it takes for ideas of proven effectiveness to enter clinical practice. This is only matched by . . . the rapid dissemination of interventions of unproven effectiveness – sometimes without formal identification of possible harm' (Bandolier 1996).

Sore nipples

In the early days of breastfeeding, sore nipples are almost always the result of incorrect attachment. If the baby has not been enabled to take a good mouthful of breast so that the nipple reaches the junction of the hard and soft palate, the baby's tongue will compress the nipple against the hard palate as he feeds (Figure 24.4).

Blanching nipples

Some women may experience intense nipple pain after a feed with an obvious change in the nipple from its normal pink to a pinched, white colour. Although it is prevalent in women who have a history of Raynaud's phenomenon, it is usually a sign that the nipple is being traumatized as a result of incorrect attachment.

Damaged nipples

Repeated compression of the nipple will usually result in damage. Depending on the design of the breast, the damage may be at the tip or the base of the nipple.

Treatment of these problems involves observing and correcting the attachment. Feeds should subsequently be pain free. There may be transitory pain at the very beginning of the feed until the nipple is healed as the damaged tissue stretches to form the teat within the baby's mouth. Damaged nipples heal very quickly once the cause is removed.

The frequently repeated advice to expose nipples to the air to aid healing is not supported by research. There is evidence that a superficial, clean wound will heal more rapidly if it is kept moist (Winter and Scales 1963); this is now the basis of modern wound healing (Alper 1983; Anon 1988). To achieve this, small squares of sterilized, paraffin-impregnated gauze placed over the nipple (and under a breast pad) prevent the damaged area from drying out. If the damaged area has become superficially infected, paraffin gauze which is impregnated with fucidic acid may help. Although there is good theoretical basis for this, the use of paraffin gauze has not been evaluated.

There is no evidence to support the use of any creams, sprays, or ointments, antenatally or postnatally, to prevent or treat nipple soreness (Inch and Renfrew 1989).

Poor attachment does not always result in pain and damage. Thus the absence of pain does not necessarily indicate that the attachment is correct. If the baby is unsettled or fussing at the breast, attachment should also be checked.

Antenatal preparation of the breasts for breastfeeding is unnecessary. Attempts to improve breastfeeding outcomes by antenatal breast expression, toughening the nipple epithelium, or trying to improve nipple protractility by the use of shells or stretching 'exercises' have all been shown to be of no value (Inch 1987, 1989; Alexander 1990; Alexander *et al.* 1992; MAIN Trial Collaborative Group 1994).

(a)

(b)

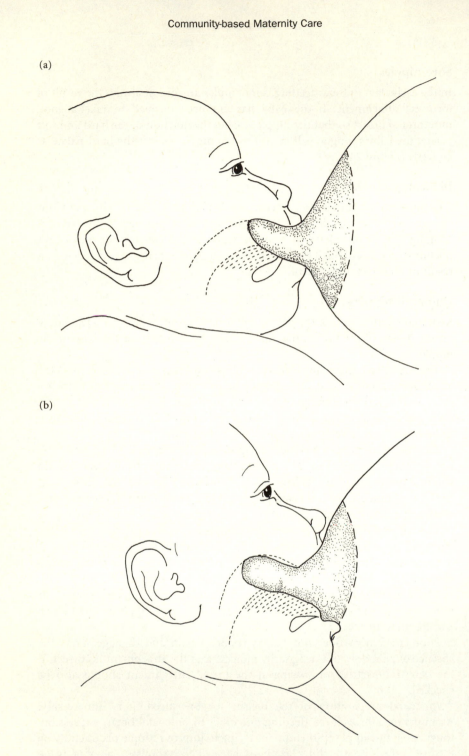

Figure 24.4 *(a) poor attachment; (b) good attachment.*

Engorgement

As the placental hormones recede, the breasts become active. The blood supply increases and the mother may experience some discomfort (vascular engorgement). This subsides as milk is produced provided that its removal is efficient, the baby is correctly attached, and feeds are unrestricted.

If milk is not removed efficiently, the breasts may become overfull (milk engorgement). It may be possible to resolve this if the mother receives skilled help with attachment, although it will be difficult for the baby to create an effective teat from tense, oedematous breast tissue. Gentle hand expression or the use of an effective electric breast pump may be used to encourage the milk to flow and soften the tissue to the point where the baby can be correctly attached.

Mastitis

Mastitis (inflammation) is usually the result of inefficient 'milking' of the breast. In most cases it occurs on the side opposite the mother's preferred side for holding (Inch and Fisher 1995).

Milk production is a continuous process. If milk removal does not keep pace with production, the pressure within the ductal system will rise. While the milk is contained within the ducts, the mother may be aware of lumpy, painful areas in the breast but no inflammation. This is sometimes referred to as 'blocked ducts'.

If the pressure rises, milk is forced into the surrounding breast tissue. Here it provokes an acute and localized inflammatory response. If the escaped milk also enters the bloodstream it causes fever and flu-like symptoms. At this point it should still be possible to resolve the situation by improving milk removal by improving attachment – possibly in conjunction with effective hand or mechanical expression.

Routine use of antibiotics should be avoided as they expose both mother and baby to their potential side-effects and predispose them to nipple/oral thrush (p. 444). Although antibiotics may appear to resolve the condition, this is usually by virtue of their anti-inflammatory (Spector and Willoughby 1974; Dewdney 1981; MIMMS 1994) rather than their antibacterial properties, since most mastitis is not caused by infection (Thomsen *et al.* 1984; Matheson *et al.* 1988).

A pragmatic approach might be to give the mother an antibiotic but to advise her not to take it unless the condition fails to respond to more conservative measures. On no account should a woman with mastitis be advised to stop breastfeeding as this will increase her chance of developing an abscess (Newton 1950; Marshall *et al.* 1975; Thomsen *et al.* 1984).

Blocked ducts

Very occasionally, a ductal opening in the nipple tip may become obstructed by white granules or a milk-filled blister. These are not a consequence of poor attachment. White granules appear to be caused by the aggregation and fusion of casein micelles to which further materials become added (Cowie *et al.* 1980). This hardened lump may obstruct a milk duct as it slowly progresses to the nipple where it may be removed by the baby during a feed or expressed manually (New Generation 1982). The milk-filled blister may also resolve by the baby feeding or it may be removed with a clean fingernail, rough flannel, or sterile needle. True blockages of this sort tend to recur but once the woman understands how to deal with them, progression to mastitis can be avoided.

Deep breast pain

Some women report deep breast pain during or after feeds. In most cases this responds to improvement in breastfeeding technique and is thus likely to be due to raised intraductal pressure caused by inefficient milk removal. Although it may occur during the feed, it typically occurs afterwards, and thus can be distinguished from a strong let-down reflex (see below). Very rarely, deep breast pain may be the result of ductal thrush infection. This will be unaffected by improved feeding technique and responds to systemic anti-fungal preparations (Amir 1991).

Breast abscess

An abscess may occur rapidly following direct infection, usually from a damaged nipple. It may also occur when non-infective mastitis is not treated promptly. When an abscess has formed, a fluctuant mass can be felt in the breast and can be detected by ultrasonography (Bertrand and Rosenblood 1991).

Breastfeeding should continue unless pus drains from the nipple, in which case the affected breast should be expressed (if possible) and the milk discarded until the mother is able to resume full breastfeeding. Previously, treatment consisted of surgical incision and antibiotics. Dixon (1988) described aspiration of abscesses with syringe and needle, and this is now the first-line treatment; it can be performed on an out-patient basis and causes no breast disfiguration (Dixon 1994).

Thrush

This is an occasional cause of sore nipples although the incidence seems to be increasing. It is commoner in women who have received antibiotics (Amir 1991). It can be distinguished from the soreness of poor attachment by observation of feeding technique, and often occurs after a period of trouble-free feeding. It commonly occurs bilaterally and is usually evenly distributed around the nipple and possibly the areola. The nipple pain intensifies during the feed and continues for some time between feeds. The nipple and areola are often pink and shiny. In some cases the baby may also have clinically obvious oral or peri-anal thrush. There is often a history of recent antibiotic use.

If thrush is suspected, mother and baby should be treated simultaneously with topical preparations to prevent reinfection. Clotrimazole should be avoided as it may cause skin irritation on the nipple.

Very rarely, the lactiferous ducts become infected, giving rise to deep breast pain (see above). Systemic treatment will be needed. Poor technique and nipple thrush may coexist.

Let-down or milk ejection reflex

Although all lactating women will be subject to the effects of oxytocin release, not all women are aware of it in their breasts, although in the early days they may be aware of its effects on the uterus. However, once lactation is established, some women will experience a brief shooting or tingling sensation in the breast as the feed begins. This is normal.

Let-down difficulties

Stress has often been regarded as a cause of feeding problems, and mothers are frequently exhorted to 'relax'. However, a breastfeeding mother is most unlikely to have problems with her let-down reflex. In nearly 4000 out-patient referrals to two breastfeeding clinics there have been no confirmed cases of let-down inhibition (Fisher and Inch, personal communication; Woolridge, personal communication).

Furthermore, if impaired let-down was the cause of a breastfeeding problem, the administration of oxytocin should overcome it. Yet in none of 800 plus subjects examined in the context of randomized controlled trials (Inch and Renfrew 1989) could the administration of oxytocin be shown to be of benefit in women suckling normally. Although one small study demonstrated that the frequency of the oxytocin pulses could be reduced in 'stressed' lactating women, this made no difference to the amount of milk the baby obtained (Ueda *et al.* 1994).

'Insufficient' milk

Mothers whose babies are feeding frequently, feeding for long periods but are unsatisfied after feeds and sometimes not gaining weight may well believe (or be told) that the cause is insufficient milk. In the early days of lactation this is most unlikely since most women are inherently capable of breastfeeding twins, but as time passes without correcting the cause of the problem, reduced milk removal may result in milk production being reset at a lower level. This is yet another reason for ensuring that attachment is optimal before the mother leaves the care of the midwife.

The following check-list may help to identify those women who need extra help:

A mother who is experiencing any of the following:

- pain – except possibly fleeting discomfort at the beginning of a feed
- breasts – engorged
- nipples – damaged
          – compressed when the baby comes off (white 'line' visible)

or whose baby is:

- not coming off the breast spontaneously
- restless at the breast
- not satisfied after the feed
- taking a long time to feed (i.e. regularly more than 30–40 minutes)
- feeding very frequently (i.e. more than 10 feeds in 24 hours)
- feeding very infrequently (i.e. fewer than three feeds in the first 24 hours or fewer than six feeds in 24 hours at 24–48 hours old)
- still passing meconium at 36–48 hours.

In the early days, it is much more likely that the baby is not obtaining the milk that is in the breast rather than there being an inadequate supply. Attention paid promptly to the technique of breastfeeding (p. 439) for any mother with any of the above problems will avoid true insufficiency.

Problems with the babies

In the baby, poor attachment may give rise to:

- restlessness at the breast
- prolonged feeds
- very frequent feeds
- very infrequent feeds
- colic
- liquid stools
- excessive flatus
- possetting
- breast rejection.

In addition, babies may be growing but unhappy, growing slowly, not growing at all, or even losing weight.

Colic

Colic is a vague term often used by mothers to describe a baby who cries as if in pain whilst drawing up his knees. If the baby also has explosive stools and passes a lot of wind, the colic may be due to inappropriate breast usage (Woolridge and Fisher 1988). If the mother is timing the feeds, or taking the baby off the first breast to ensure that he feeds from the second, she should be advised not to restrict the feeds but to allow the baby to finish the first breast first and come off spontaneously before being offered the second, which he may or may not require. It does not matter if the baby takes one or two breasts at a feed; the mother needs only to start on alternate breasts. If there is no improvement within 24 hours, the feeding technique may need improving with help from a midwife.

Poor feeding technique may also result in the above symptoms. If the baby is poorly attached, most of the milk that he gets is a result of the mother 'pushing' it to him via the let-down reflex. He may receive a lot of milk all at once and may be restless at the breast or even come off spluttering because he is unable to control the flow in the way that he would if he had a better mouthful of breast.

The baby may feel engulfed by the milk and try to avoid repeating the experience by crying as he approaches the breast. If the mother is also flexing his head as he comes to the breast because she is concentrating on his top lip instead of his bottom lip as she tries to attach him, he may be unable to breathe because his nose reaches the breast first and is compressed by it. This experience will reinforce his reluctance. If this is not addressed, it may become breast rejection, leading to great distress in both mother and baby.

If the baby can tolerate the ejected milk flow, he will consume a large volume, usually taking from both breasts, in an effort to obtain sufficient calories. The calorific value of ejected foremilk is much less than would be obtained from the mixture of foremilk and higher-fat hindmilk obtainable if he were well attached. Inability to form an adequate teat from the breast tissue prevents the baby using his tongue to actively remove milk from the ducts. Thus, no matter how long he stays at the breast the feed does not satiate him and he does not release the breast spontaneously. His mother may remove him or he may 'fall asleep' at the breast only to be awake and hungry again soon.

If the baby is having to consume much larger volumes of milk than he would if he were well attached, he may posset large amounts after the feed. Much larger volumes of milk are also passing through his gut and the bacteria resident there ferment the larger than normal quantity of lactose, giving rise to distressing gastrointestinal symptoms (colic, liquid stools, and excessive flatus).

The frequent feeds may also cause the mother to produce more milk than she really needs since she will stimulate prolactin release each time she feeds as well as removing large volumes of milk. The health professional may thus be presented with a seeming paradox – a mother with an abundant (or even overabundant) milk supply and a baby who is 'never satisfied'.

If the baby can consume and retain enough low-fat foremilk he will grow; if he cannot his weight will reflect this fact. In an apparent attempt to conserve energy, poorly growing infants may sleep for long periods and feed infrequently. Poor milk removal and infrequent breast stimulation may ultimately cause the mother's milk supply to reduce in volume.

In most instances the problems are resolved by improving the attachment (Figure 24.5). If the baby is not growing it may be necessary for the mother to express milk from her breasts after she has fed him and use her own milk to 'top up' the intake (Figure 24.6).

Colic and dietary sensitivity

The distressing colic symptoms outlined above are most likely to be due to poor attachment. Thus the first step to resolving the problem is to observe the mother's feeding technique.

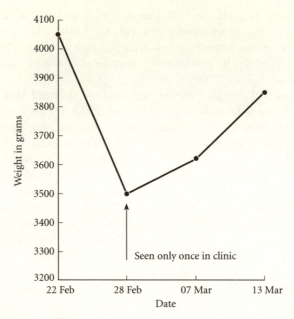

Figure 24.5 *Referred because of failure to thrive. Explanation of the principles of attachment is needed. Improvement in baby's behaviour becomes apparent within 24 hours.*

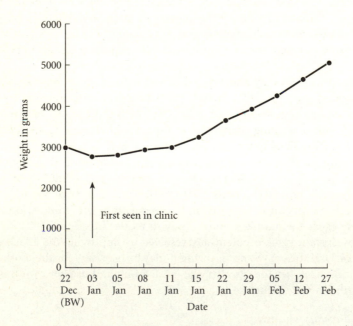

Figure 24.6 *Referred because of static weight and below birthweight at two weeks. Seen in clinic on six occasions; lent breast pump for one week; attention to technique.*

In the few cases in which the colic persists in spite of good attachment, it may be that the baby is reacting to elements of the mother's diet, particularly if there is a family history of allergy or atopic disease. The most likely substance is cows' milk protein, although eggs and wheat are sometimes responsible (Evan *et al.* 1981; Jacobsson and Linberg 1983; Cant *et al.* 1986). The mother should be advised to omit cows' milk and related products from her diet for at least a week.

If the changes in the child's symptoms warrant their permanent exclusion, she may need dietetic help to meet her own nutritional needs. Dimethicone, which is often prescribed for babies with colic, has not been shown to be of value (Metcalf *et al.* 1994).

Giving expressed milk

If it is necessary to give a breastfed baby his mother's milk by indirect means, this can be accomplished by various methods: syringe, dropper, spoon, cup, bottle, or soft-spouted beaker, depending on the baby's age and the reason for feeding. Staff in Baby Friendly hospitals will encourage the use of cups, appropriate for one or two feeds for very young babies requiring small amounts; it allows them to remain more in control of their intake and consume only what they need.

However, for longer-term use, while the mother is expressing milk for her term baby to maintain her milk supply and ensure adequate nutrition for the baby, and dealing with the problem of poor or difficult attachment, a feeding bottle may be more satisfactory. It is quicker, less wasteful than cup feeding, and in most cases more acceptable to the mother.

There is currently concern that if a baby feeds from a bottle he will not 'remember' how to feed from a breast. This is often referred to as '*nipple confusion*'. There is no evidence to support this (Neifert *et al.* 1995; Fisher and Inch 1996).

The normal term baby is born with a rooting reflex because feeding is a biological imperative. In a normal baby, turning the head in response to a touch of the cheek, opening the mouth wide, and putting the tongue down and forward (gaping) are reflex actions. With a deep mouthful of breast the stimulus of the palate triggers sucking with rhythmical cycles of compression applied to the breast by the tongue.

There is no evidence to support the view that the baby may forget how to do this if he is given something else to suck. The baby sucking on a bottle teat seen on ultrasound seems to be exerting a piston-like action with his tongue, but this may just be the effect of the rhythmical tongue action against a much less yielding surface (Neil, personal communication). It is probable that the apparent differences in the sucking are superficial, and the baby is using the same action but the effect is different against different surfaces.

There is no evidence to suggest that a normal baby may have a limited ability to adapt to various oral configurations, or that if 'the first feed after birth is given by bottle, that the artificial teat may be imprinted in the infant and make subsequent attempts at breastfeeding more difficult' (Neifert *et al.*

1995). There is no evidence to suggest that 'imprinting' occurs in humans to any degree.

There are undoubtedly conditions that may make it difficult for the baby to make an effective teat from the breast; but these difficulties are likely to be evident whether or not the baby is given a bottle-feed. Furthermore, babies who have never been attached to the breast correctly, or who have been 'manhandled' by unskilled helpers, may exhibit distress at the breast or 'switch off' and refuse to feed. If this situation is 'resolved' by giving a bottle, this pattern may be repeated on the next occasion and the baby will again refuse the breast. This baby has never been to the breast and is not 'confused'; he is manifesting his distress. This may be interpreted by some as an apparent 'preference'. In such circumstances the baby might easily express a preference for a cup (Lang 1996). If, however, the distressed baby has his hunger assuaged by some of his mother's milk (from a bottle), he may then be sufficiently calmed to allow a skilled carer to attach him to the breast correctly and gently.

If the baby cannot be attached to the breast adequately/successfully by his mother, the priorities are that the mother makes milk (by expressing) and that the baby receives it (by bottle). This gives the mother *time*, and the baby can be offered the breast, with help, at each available opportunity until she can do it herself. In no instance in these circumstances has any of the babies seen in the Oxford Breastfeeding Clinic ever refused the breast, even when breastfeeds have been separated by several days of exclusive bottle-feeding. From 1991 to date the Oxford Breastfeeding Clinic has seen nearly 3000 mothers and babies.

It is not yet known whether it will do more harm than good to deprive a baby who cannot yet feed from the breast the opportunity to *suck* at all. Alternative methods of feeding term babies should only be explored via randomized controlled trials.

Other practical issues

Maternal diet

As a general rule, breastfeeding mothers can eat anything they like while they are breastfeeding. Various folklore prohibitions do not stand closer examination as in the main whatever is prohibited in one culture is consumed as a staple food in another, with no ill effects on the baby!

Maternal food intake

Metabolic efficiency seems to be enhanced during lactation and mothers are able to meet their own and their infants' needs on as little as 1600–1800 calories per day (Illingworth *et al.* 1986). This finding explains why the actual calorie intake of well-nourished mothers has been found to be consistently below the previously recommended intake (Whitehead *et al.* 1981; Butte *et al.* 1984) and why giving food supplements to undernourished women does not result in increased growth in their infants (Delgado *et al.* 1982; Prentice *et al.* 1983).

Maternal fluid intake

Increased fluids do not result in increased milk output, nor will reduced fluids reduce milk volume (Olsen 1940; Illingworth and Kilpatrick 1953; Dearlove and Dearlove 1981; Dusdieker *et al.* 1985). Mothers need only be guided by their thirst.

Rest vs exercise

There is no basis on which to recommend that breastfeeding mothers should rest in order to make milk. Aerobic exercise performed for 45 minutes at a time, four to five days per week, for 12 weeks (beginning at six weeks post-partum) had no adverse effect on lactation and significantly improved the cardiovascular fitness of the mothers (Dewey *et al.* 1994).

Additional fluids for exclusively breastfed babies

Babies who consume enough breast milk to satisfy their energy needs will easily meet their fluid requirements, even in hot, dry climates (Almroth 1978; Armelini and Gonzalez 1979; Goldberg and Adams 1983; Brown *et al.* 1986; Almroth and Bidinger 1990; Sachdev *et al.* 1991; Ashraf *et al.* 1993).

Extra water will do nothing to speed the resolution of physiological jaundice (Carvahlo *et al.* 1981; Nicoll *et al.* 1982). The only consistent effect of giving additional fluids to breastfed infants is to reduce the time for which they are breastfed (de Chateau *et al.* 1977; Herrera 1984; Fenstein *et al.* 1986; White *et al.* 1992).

Stools of a breastfed baby

The stools of a breastfed baby differ from those of an artificially fed baby in several respects. They will take longer to change from black to yellow but should nevertheless be starting to change by 48 hours and should be yellow by 72–96 hours if the baby has been well attached and feeding well (Salariya and Robertson 1993). The stools are much less bulky than those of an artificially fed baby and the frequency may range from once a feed to once every 12 days (Weaver *et al.* 1988; Morley *et al.* 1997). Mothers can be reassured that their healthy, breastfed baby cannot be constipated.

Breastfeeding and working

Once the milk supply is established (six to eight weeks post-partum), women returning to work and continuing breastfeeding have several options. They can feed their baby when they are at home and express milk mechanically or by hand while at work and give it to their childminder for the following day; they can have the child brought to them or go to the child at feed times (if work is close enough) or they can breastfeed at home and the childminder can give formula. In the first case, the mother will need to begin expressing after some feeds for several days before she plans to start work so that she builds up enough stored milk for the childminder to use on the first day. In the last case, if she wishes to continue with morning and evening feeds but cannot feed or express during the day, the mother will need to start dropping breastfeeds and substituting formula over the course of the weeks preceding her return to work so that milk production has reduced before she has her first long break from her baby.

Storage of breast milk

Human breast milk has impressive bacteriostatic qualities. Preterm milk can be safely stored at room temperature, even in the tropics, for up to four hours (Nwanko *et al.* 1988) and term milk for 6–10 hours (Ajusi *et al.* 1989; Barger and Bull 1987; Larson *et al.* 1984; Olowe *et al.* 1987; Sosa and Bardess 1987). Colostrum can be left even longer: up to 24 hours (Pittard *et al.* 1985).

If refrigerated, milk is safe for a further 48 hours (Berkow *et al.* 1984; Jensen and Jensen 1992), after which it should be used, discarded, or frozen. Once frozen it will keep for at least three months in a freezer with a separate door. It can be thawed either in the fridge or at room temperature. For speed it can be placed in a jug of *warm* water.

Reducing the attrition rate

Telling women that they really should breastfeed, without telling them how, is about as useful as telling them that potatoes are edible without telling them how to cook them (Palmer 1988). Although all women ought to be informed in the antenatal period of the health benefits of breastfeeding, greater emphasis needs to be placed on the fact that breastfeeding is a skill that has to be learned. It may be 'natural', but it is not *instinctive*.

An outline of the steps needed to attach the baby to the breast may well be useful, but many first-time mothers may not absorb much information about events beyond birth itself. The following points made antenatally may nevertheless be useful:

- breastfeeding has to be learnt
- you are likely to need help at the beginning – even if you have breastfed before
- breastfeeding should not hurt
- you may receive conflicting advice.

All breastfeeding women should be put in touch with sources of breastfeeding support either antenatally or as soon after birth as is practicable.

Most women start breastfeeding in hospital. Hospital policies and hospital-based practitioners will thus influence the mother at her most vulnerable. It is essential that policies and practices are soundly based and harmful ones are abandoned (see Further reading). The drive to achieve Baby Friendly status may assist this process.

What individual practitioners can do

More post-partum care is being provided in the community. Many mothers leave hospital within six hours and from that moment they will turn to midwife, GP, and health visitor for help.

Each practitioner should consider who else within their sphere of influence is giving advice to breastfeeding mothers and whether the advice is correct and consistent.

Research-based texts and videos for women are available (see Further reading). The development of a group breastfeeding policy based on these, which could be given to mothers, may reduce the amount of conflicting advice.

Validated study days on breastfeeding, and the breastfeeding training of health professionals by hospitals seeking Baby Friendly status, may be additional sources of good information.

Health professionals need to be aware of the undermining that may go on around the breastfeeding mother – her own mother or other relatives or friends may not have breastfed successfully. Professionals themselves may not have had a positive personal experience of breastfeeding (Crawford 1992). It is an emotional business; health professionals need to acknowledge their own feelings if they are to be of help.

Support groups

The National Childbirth Trust, La Leche League, and the Association of Breastfeeding Mothers are the three main lay breastfeeding organizations. An up-to-date list can always be obtained by telephoning the national number. Lay counsellors/leaders provide 'informed' mother-to-mother support and advice (see later – Other resources).

The National Infant Feeding Specialist Group (comprising mostly mid-wives) has about 40 members across the country. If there is one locally, it could be used as a resource for breastfeeding problems (see Other resources).

Some midwives run drop-in breastfeeding sessions/clinics in health centres or hospital departments.

There is a Breastfeeding Awareness Week (third week in May) – surgeries and health centres should emphasize and utilize it.

Within a practice, no breastfed baby should be discharged from midwife care until he has regained his birthweight on breast milk alone.

Initial and sustained breastfeeding is a baby's birthright; the more it is achieved, the better the health of the nation.

Other resources

Keeping Abreast. Newsletter of the National Network of Breastfeeding Coordinators. 113 Hindes Road, Harrow HA1 1RS.

National Childbirth Trust. Breastfeeding promotion group. London W3 6NH.

La Leche League. BM 3424, London WC1N 3XX.

Association of Breastfeeding Mothers. 26 Holmshaw Close, London SE26 4TH.

Infant Feeding Specialist Group. Tel: 01372 745266 or 01865 221695.

References

Ahn, C. H. and MacLean, W. C. (1980). Growth of the exclusively breastfed infant. *American Journal of Clinical Nutrition,* 33, 183–92.

Ajusi, J. D., Onyango, F. E., Mutanda, L. N., *et al.* (1989). Bacteriology of unheated breast-milk stored at room temperature. *East African Medical Journal,* 66, 381–7.

Alexander, J. (1990). Antenatal preparation of the breast for breastfeeding. In: *Antenatal care: a research-based approach* (ed. J. Alexander, V. Levy, and S. Roch). Macmillan Education, London.

Alexander, J., Grant, A., and Campbell, M. (1992). Randomized controlled trial of breast shells and Hoffman's exercises for inverted and non-protractile nipples. *British Medical Journal,* 304, 1030–2.

Almroth, S. G. (1978). Water requirements of breastfed babies in a hot climate. *American Journal of Clinical Nutrition,* 31, 1154–7.

Almroth, S. and Bidinger, P. D. (1990). No need for water supplementation for exclusively breastfed infants under hot and arid conditions. *Transactions of the Royal Society of Tropical Medicine and Hygiene,* 84, 602–4.

Alper, J. C. (1983). Moist wound healing under a vapour-permeable membrane. *Journal of the American Academy of Dermatology,* 8(3).

Amir, L. (1991). *Candida* and the lactating breast: predisposing factors. *Journal of Human Lactation,* 7(4), 177–81.

Anon (1988). Current concepts and approaches to wound healing. *Critical Care Medicine,* 16(9).

Armelini, P. A. and Gonzalez, C. F. (1979). Breastfeeding and fluid intake in a hot climate. *Clinical Pediatrics,* 18, 425–6.

Arneil, G. and Stroud, C. (1984). Infant feeding. In: *Textbook of paediatrics Vol. 1* (3rd edn) (ed. J. O. Forfar and G. Arneil), pp. 259–77. Churchill Livingstone, Edinburgh.

Ashraf, R. N., Jalil, F., Aperia, A., and Lindblad, B. S. (1993). Additional water is not needed for healthy babies in a hot climate. *Acta Paediatrica,* 82, 1007–11.

Bandolier (1996). *Journal of Evidence-based Medicine* (Oxford and Anglia Region), 3(2), 24.

Barger and Bull (1987). A comparison of the bacterial composition of breast milk stored at room temperature and stored in the refrigerator. *International Journal of Childbirth Education,* August, 29–30.

Berkow, S., Freed, L., Hamosh, M., *et al.* (1984). Lipases and lipids in human milk: effects of freeze-thawing and storage. *Pediatric Research,* 18, 1257–62.

Bertrand, H. and Rosenblood, L. K. (1991). Stripping out pus in lactational mastitis: a means of preventing breast abscess. *Canadian Medical Association Journal*, **145**(4), 299–306.

Borresen, H. C. (1995). Rethinking current recommendations to introduce solid food between four and six months to exclusively breastfeeding infants. *Journal of Human Lactation*, **11**(3), 201–4.

British Paediatric Association (1994). Guidelines for the establishment and operation of human milk banks in the UK. BPA, London.

Brown, K. H., Creed de Kanashiro, H., Aguila, R., *et al.* (1986). Milk consumption and hydration status of exclusively breastfed infants in a warm climate. *Journal of Pediatrics*, **108**(1), 677–80.

Butte, N., Garza, C., O'Brian Smith, E., and Nichols, B. (1984). Human milk intake and growth in exclusively breastfed infants. *Journal of Pediatrics*, **104**, 187–95.

Campbell, C. (1996). Breastfeeding and health in the western world. *British Journal of General Practice*, **46**, 613–17.

Cant, A. J., Bailes, J. A., Marsden, R. A., and Hewitt, D. (1986). Effect of maternal dietary exclusion on breastfed infants with eczema: two controlled studies. *British Medical Journal*, **293**, 231–3.

Carvahlo, M., Hall, M., and Harvey, D. (1981). Effects of water supplementation on physiological jaundice in breastfed babies. *Archives of Diseases in Childhood*, **56**, 568–9.

Chavasse, J. (1906). *Advice to mothers* (16th edn). J. & A. Churchill, London.

Chetley, A. (1986). *The politics of babyfood – successful challenges to an international marketing strategy.* Francis Pinter (in which he quotes the WHO's provisional summary record of the 8th meeting of Committee A, 33rd World Health Assembly: Document No. A33/A SR/8; Geneva, 17th May 1980, p.11.

Cohen, R. J., Brown, K. H., Canahuati, J., Rivera, L. L., and Dewey, K. G. (1994). Effects of age on introduction of complementary foods on infant breast milk intake, total energy intake, and growth: a randomized intervention study in Honduras. *Lancet*, **343**(8918), 288–93.

Cowie, A. T., Forsyth, I. A., and Hart, I. C. (1980). *Hormonal control of lactation.* Springer Verlag, Berlin.

Crawford, J. (1992). Understanding our own breastfeeding experiences. *JBL Newsletter* no. 4, 1st June, 1–2.

Dearlove, J. and Dearlove, B. (1981). Prolactin, fluid balance, and lactation. *British Journal of Obstetrics and Gynaecology*, **88**, 652–4.

de Chateau, P., Holmberg, H., Jakobsson, K., and Winberg, J. (1977). A study of factors promoting and inhibiting lactation. *Developmental Medicine and Child Neurology*, **19**, 575–84.

Delgado, H., Marmtorell, R., and Klein, R. (1982). Nutrition, lactation, and birth interval components in rural Guatemala. *American Journal of Clinical Nutrition*, **35**, 1468–76.

Department of Health (1994). *Weaning and the weaning diet.* Report: Health and Social Subjects no. 45. HMSO, London.

Department of Health (1995). *Breastfeeding: good practice guidance to the NHS.* 0573 2RP 34K. July 96 (12).

Dewdney, J. M. (1981). The effects of antibacterial antibiotics on immune reaction and host resistance to infection. In: *Immunological and clinical aspects of allergy* (ed. M. Lessof), pp. 407–27. MTP Press.

Dewey, K. G., Lovelady, C. A., Nommsen-Rivers, L. A., *et al.* (1994). A randomized study of the effects of aerobic exercise by lactating women on breast milk volume and composition. *New England Journal of Medicine*, 330(7), 449–53.

Dixon, J. M. (1988) Repeated aspiration of breast abscesses in lactating women. *British Medical Journal*, 297, 1517–18.

Dixon, J. M. (1994). ABC of breast diseases: breast infection. *British Medical Journal*, 309, 946–8.

Dusdieker, L., Booth, B., Stumbo, P., and Eichenberger, J. (1985). Effects of supplemental fluids on human milk production. *Journal of Pediatrics*, 105, 207–11.

Enkin, M., Keirse, M., Renfrew, M., and Neilson, J. (1995). *A guide to effective care in pregnancy and childbirth* (2nd edn). Oxford University Press, Oxford.

Evans, R., Fergusson, D., Allardyce, R., and Taylor, B. (1981). Maternal diet and infantile colic in breastfed babies. *Lancet*, i, 1340–2.

Fenstein, J., Berkelhamer, J., Gruszka, M., *et. al.* (1986). Factors related to early termination of breastfeeding in an urban population. *Pediatrics*, 78(2), 210–15.

Fisher, C. and Inch, S. (1996). Nipple confusion – who is confused? *Journal of Pediatrics*, 129(1), 174–5.

Forsyth, D. (1913). Breastfeeding: the consumption of breast milk. *Lancet*, 14th June, 1656–7.

Foster, K., Lader, D., and Cheesbrough, S. (1997). *Infant feeding 1995*. The Stationery Office, London.

Goldberg, N. M. and Adams, E. (1983). Supplementary water for breastfed babies in a hot and dry climate – not really a necessity. *Archives of Diseases in Childhood*, 58, 73–4.

Herrera, A. J. (1984). Supplemented versus unsupplemented breastfeeding. *Perinatology–Neonatology*, 8, 70–1.

Hitchcock, N. E., Gracey, M., and Owles, E. N. (1981). Growth of healthy breastfed infants in the first six months. *Lancet*, 2, 64–5.

Howie, P., *et al.* (1990). Protective effect of breastfeeding against infection. *British Medical Journal*, 300, 11–16.

Illingworth, P. J., Jong, R. T., Howie, P. W., *et al.* (1986). Diminution in energy expenditure during lactation. *British Medical Journal*, 292, 437–41.

Illingworth, R. S. and Kilpatrick, B. (1953). Lactation and fluid intake. *Lancet*, ii, 1175–7.

Inch, S. (1987). Difficulties with breastfeeding: midwives in disarray? *Journal of the Royal Society of Medicine*, 80, 53–7.

Inch, S. (1989). Antenatal preparation for breastfeeding. In: *Effective care in pregnancy and childbirth* (ed. I. Chalmers, M. Enkin, and M. J. N. C. Keirse). Oxford University Press, Oxford.

Inch, S. (1991). *Oxford Infant Feeding Survey*. Available from the Breastfeeding Clinic, Level 5, Women's Centre, Oxford Radcliffe Hospital, Headington, Oxford OX3 9DU.

Inch, S. and Fisher, C. (1995). Mastitis: infection or inflammation? *Practitioner*, **239**, 472–5.

Inch, S. and Garforth, S. (1989). *Establishing and maintaining breastfeeding*. Oxford University Press, Oxford.

Inch, S. and Renfrew, M. J. (1989). Common breastfeeding problems. In: *Effective care in pregnancy and childbirth* (ed. I. Chalmers, M. Enkin, and M. J. N. C. Keirse). Oxford University Press, Oxford.

Jacobsson, I. and Linberg, T. (1983). Cows' milk proteins cause infantile colic in breastfed infants: a double-blind crossover study. *Pediatrics*, **71**(2), 268–71.

Jensen, R. and Jensen, G. (1992). Speciality lipids for infant nutrition. I. Milks and formulas. *Journal of Paediatric Gastroenterology and Nutrition*, **15**, 232–45.

King, F. T. (1913). *Feeding and care of the baby*, p.36. Society for the Health of Women and Children, London.

King, M. T. (1934). *Mothercraft*. Whitcombe and Tombs Ltd, Sydney and Melbourne.

Lang, S. (1996). *Breastfeeding special care babies*. Baillière Tindall, London.

Langmead, F. (1916). Breastfeeding. In : *Mothercraft*, p.74. The National League for Physical Education, London.

Larson *et al.* (1984). Storage of human breast milk. *Infection Control*, **5**, 127–30.

Liddiard, M. (1924–1954). *The mothercraft manual*. J. & A. Churchill, London.

Lucassen, P. L. B. J., Assendelft, W. J. J., Gubbels, J. W., van Eijk, J. T. M., van Geldrop, W. J., and Knuistingh Neven, A. (1998). *British Medical Journal*, **316**, 1563–9.

MAIN Trial Collaborative Group (1994). Preparing for breastfeeding: treatment of inverted nipples and non-protractile nipples in pregnancy. *Midwifery*, **10**, 200–14.

Marshall, B. R., Hepper, J. K., and Zirbel, C. C. (1975). Sporadic puerperal mastitis: an infection that need not interrupt lactation. *Journal of the American Medical Association*, **233**(13), 1377–9.

Matheson, I., Aursnes, I., Horgen, M., Aabo, O., and Melby, K. (1988). Bacteriological findings and clinical symptoms in relation to clinical outcome in puerperal mastitis. *Acta Obstetrica et Gynecologica Scandinavica*, **67**, 723–6.

Metcalf, I. J., Irons, T. G., Lawrence, D. S., and Young, P. C. (1994). Simethicone in the treatment of infant colic: a randomized, placebo-controlled, multicentre trial. *Pediatrics*, **94**, 29–34.

MIMMS (Monthly Index of Medical Specialities), September 1994, p.248.

Moon, J. L. and Humenick, S. S. (1989). Breast engorgement: contributing variables and variables amenable to nursing intervention. *Journal of Obstetrical, Gynaecological and Neonatal Nursing*, **18**, 309–15.

Morley, R., Abbott, K. A., and Lucas, A. (1977). *Child: Care, Health and Development*, **23**(6), 475–8.

Myles, M. (1956). *Textbook for midwives* (2nd edn), p.490. Livingstone Ltd, Edinburgh and London.

Neifert, M., Lawrence, R., and Seacat, J. (1995). Nipple confusion: towards a formal definition. *Journal of Pediatrics*, **126**, 5125–9.

New Generation (1982). 'Blocked ducts' and 'blocked ducts revisited'. *New Generation*, 1(1), 16–17 and 1(4), 16–19.

Newton, M. (1950). Breast abscess as a result of lactation failure. *Surgical and Gynecological Obstetrics*, **91**, 651–5.

Nicoll, A., Ginsburg, R., and Tripp, J. (1982). Supplementary feeding and jaundice in newborns. *Acta Paediatrica Scandinavica*, **71**, 759–61.

Nwanko, M. U., *et al.* (1988). Bacterial growth in expressed breast milk. *Annals of Tropical Pediatrics*, **8**, 92–5.

Olowe, J. A., *et al.* (1987). Bacteriological quality of raw human milk: effect of storage in a refrigerator. *Annals of Tropical Paediatrics*, **7**, 233–7.

Olsen, A. (1940). Nursing under conditions of thirst or excessive ingestion of fluids. *Acta Obstetrica et Gynecologica Scandinavica*, **20**, 313–43.

Palmer, G. (1988). *The politics of breastfeeding*. Pandora Press, Allen & Unwin, London.

Patterson, D. and Smith, J. F. (1926–1955). *Modern methods of feeding in infancy (and childhood)* (10 edns). Constable & Co. Ltd, London.

Pittard, W. B., *et al.* (1985). Bacteriostatic qualities of human milk. *Journal of Pediatrics*, **107**, 240–3.

Prentice, A., Whitehead, R., and Roberts, S. (1983). Dietary supplementation of lactating Gambian women. 1. Effect on breast milk volume and quantity. *Human Nutrition and Clinical Nutrition*, **37**(c), 53–64.

Pritchard, E. L. (1904). *The physiological feeding of infants*. Henry Kimpton, London.

Ross, S., Loening, W., and van Middlekoop, A. (1983). Breastfeeding – evaluation of a health education programme. *SA Medlese Tydskrif Deel*, **64**, 356–62.

Sachdev, H. P., Krishna, J., Puri, R., *et al.* (1991). Water supplementation in exclusively breastfed infants during summer in the Tropics. *Lancet*, **337**(8747), 929–33.

Salariya, E. M. and Robertson, C. M. (1993). The development of a neonatal stool colour comparator. *Midwifery*, **9**, 35–40.

Sarjeant, H. (1905). *Hints for infant feeding*, p.4. Elliot Stock, London.

Sosa, R. and Barness, L. (1987). Bacterial growth in refrigerated human milk. *American Journal of Diseases in Childhood*, **141**, 111–12.

Spector, W. G. and Willoughby, D. A. (1974). *Inflammation: useful and non-useful*. *Folia traumatologica*, p.15. Ciba-Geigy Ltd, Switzerland.

Thomsen, A. C., Espersen, T., and Maigaard, S. (1984). Course and treatment of milk stasis, non-infectious inflammation of the breast, and infectious mastitis in nursing women. *American Journal of Obstetrics and Gynecology*, **149**(5), 492–5.

Ueda, T., Yokoyama, Y., Irahara, M., and Aona, T. (1994). Influence of psychological stress on suckling-induced pulsatile oxytocin release. *Obstetrics and Gynaecology*, **84**, 259–62.

Vincent, R. (1904). *The nutrition of the infant*. Baillière, Tindall, and Cox, London.

von Kries, R., Shearer, M., McCarthy, P., *et. al.* (1987). Vitamin K1 content of maternal milk: influence of the stage of lactation, lipid composition, and vitamin K1 supplements given to the mother. *Paediatric Research*, **22**, 513–17.

Weaver, L. T., Ewing, G., and Taylor, L. C. (1988). The bowel habits of milk-fed infants. *Journal of Pediatric Gastroenterology and Nutrition*, **7**, 568–71.

White, A., Freeth, S., and O'Brien, M. (1992). *Infant feeding 1990*. OPCS Social Survey Division, HMSO, London.

Whitehead, R., Paul, A., Black, A., and Wiles, S. (1981). Recommended dietary amounts of energy for pregnancy or lactation in the UK. In: *Protein energy requirement of developing countries – evaluation of new data* (ed. B. Torun, V. Young, and W. Rang), pp.259–65. United Nations University, Tokyo.

Winter, G. D. and Scales, J. T. (1963). The effect of air drying and dressings on the surface of a wound. *Nature*, **5 Jan.**, 91–2.

Woolridge, M. (1986). The aetiology of sore nipples. *Midwifery*, **2**, 172–6.

Woolridge, M. W. and Fisher, C. (1998). Colic 'overfeeding' and symptoms of lactose malabsorption in the breastfed baby: a possible artifact of feed management? *Lancet*, **ii**, 382–4.

Further reading

Alexander, J., Levy, V., and Roch, S. (eds.) *Midwifery Practice* series: *Antenatal care* and *Postnatal care* (research-based information on breastfeeding). Macmillan Education, London.

Breast or bottle? A pair of leaflets for pregnant women and health professionals. MIDIRS & the NHS Centre for Reviews and Dissemination.

Renfrew, M. J., Fisher, C., and Arms, S. (1990). *Bestfeeding: getting breastfeeding right for you*. Celestial Arts, California. Available from Airlift Books, London.

Renfrew, M. J., Ross McGill, H., and Woolridge, M. W. (1998). *Enabling women to breast feed – a review of the evidence*. The Stationery Office, London.

Royal College of Midwives (1991). *Successful breastfeeding* (2nd edn). Churchill Livingstone, London.

Royal College of Midwives comparison chart (breast milk compared with alternatives). Available from the Royal College of Midwives (Welsh Board) Brandy Cove Suite, Henley House, Queensway, Fforestfach, Swansea, SA5 4EL.

Videos

Breast is best (from Norway). BMA, 23, St Andrew's St, Cambridge, CB2 3AX.

Breastfeeding: coping with the first week. (1996). Mark-It TV, Bristol BS12 6UX.

Breastfeeding: dealing with the problems. (1977). Mark-It TV, Bristol BS12 6UX.

Helping a mother to breastfeed – no finer investment. (1990). Healthcare Productions Ltd, London SE1 8EN.

Note: We acknowledge that babies are either male or female, but as all mothers are female, we have, for the sake of clarity, referred to the baby as he or him throughout.

SECTION FIVE

CONCLUSIONS

CHAPTER TWENTY-FIVE

Community-based maternity care in the new millennium

Geoffrey N. Marsh and Mary J. Renfrew

Working on this book has been a major learning exercise for us. As we read the chapters that our contributors sent, we found that we learned much that was new to us about developments in community-based maternity care. We have also benefited from our discussions and work with each other. The combination of perspectives of an experienced GP who has cared for nearly 2000 child-bearing women with an academic midwife who believes in the key role of midwifery in the community as well as the fundamental importance of evidence-based care was not always straightforward, but it was always valuable. We knew when we started out that this book would be for other people – principally midwives, GPs, and obstetricians. It became, also, a mind-expanding exercise for us.

Our enormous task for the next few pages is to try and distill the wisdom and analyses of our contributors – much of it new to us, some of it time-honoured, and some of it iconoclastic. From it, we will try to paint a picture of how maternity care could be, should be, and even perhaps will be in the early part of the third millennium. There will be no new references except to the relevant chapters in the book: each one is more than adequately referenced. In particular, we will try to highlight ideas and information that are important for GPs and midwives in everyday clinical practice; they will still be there long into the third millennium, and it is impossible to imagine maternity care without them. So in the future as the midwife and GP go to their health complex, surgery, or clinic, variably situated in skyscraper, supermarket, railway or bus terminal, suburban street, or market square, they will feel better armed to develop appropriate changes in their own setting. They will also be reinforced in their determination to preserve qualities and styles of care that they have practised possibly for years, which no amount of 'new thinking' can undermine or devalue. For our chapter contributors have emphasized the importance of retaining practices that work well, in addition to introducing new ones.

The mother, the midwife, and the GP

In Chapter 2, Gavin Young makes a strong case for maternity care which is based in the community, including a cogent case for home birth, if that is what women wish. He also emphasizes that care for the great majority of women will be at local, often small, health centres, frequently far away from hospitals and institutions, and usually close to their own homes and familiar to women. In the foreseeable future the great majority of women will no longer look to the hospital for their care before or after birth, and the choice to labour and give birth at home or in a local community-centre setting will be a real one.

In the remainder of the first section, we encouraged commentary on the roles of the four major participants in maternity care: the woman, the midwife, the GP, and the specialist obstetrician. We now analyse, review, and place our own emphasis on the varying important options and ideas that have been discussed.

Women themselves

All pregnant women would like their care to be as 'normal' as possible. Even women classed as 'abnormal' or having 'high-risk pregnancies' by clinicians would like most of their care in the community and would like their antenatal and postnatal care in a friendly and familiar setting. We believe that women with 'high-risk' pregnancies are just as much, if not more, in need of normal care from their local community-based primary maternity care team than their 'low-risk' sisters. Women with problems should not routinely be sent off to unknown specialists at distant and unfamiliar centres when they are already feeling vulnerable by being 'at risk'. Occasional visits will be necessary, of course, but their routine, personalized care should still be available for the most part in their community-based centre or in their own home.

Both Jo Garcia and Gavin Young (Chapters 6 and 2) emphasize that women want good communication which leads to clear understanding. They want attention to their emotional and psychological as well as their physical well-being. There is evidence that GPs and midwives are particularly good at providing this kind of care, which could be a major reason why they score so highly in the 'satisfaction stakes'.

Continuity of care throughout pregnancy by the same people who know each other, respect each other, and say the same things is much appreciated and we anticipate an even greater emphasis on this in the years ahead. Attention to the common, distressing though not life-threatening illnesses of pregnancy (Chapter 20) with reassurance, comfort, and even cure from a GP or midwife who women know will continue to be an important concept in the future.

Jo Garcia (Chapter 6) finds that women want their GP involved in their maternity care. A minimal scenario for the millennium should be the choice of continuity of care by GP, midwife, and health visitor, all of whom the woman knows. This is the fundamental primary maternity care team. In the more comprehensive and elaborate teams discussed later, continuity of care will need careful organization.

In an era of increasing emphasis on the need for women to make informed choices we must remember, as Jo Garcia notes in Chapter 6, that some women prefer and are happy with care-givers making decisions for them. The commonly posed question 'what do *you* advise?' to midwives or doctors still occurs frequently and seems sensible, even if currently thought old-fashioned. Is it not reasonable that many women demur from taking too much responsibility for decisions about their care? We may prefer it if women are more active in making decisions and seeking information, but asking their care-givers to advise their decisions should be respected as some women's choice.

Gavin Young emphasizes that despite his 'heresy' regarding safety not being the be all and end all of maternity care, we must not, as professional carers, be lulled into taking safety for granted. It requires high clinical standards and constant vigilance. New problems and threats will emerge in the future and women will expect high-standard clinical responses from their carers. New tests and therapies will be discovered and if their use is evidence based, women will expect to be offered them. Women expect safety to be given the highest priority.

Midwives for the millennium

It is apparent from Chapter 3 that midwives are now autonomous professionals and have the respect of their colleagues. This has resulted firstly from a long-continued respect by GPs who have always been aware of midwives' quality care at home births, even in an era when technology was rampant and hospitalization for drips and monitors was becoming routine. Secondly, respect has flowed from mothers (and often their partners) who knew who was 'really' there and was tending them through virtually every labour, be it normal or abnormal. Thirdly, it has come from specialist obstetricians who, with approximately 90% of labouring women in their delivery suites, realized that without midwives to take responsibility for around 70–80% of them, they would be lost. Finally, it has come from Government committees and working parties and the Royal Colleges in documents repeatedly referenced in many of the chapters in this book.

Midwifery care has been changing and developing as the role has developed over the years. There is a decreasing emphasis on ritual and traditional practices and an increasing awareness of the need to base care on the needs of the individual woman and baby, and on knowledge derived from research. Midwives have tried hard to find ways of offering more continuity of care to women, working in small teams, or offering one-to-one care, or working as independent midwives. Sadly, it has been the case that striving to achieve continuity of carer through pregnancy and birth has sometimes resulted in workload problems for midwives and a decline in postnatal care. Organizing continuity of care for large numbers of women is a continuing challenge as we seek to find ways of offering women appropriate care that suits their needs, is locally available, and is sustainable and cost-effective. Research is still needed to help assess the best ways of organizing services, especially for women with special needs.

As midwifery care has developed and changed, so has midwifery education. Recent years have seen the move of midwifery education into universities and the development of direct-entry degrees. This move should be welcomed as it enhances the opportunities for midwives to learn in a questioning environment and to use information resources to the full, and it also offers opportunities for multidisciplinary education. Midwives working in the community have a crucial role in education as direct-entry programmes increasingly encourage students' early clinical experience to be based in the community.

So the future looks good for midwives – they have been empowered and we see them firmly in the maternity driving seat in the next millennium. But as they take over most antenatal and postnatal care, continue to be responsible for about 80% of births – up to 10% of which may be at home by the year 2010 – we must guard against euphoria or complacency. Other people will continue to have roles in the child-bearing process, and some of these will develop further. The woman herself, of course, will largely ordain her own care – 'the prime carer for the pregnant woman and her unborn baby is the woman herself' (Keirse). Her partner may wish to be involved and can have a fundamentally important role. The general practitioner has a psychosocial expertise with families and a long-continued knowledge of the mother and ultimately the baby, and expertise in diagnosing and treating pathology in pregnancy and after birth (Chapter 20). There is evidence in Chapter 4 , for example, that transfer rates to specialist care are less if GPs are involved. And midwives will need to continue to work closely with the small cadre of trained GP obstetricians as well as specialist obstetricians so that they refer readily and promptly when normal pregnancy, labour, or the puerperium go awry. Midwives will need an increasingly flexible attitude to the involvement of health visitors whose expert knowledge of health promotion, health education, and baby care is likely to be greater than their own. And finally, lay groups and other professionals – breastfeeding counsellors, psychologists, and physiotherapists – all have expertise to offer. The more confident and competent the midwife, the more she will wish to use the help of others. So it becomes apparent that in some form or another, there is a need for teamwork.

Teamwork

There are so many different professionals needed in many contrasting settings – from inner cities to leafy suburbia, from town high streets to remote rural areas. So their ways of working together, coordinating care, eradicating duplication, and avoiding contradictions will vary too. The organization of comprehensive and effective teamwork will be and should be different from setting to setting. Tony Dowell and Helene Price (Chapter 5) remind us that the primary care team based in a general practice has been evolving since 1968 at least, and the majority of women in the UK receive their care from members of this team. They highlight the variations and emphasize the effective characteristics of any multidisciplinary team. Variety will be the spice of life for teams in the new millennium; there is not, nor ever should be, a single blueprint for the maternity care team. However, we do believe that the isolated professional working alone, or the single professional group (be they all midwives, all GPs, or all specialists), will have too narrow a focus for the needs of their clients. We reiterate the paradox – the greater the knowledge of a professional carer, the more he or she will realize how much they depend on professionals from other disciplines in order to meet the total needs of the child-bearing woman. As well as offering more comprehensive care, contact with colleagues from disciplines other than their own will be a learning experience, widening their perspectives and adjusting the relative importance of what needs to be done.

So we anticipate multidisciplinary teams, with a varied composition depending on local needs and circumstances, as the caring groups of the future. There is evidence in Chapter 5 that women themselves value different professionals working together. The team may be simply the woman, her family (if that is what she wishes), a midwife, a GP, and a health visitor – the primary maternity care team – in a remote, rural area, but even this small team is likely to have computer links to their fellow team members many miles away. Alternatively, it may be a complex primary maternity care team including the woman, her partner, her family, the midwife, the GP, health visitor, obstetrician, family planning nurse, physiotherapist, social worker, counsellor, community psychiatric nurse, dietitian, practice nurse, complementary medical therapists, manager/administrator, research assistant, audit clerk, records managers, secretary, receptionist, and lay personnel such as National Childbirth Trust teachers and breastfeeding counsellors (and students of all these groups). Increasingly, they will work with electronic links with each other and with laboratory and diagnostic services.

The midwife, as well as being the prime carer, will be a major coordinator of her multidisciplinary team. Her work volume and relative importance to individual women will usually be considerably greater than that of the other team members; she will be the major carer. She will be cognisant and respectful of the skills and knowledge of others. Much of her role will be unique to her and her midwife colleagues but she will need to know when to involve her other professional colleagues. Her work as coordinator will be considerable and will overlap with the erstwhile coordinator, the general practitioner.

General practitioners

A thousand and one anecdotes and the evidence from Lindsay Smith and David Jewell in Chapter 4 suggest that GPs are giving up, and in many areas have already given up, maternity care almost completely. They 'leave it to the midwife', say 'she [the midwife] is the expert', and that they are 'too busy', 'too tired', 'out of date', 'not interested', 'no facilities', and 'the money isn't worth it' – these are the messages in Chapter 4. Yet many people are convinced that there is an important role for GPs. The role of the midwife is now clearly defined and developing effectively. This section on the role of the GP will be longer as we try and work out what the role of the GP could and should be in the coming years.

There can be, and frequently is, an important relationship between patients and their GPs. One of the special characteristics of the health care system in the United Kingdom – noted particularly by American visitors – is that virtually everybody knows the name of 'their' GP and where he or she practices. There is a tradition of personal doctoring – albeit under strain in many large and inner-city practices – that runs deep in British society, and is possibly especially noticeable when a woman is pregnant. It is considered to be perfectly normal at present that when a woman is pregnant, particularly for the first time, she usually goes first to her GP to tell her. The GP may well have provided several years of care, perhaps even the whole of her lifetime to date. The care could well have included, for example, menstrual problems, sexual anxieties, cervical smears, contraception, gynaecological problems, anxieties about fertility, and preconception advice, all of which are relevant to care in pregnancy. These may well be set against a background of consultations for the minor illnesses of childhood and teenage years. The GP has probably also cared for her other children and her partner, and knows her family circumstances. If this is the case, the doctor 'knows' the woman, and it seems logical to us that in such circumstances it is to the GP that the pregnancy should be made known if that is what the woman wishes; although of course it is appropriate also to talk first with the midwife, if women wish to do that.

The role of the GP in antenatal care

Many GPs are, and increasingly will be, signposts to the team of fellow professionals that surround them. The midwife will of course become involved immediately and will become the major carer during the pregnancy and after the birth (we will consider intranatal care later). But the GP cannot abandon her interest in the woman or her pregnancy. There is still, for example, a need for a general physical examination and knowledge and understanding of how previous illnesses and history of family problems might impact on the woman's physical and emotional well-being. Midwives are not expected to detect heart murmurs nor understand the relevance of the latest asthma therapy in pregnancy, nor will they know necessarily, as their GP may do, of any psychosocial or psychosexual problems in the mother's background which may impact significantly on her health and well-being. And even for the large majority of women who are perfectly healthy and have a normal family background, there may be a desire that their GP be involved in their care (see Chapters 2 and 6). If we support women's choice, there is evidence that many women will choose to have their GPs involved in their maternity care.

We believe that there is often a 'special relationship' between the pregnant woman and her GP – just as there is between her and her midwife – that needs to be respected. It is, of course, more difficult in large, urban practices where the population is more mobile and where people are often seen by a number of different GPs. But in circumstances where such care is possible – and even in adverse situations it can be achieved – this relationship should be respected and encouraged.

There is no doubt that the month by month and week by week routine care, reduced to a more efficient and cost-effective system as Marion Hall and Janet Tucker suggest in Chapter 19, will be coordinated and carried out by a midwife. It is likely that structured attendance – 'structured' because it is more likely to take place – will continue to be a fundamental component of good general practice and good maternity care. How often visits with the GP should take place in addition to visits with the midwife will vary according to the individual needs and wishes of each woman, her midwife, and her GP, but for the majority of normal women we would suggest one visit in the first trimester, another in the second, and one or two in the third. For women with problems, and especially those who require hospital-based specialist care, the number of GP attendances may be much greater. Thus the 'special relationship' will flourish and a psychosocial bond be effected that will strengthen the GP's care of the mother, her partner, the baby, and their family, possibly for many years.

GPs also need to know about the progress of the woman's pregnancy because being pregnant does not preclude coincidental or pregnancy-related illness. Chapter 20, on illnesses women experience in pregnancy, is written appropriately by three GPs and a midwife. We believe it to be essential that the GP who attends a pregnant woman who is sick has had some contact with her before the illness developed. The GP in his or her surgery, at the health complex, 'night centre', or in the woman's home will need to comprehend the midwives' antenatal record and have sufficient general knowledge of antenatal care to be able to put her diagnosis and therapy into the appropriate context of the pregnancy. When the pregnant woman is sick, she turns to her doctor – it is a role unique to general practice.

Women who have had children already may make different choices about their care. Many multigravid women go straight to the midwife they know – they have met her in their previous pregnancy and they are aware of who is the major care provider. We believe that midwives should suggest that all multigravid women also see their general practitioner and encourage a system of structured antenatal attendances with the GP. We have suggested that three attendances is probably the minimum for the primigravid woman, and perhaps two would be a minimum for multigravid women.

Midwives are likely to welcome GP availability at antenatal sessions. The GP needs to be available for the diagnosis and treatment of the various illnesses that may present – urinary tract infections, upper respiratory tract infections, phlebitis, non-specific abdominal pain, difficult backache (see Chapter 20 for more) – but women will also welcome the support of informed and interested GPs regarding any anxieties that occur in their month by month care. The GP has a special expertise in tolerating, and temporizing over, the uncertain. The slightly different perspective that the GP and midwife have broadens each other's horizons.

Abandoning the stimulating psycho-socio-clinical challenges and opportunities for GPs in their involvement in antenatal care could ultimately have grave consequences for the whole of general practice. Maternity care is not unique in being multidisciplinary. Psychiatric and paediatric care are similarly structured specialties. If GPs are prepared to abandon antenatal and postnatal care entirely to midwives, health visitors, specialist obstetricians, and family planning nurses, is there not a parallel case to be made for the abandonment of psychiatric care to community psychiatric nurses, psychogeriatric nurses, psychologists, social workers, and psychiatrists, and paediatric care to paediatric nurses, health visitors, social workers, and community paediatricians?

The role of the GP after birth

To keep the GP in touch with normal progress and postnatal care, to help identify problems and to continue the relationship with the family and the new baby, a routine home visit to mother and baby soon after birth seems sensible. Even if the baby has been comprehensively examined in hospital, the GP will need to carry out a further check about six days after birth (Chapter 23). There are now a small number of programmes to train midwives to carry out this baby check, but the number of midwives trained is limited at present. Knowledge gained from such visits about the birth, the well-being of the mother and the baby, and the developing family relationships will stand the GP in good stead as the baby grows. Many women, and their partners, will also enjoy the opportunity to talk about the birth and their baby with their GP.

The role of the GP in labour and birth

We hope that in the new millennium the general practitioner who has been involved in the antenatal care and will be involved in the postnatal and later care of the family would make time to visit the woman in labour if she would like this and it is geographically feasible. No special obstetric expertise is needed – the support will be primarily psychosocial. It could take place at home (it will increasingly do so), in a midwife unit, or in a specialist hospital. It need not take long. Compared with many of the mundane 'home visits' and surgery consultations that a general practitioner undertakes, a brief attendance at the imminent arrival of a new person into the world with all the profound physiological processes and upheavals that are taking place is of far greater interest and importance. When attendance at the actual moment of birth takes place – either fortuitously or by design – there is an opportunity for sharing in a profound 'health moment' of both mother, father, and baby. Such events occur relatively infrequently in an average-sized practice and we believe the benefits of attendance are likely to be ample reward for the short time spent; and the antipathy that many midwives currently have towards their general practitioner colleagues may disappear once they appreciate the value of the GP's psychosocial supportive role. We emphasize that the midwife is in charge of the labour and the responsibilities for clinical care are hers so we have no medico-legal nightmares about the GP's psychosocial involvement. To pre-empt legal problems, the role can be clarified to the woman during the pregnancy.

There will remain a small number of general practitioners who wish to be more involved in childbirth and many of them will have a GP unit or GP beds in a consultant unit or be welcome at midwife-run units as informed and helpful clinical colleagues. But after studying Chapter 4, we feel that their numbers will be small and most GPs will have a psychosocial role only. But we respect it and commend its practice, and evaluation, in the new millenium.

Health visitors

Critics of this book will note that there is no chapter by a health visitor, nor one examining her work. The health visitor is, however, mentioned frequently in the chapters; she plays an essential part in maternity care, although her role is less central.

In the new millennium we would hope to see health visitors having the opportunity for routine consultations with all pregnant women, and that a more seamless handover from the midwife be developed. We strongly support variation in the organization of care between and within practices and teams, and believe that there will be a range of ways in which health visitors will be involved in different circumstances. The health visitor's special orientation on preventative care and health promotion, and her monitoring of the progress of the baby, needs no emphasis from us and we are sure this will continue. Health visitors are increasingly responding to needs by developing a flexible approach to the care they provide for different families – less care for some in order to provide time for more care for others. We have one special plea: that health visitors attend as much to the well-being of women in their routine 'baby' clinics as they do to babies. Women are the primary care-givers for their babies and if they are well cared for it is likely that they will be helped to care well for their babies. Baby clinics are a valuable opportunity for routine contact with women. Some health visitors already use their clinics to assess the health of both mother and baby, but more could be done to use this opportunity to address women's emotional well-being, including organizing mother-to-mother support (Chapter 18) and providing support for breastfeeding women (Chapter 24). The number of women not starting to breastfeed, or discontinuing soon after birth, is unacceptably high. Health visitors could have a crucial role in improving that.

Specialist obstetricians

Obstetricians are much less likely now to wish to embrace the whole of maternity care as they see and appreciate the quality of care provided by midwives in hospital and in the community, and by the primary maternity care team. Accordingly, and the case is made in Chapter 5, specialist obstetricians are increasingly unlikely to see women without complications unless women wish this, and they will be able to give more care to women with clinical problems. This will justify their expertise and provide the clinical satisfaction that any specialist seeks and should expect from his or her work. Women will be referred directly from the midwife or GP, and ideally from both working together. One of the major aims of obstetric care will be to work towards returning the woman to normal care by midwife and GP, if this is possible. The congestion at specialist antenatal clinics which caused such difficulty for women in the 1970s, '80s and early '90s is resolving as antenatal care is increasingly carried out in the community. But once women are referred to hospital clinics with a problem, they are rarely transferred back out of the system, even though their 'problems' may have been found to be of little significance or have been resolved. Instead, once discharged back to community care, guidelines for re-referral should be part of the expertise of good specialist care. The specialist obstetrician in the new millennium should be running small clinics attended by skillfully selected women with major problems for whom he or she can provide ample time and exemplary care. Such care may not necessarily be provided in the hospital – we have been encouraged by the mention in the book of outreach clinics provided by obstetricians to provide secondary care in the community.

Contemporary issues

In Chapter 7, Peter Selman and Erica Haimes discussed our rapidly changing society, and we see no reason for believing that things are going to slow down. All midwives and GPs know – their day-to-day consultations already make it very apparent – that mum, dad, and children are no longer the 'normal family'. That family still exists and it should be respected, preserved, and promoted if possible. It is still probably the most common family unit in British society, but the recent statistics have highlighted the increasing occurrence of other family types or family units. Marital and cohabitation breakdown has become the norm. Whether or not such instability is a 'good thing', all the people involved, adults and children, need support and not critical value judgements.

Partly as a result of trying to sustain the financial viability of the family, working mothers have also become a norm. In addition, the majority of women regard an occupation or career outside the home as theirs by right, and often defer child-bearing until they have spent several years working. This is set in the hostile social context, however, of sparse and expensive child-care provision, and of meagre financial support around pregnancy and after birth (Chapter 7). Single women, especially, find it almost impossible to find or to keep jobs where they can afford to pay for good-quality child care. And the under-16s appear to have virtually no maternity rights – this group urgently needs more thought, attention, and support. The concept that they are 'the family's responsibility', although perhaps understandable in principle, frequently does not materialize in practical terms. Midwives and GPs need to plan care provision particularly carefully and in a very holistic way for these often troubled, teenage pregnant girls. The midwife is likely to need the support of all the relevant members of the multidisciplinary maternity care team, including GPs, social workers, health visitors, and family planning nurses. The number of routine antenatal attendances should probably also be increased rather than decreased with this group, despite the often very normal clinical progress of the pregnancy. In our future plan for comprehensive care, the psychosocial and economic needs of this group need particular attention. Mary Hepburn includes them in Chapter 12 as 'women with special needs' and we wholeheartedly agree with her assessment of their difficulties and needs.

In parallel with this, one of the major challenges for the primary health care team, and especially for the GP, midwife, and family planning nurse, is the prevention of unwanted teenage pregnancies. Studies described by Selman and Haimes in Chapter 7 suggest that most teenage pregnancies are unwanted and, importantly, that non-use of contraception is not primarily one of poor motivation. So GP-based contraception is currently not reaching this group. Family planning aimed at and getting to teenagers is vital. This includes the ready availability of the 'morning-after pill'. Michael Maresh in Chapter 9 suggests that the prevention of teenage pregnancy is an eminently suitable topic for audit in a general practice. This is a challenge that, if met, would bring enormous benefits and happiness to individual young people, their parents, the maternity services, and society as a whole. As an obvious entree to the provision of formal contraception, such advice should be a high priority at postnatal clinics, post-abortion checks, and following requests for the morning-after pill. There is also a need for requests for such prescriptions to be handled appropriately by receptionists, who should be seen as members of the multidisciplinary team.

Another high-risk group, albeit often with clinically normal pregnancies, are lone parents. Their numbers are increasing and they especially need a multidisciplinary, holistic, team approach as they deal with the emotional, psychosocial, and financial challenges of child-bearing and child-rearing without the support of a partner.

For couples who wish to have children but who have problems conceiving, the GP will also need to have a comprehensive knowledge of 'fertility problems' and, as importantly, 'fertility solutions'. She will need to know which services are available locally and regionally and whether they are NHS-funded or private. GPs may wish to use their own counselling skills or request specialist help from trained counsellor colleagues who are increasingly present in multidisciplinary primary health care teams. Couples' needs will vary; some will ultimately be successful in achieving a pregnancy but others will remain on prolonged, NHS-funded waiting lists, and there will always be increasingly anguished childless couples who have to face painful decisions about whether or not to discontinue treatment.

Sara Twaddle and Denise Young make a convincing case that there is not a great deal of evidence to support radical changes in programmes and personnel in maternity care for reasons of cost. It is indeed startling how little is known about the cost of NHS maternity care. Care must go on in the meantime, however, and decisions need to be made about the organization of services in the absence of complete data on costs. We have identified the small areas of evidence-based change that could be made almost immediately – indeed, many are probably being made already. More adventurously, we have looked for straws in the wind and tried to make some reasonable guesses. We feel somewhat supported in this by the fact that many of the conventional routines and practices of present-day maternity care have never been examined cost-effectively. So, within reason, it would be permissible to move to another system which appears less expensive so long as it did not worsen clinical outcomes.

As a generalization it seems to us that antenatal care is cheaper when delivered away from institutions. This reflects the spirit of our book: community-based, relatively small, health complexes and centres near women's homes. The objection that fixed hospital costs may not change immediately is cogent, but if community-based care proves satisfactory, and we believe it will, then within the first decade of the new millennium looms the possibility of the contraction of hospital buildings and the move of staff into the community.

With regard to the recent trend – very variably implemented – of reducing the number of antenatal attendances by women to their carers, we are unsure, as are Sara Twaddle and Denise Young, about the answer to their question 'is the reduction in cost worth the reduction in psychological outcomes?' However, they reference only one study that found that there was a deterioration in psychological outcomes so the case is not conclusively proved. We believe a major challenge to a comprehensively community-based system of the future would be for midwives and GPs to be perceptive enough to identify women at risk of psychological problems and to offer an appropriate number of visits.

There is some evidence that much antenatal in-patient care for conditions such as hypertension, placenta praevia, and multiple pregnancies could be given by attentive midwives and GPs prepared to make home visits on a fairly frequent and coordinated basis. The use of the telephone and appropriate technologies (Chapter 19) in selected cases could make this easier. Selection of women for home-based care would not just be determined by the clinical condition but also the psychosocial issues with which the community midwife and GP would be familiar.

We are forced to conclude from Chapter 8 that home births are not necessarily cheaper; certainly until the proportion of them rises to levels which are probably unattainable. It seems that if women chose home births then the health service will cost more, though for the foreseeable future the small number of women having home births would make such increases in cost insignificant. There are no other grounds for restricting women's choice to give birth at home.

It seems clear that prophylactic antibiotics after Caesarian section reduce complications and cost; the decision to use these will rest usually with the specialist obstetrician, but primary care-givers will want to be sure that women are offered care that will reduce postnatal complications.

Earliest possible postnatal discharge from hospital of mother and baby would seem to us to be a way of reducing hospital running costs considerably and possibly, ultimately, capital costs. Care should be taken, however, to ensure that women who would benefit from a longer stay are not sent home prematurely. Some women will benefit from a longer stay in hospital, and decisions should be based on women's individual needs. Once home, the routine schedule of postnatal visits in the first 10 days should be questioned; many women will need less, others more. Flexibility of care in that 10-day period, with care tailored to individual need, is likely to prove cheaper than standard care for all women.

We support the view in Chapter 9 that audit, like care, should be woman centred. This will be an overriding principle in the new millennium. Having said that, we would emphasize, as do the chapter writers, that those undertaking audits must find them interesting. That the results can be readily implemented is another 'must'. At the more basic level, routine recording of care should be done in a way that lends itself to audit but, most important, the actual auditing should be done by 'auditors'. Such people are often called 'audit clerks' or even 'research assistants', and we would hope that by the year 2010 no large community-based health complex will be without them and that the budgets of such establishments should automatically include a sum for their payment.

There are many challenging ideas for audit in Chapter 9 but we are particularly supportive of audits of contraception and the prevention of unwanted pregnancy (especially in teenagers), breastfeeding, and postnatal depression. Such topics are rooted in the community and need community-based care.

It becomes clear to us from Jo Alexander and Lindsay Smith's chapter (Chapter 10) that unidisciplinary teaching has led to, and continues to lead to, unidisciplinary working. The philosophy of our book is community-based *multidisciplinary* care, so we applaud their arguments for the need for integrated, interprofessional education. The challenge for the educators of the new millennium is to provide medical students, GP registrars, student midwives, practising midwives, and GPs with multidisciplinary basic and postgraduate training. If a medical or nursing student graduates without having seen a baby born normally, for example, there will be a gap in her or his knowledge and experience and a sad unawareness of a profoundly important physiological process. One way of reinforcing this is for there to be consumer involvement, not only in the planning of teaching but also in its delivery. Consumers above all will demonstrate their multiple needs and hence the need for a multidisciplinary approach. That the training should be given by people working in the setting of integrated care goes without saying.

Such integration should eliminate the duplication of educational facilities and teachers (possible economies here) and the contradiction of ideas and practices that currently so commonly occur. It should lead to an under-standing of the differing philosophies of different carers. It should ultimately produce a seamless, holistic care.

We are encouraged by Lindsay Smith's evidence that exposure to GP maternity care is the best way of encouraging GPs in training to practise it later. However, we would go further. We feel that all GP registrars should try to attend a birth, especially a home birth, with their trainer, whether she is merely doing the more usual psychosocial support or is more deeply involved as a GP obstetrician. GP registrars may, as a result of this, wish to be present at the labour and perhaps occasionally the birth of women they care for where this is geographically feasible, and if women wish this.

Finally, we would agree that there needs to be a benchmark diploma set jointly by the Royal College of Obstetricians and the Royal College of General Practitioners – and we would also include the Royal College of Midwives – for GPs wishing to be fully involved in intranatal care.

Clinical challenges

The coexistence of multiple problems in the same women becomes apparent in Chapter 11 and is reinforced in Chapter 12 which considers women with special needs. Hence there is considerable overlap in these two chapters, not only about the problems faced but also the solutions proposed. We make no apology for this. We believe that overcoming the worsened 'maternity morbidity' arising from these problems is a major challenge of the third millennium. Chapter 12 makes depressing reading and is indeed a serious criticism of the 'achievements' of the 20th century. There are, of course, social and political dimensions to the solutions, but there are still clinical areas that only carers – and especially community-based carers – can overcome. Chapters 11 and 12 are full of suggestions and ideas and would form excellent starting points for multidisciplinary workshops.

Awareness of the problems is an important first step but Mary Hepburn states (Chapter 12) that we have been increasingly aware of inequalities in health for over 10 years and not a great deal has been done. GPs and midwives see the effects of social inequalities since these pervade all aspects of their care, and they are witness to the struggles of families to escape these. They are also aware of families that have just 'given up' and they know of those that have descended to dishonesty and criminal behavior as their solution.

Both chapters emphasize that the solution lies best in a multidisciplinary approach. No one carer can possibly embrace even an awareness of, never mind solutions to, the multiple problems that such women have. Paradoxically, although the care will need to be offered by many people, it needs to follow an individualized programme resulting from one-to-one discussion with a lead coordinating person. This 'lead carer' must be prepared to involve others and to undertake a managerial as well as a clinical role in the pregnancy. The midwife and possibly the GP are the people best situated to provide this, although flexibility of organization and provision of care may occasionally result in other people being the 'lead carer'. Good, up-to-date information is necessary regarding benefits, support groups, link workers, interpreters, and other forms of support. Chapters 11 and 12 outline this.

Vital to this kind of care is a non-judgemental attitude by all the carers. Implicit is the ability to listen, to note particularly the psychological needs and be well versed in counselling skills to meet these. It goes without saying that readers of this book will know firsthand how much effort and personal cost is involved in providing this care, often with frustratingly poor outcomes. But it must be done – providing high-quality care for women with special needs is vital.

A frequent sequel to these problems is the baby being born too soon and/or too small, and it is appropriate that Chapter 14 deals with that. Seventy one per cent of babies born at 26 weeks or less have a moderate to severe handicap compared with only about 5% at 30–32 weeks – this makes prolonging pregnancy a major challenge. But there are no easy answers and it is clear that a range of scientific advances are still necessary to support our goal of reducing preterm birth. Women in deprived circumstances, those who smoke, and those who have already had a preterm baby are most at risk. More frequent antenatal attendance, including efforts to address the multiple problems, may be helpful, if this is feasible. Antibiotics for asymptomatic bacteriuria and serial symphysial fundal height measurements by the same observer to detect intrauterine growth retardation appear valuable. Antibiotics as an aid to preventing preterm labour may well become important. Doppler studies of umbilical artery blood flow have potential.

One response to the problems of prematurity and/or small size has been 'technology'. Jim Neilson's chapter (Chapter 13) emphasizes the importance of evaluating technology just as drugs are evaluated. Many technologies have not proved of value, particularly when they become routinized and used indiscriminately. Their use in specific instances for definite risk seems to give much better results. It would also seem to us that by 2005 it is possible that most of the present 'technologies' will have been improved or abandoned; and we hope that their replacements will have been more carefully evaluated.

There are two overriding messages in Chapter 13: if a woman is having a low-risk pregnancy then 'technology' has little to offer; and investment of funds in 'people' – carers of one sort or another – is a better buy than the latest machine.

We have also included as a 'clinical challenge' Chapter 15 which orientates around a fascinating theory that causes of premature mortality have their roots in the nutrition of the fetus and infant. If this is true – and Louise Parker produces strong evidence – then they should be preventable. Just as diet and lifestyle are important in childhood for the developing adult, they are probably even more important during pregnancy. There are practical suggestions in the chapter regarding preconception advice about diet, nutrition, smoking, and alcohol. Although evidence is lacking about specific behaviours, some general recommendations are likely to be helpful. Women who are underweight as a result of dieting should increase their weight before becoming pregnant. The overweight should not be dieting when they become pregnant. A healthy diet, good exercise, moderate alcohol, not too much stress are broad-brush descriptions, but if women are able to follow these recommendations, the growth and development of the fetus and infant will be improved. Health promotion with some groups is challenging, however, as it can imply value judgements of people's different ways of life, and this is a challenge we should address carefully. Looking at the needs of women from groups where changes in lifestyle are probably most difficult to make, and where the greatest benefits are likely to be achieved, runs through Chapter 15 and it turns us full circle to the beginning of the section.

Clinical care

This is not a textbook. It does not tell anyone how to apply a ventouse, nor the indications for Caesarian section. Nevertheless, high-quality clinical care is vital, be it institution or community based. It must never be taken for granted; women expect high-quality care and they say so in surveys. We therefore thought it necessary to highlight certain clinical areas and ask appropriate contributors to deliberate on the current problems and the future. The chapters largely speak for themselves and the following notes are points that struck us most forcibly. For those who start reading a book by reading the final chapter, we hope it will stimulate them to turn back for the detail!

The Modell's account of preconception care, congenital disorders, and the new genetics (Chapter 16) was largely new to us and we suspect to most GPs and midwives. It seems to us that this sort of care is at the stage that antenatal care was in the 1930s, only being taken up by the motivated, articulate, worried well. As we discussed above, an important challenge is for GPs and midwives to provide this facility for the entire community and particularly for the groups who have most to gain. It is not clear how to do this best, however – preconception care is only possible if you plan to become pregnant, yet those with unplanned pregnancies may benefit most from the advice. Practice-based preconception clinics, although laudable forums for up-to-date advice and providing an opportunity for discussion with informed care-givers, may therefore not reach those most in need. Ad hoc advice during consultations, such as is advocated by the Modells, is valuable but such advice is often incomplete and can be inaccurate.

Two statistics leapt off the page: first, '30% of babies who get herpes die'. With the rising prevalence of this infection we see an impending problem and challenge; Chapter 20 deals with it clinically. Second, that 'miscarriage prevents the birth of most infants with chromosomal abnormalities, especially the more severe ones' is striking and can be a comfort to couples coping with miscarriage – about 20% of pregnancies. It is apparent from James Walker and Nigel Simpson's chapter (Chapter 17) that the understanding of the physiology of pregnancy continues to develop. The evidence base for many antenatal procedures is weak. Routine weighing, for example, has no clinical value. Many GPs and midwives, however, have encountered women who wish to be weighed: 'I want to get my body back to normal as quickly as possible after the baby', and care should be taken before one restriction (all women should be weighed) is replaced with another (no women should be weighed).

We are delighted to find that Sarah Clement and Sandra Elliott's chapter (Chapter 18) on psychological health before, during, and after childbirth is the longest in the book. Now that the physical health of women in UK maternity care is good, it is not surprising that the relative importance of psychological health increases. It was some reassurance to read that 58% of women in a large study felt 'reasonably cheerful most of the time during pregnancy'. Pregnancy is, for a lot of women, an enjoyable experience and we should enjoy the pregnancy with them. Always looking for things which might go wrong can make us a bit gloomy!

Anxiety in pregnancy is an important predictor of postnatal depression, and midwives and GPs may find this helpful in making decisions about offering postnatal support. Of particular interest is that depression is more common before than after birth. We conclude that it must be very underdiagnosed and treated – another challenge for the future. The chapter highlights the importance of counselling skills for GPs, midwives, and health visitors. Such skills are not instinctive but need to be taught and learned.

Continuity recurs again and again in this book and GPs and community midwives can, and should, offer it. That does not mean that women should be cared for by only one care-giver throughout – multidisciplinary care is often important, and there is no evidence that women are really more satisfied with care from only one person. But a limited number of carers, with efforts made to coordinate that care so that it is always consistent, should be the norm. Locally based care will enhance the opportunities for that to happen. Hospital-based care created the norm of a fragmented system where women saw impossibly large numbers of carers whom they had never met before. Community-based care from local carers protects against that scenario.

Sarah Clement and Sandra Elliott emphasize the importance of enhancing the self-esteem of women who perceive themselves as 'nobody' or 'not much use' or 'dim'. The appropriate attitude, encouragement, support, and genuine respect by midwife and GP can help to reverse these self-demeaning attitudes. They are not uncommon and community-based care during pregnancy and the puerperium can be a time to help address them. Clement and Elliott describe one study in which mothers saw understanding their emotional needs as the main priority of postnatal care yet this did not appear at all in the top five priorities of midwives. Here is a need for midwives to reorientate their care. As part of it there should be a very careful handover from midwife to health visitor with emphasis on the mother's psychological needs. Finally, 'two thirds of women who feel depressed postnatally will not seek any professional help': a sad reflection on care at present, and a challenge for the future.

In their latest views on antenatal care (Chapter 19), Janet Tucker and

Marion Hall present three tables (19.2, 19.3, 19.4) which form a protocol for minimal antenatal care. They present evidence that routine antenatal care can be offered by midwives and GPs in community settings to the benefit of many women with normal pregnancies. No routine specialist visit is necessary. Tucker and Hall conclude that the traditional 'blanket' care will disappear in the years ahead and focused close surveillance of high-risk groups will increase. Individualized programmes of care, tailored to each women's choice and need, will be the future for antenatal and postnatal care. Tucker and Hall also echo the chapter on economics – smaller numbers of antenatal visits are cheaper than larger ones. They also emphasize, and we support them, that midwives and GPs have a responsibility for cost-effective care. If they renege on that responsibility then they have no grounds to complain about shortage of funds. And again, they describe continuity of care as being the most important feature of the antenatal programme.

Having described the primary maternity care team as the best way of providing care, it is appropriate that the chapter on intercurrent illness (Chapter 20) is written by a team – three GPs and a midwife. Other teams will applaud the fact that they spend 11 pages on the diagnosis and management of common illnesses and only 6 on 'the rarities'. But then, they almost never see the rarities. That they have found it difficult to provide evidence-based advice on the treatments that they give for these common illnesses should not be surprising; there is little research on the common problems which women encounter in pregnancy. And yet care-givers have to do something – the woman is there in front of them. So they have told us what they do and what seems to work. What is also apparent from this chapter is the need for teamwork around illness, with the GP providing her unique contribution to antenatal care by diagnosing illness and prescribing for it, while the midwife provides ongoing support and midwifery care. As discussed earlier, GPs caring for women who become sick in pregnancy should be aware of that pregnancy by having carried out a limited number of routine antenatal consultations, and they should be familiar with antenatal care in general. They should be able to understand the maternity record held by the woman, and decide on appropriate management of illnesses.

Rosemary Mander's chapter (Chapter 21) on care in uncomplicated labour highlights again and again that many conventional practices have no basis in evidence. Such practices include, for example, the timing and type of observations in labour, pain control, timing of labour, and early breastfeeding; even newly introduced practices such as water birth have not been well evaluated. She also reminds us that even where evidence is available, it is not always used. As good research evidence is produced about questions that matter to women, ways of implementing that evidence should be explored. Care-givers need to be educated about ways of updating and using in practice everything that they learn. But this chapter also demonstrates how much care in labour has changed in recent decades, with some women able to make choices about posture, mobility, pain relief, and having a companion in labour. Women should no longer be routinely directed to 'push!' in second stage, and routine episiotomies should be a thing of the past. The evidence that does exist supports women-centred care in labour and at birth.

The realization that maternity care has been, and is being, under-researched is perhaps most apparent in the care of the mother after birth, and this is described by Sally Marchant and Jo Garcia in Chapter 22. They report that the Audit Commission found that virtually all women received home visits from a midwife after birth – 62% of them received either nine or 10 daily visits. This suggests that postnatal care is still provided routinely rather than on a selective basis. Do all women need a daily visit from the midwife, and would it be more beneficial to target visits for women most in need? Only two thirds of GPs from the same study did any home visits in the puerperium, suggesting a greater variation in work patterns and perhaps more selectivity; but 95% of GPs did a routine postnatal examination which again suggests working by rote.

It is apparent from Chapter 22 that illness between birth and the six-week postnatal check is not uncommon. As care becomes better in labour and there is less use of traumatic routine interventions, it is possible that some of the morbidity, particularly that of the uterus and perineum, will decrease. This could prevent postnatal morbidity and reduce the amount of postnatal care needed for these reasons. This could free time for dealing with psychological health (Chapters 11, 12, 18). A three-pronged approach by the midwife, health visitor, and GP working in a coordinated and integrated way would help to deal more effectively with these problems.

Sara Watkin and Cath Henson introduce Chapter 23 on the care of newborn babies by stating the obvious: that parents are the main carers of newborn babies. It is their second by second, minute by minute, and hour by hour care and observation that is most fundamental of all. They therefore need information from their professional carers and a healthy respect for their views. Carers have a lot to learn from parents, and they should listen to whatever parents have to say about their baby.

The good news is that 93% of babies are born at term in the UK, and between 95% and 99% of them are in good condition. So the several pages that they have written on the resuscitation of 'flat' babies is indeed a minority activity. Birth after birth will go by with neither midwife nor GP needing to be actively involved in any sort of resuscitation. Nevertheless, updating their knowledge and regular, probably annual, reassessment of skills such as airway opening techniques, mask ventilation, and external cardiac massage will be mandatory. Here there will be an enormous gulf between the 'psychosocially visiting' GP at deliveries and the GP obstetrician and the midwife who will be skilled in resuscitation, backed by rapidly responding paramedics, for whom neonatal intubation and care in transit of the sick neonate is part of their constantly-updated emergency care training. This chapter also provides an excellent comprehensive description of the commoner clinical problems and illnesses in newborns and neonates.

Sally Inch and Chloe Fisher (Chapter 24) describe the very low breastfeeding rates in the UK. That the criteria for a 'Baby Friendly Hospital' award is to be as low as 50% of women breastfeeding on discharge confirms both the low levels and the low national aspirations. We unashamedly gave a whole chapter to breastfeeding – we feel justified in this in that the morbidity of babies arising from its failure dwarfed other morbidity figures in this book.

Given the small but significant recent increase in the numbers of women starting to breastfeed, it is not impossible that by 2010 the majority of babies will be breastfed at least in the early weeks. Supporting women to continue to breastfeed is a major challenge for the health service. The paradox, and a problem that we must address with urgency, is that women from lower social class backgrounds are those less likely to breastfeed, and their babies are therefore those least likely to gain from the short and long-term health benefits. This perpetuates the existing inequalities in health. Without addressing that paradox we may be dealing with ongoing inequalities in health for generations yet to come.

Again, a team approach is needed. Midwife, GP, and health visitor should meet annually to discuss audit reports of breastfeeding rates in their practice and in local hospitals. From this, goals can be set and care targeted where it is most needed, including more coordinated antenatal and postnatal care for breastfeeding women. This could involve not only the three major professional carers but lay support workers, breastfeeding counsellors, and breastfeeding peers.

Chapter 24 is full of wisdom at a clinical level about how to breastfeed. We were reminded that breastfeeding may be 'natural' but it is not 'instinctive' – it has to be learned. Simply learning, understanding, and teaching the principles of pain-free, effective feeding, including positioning and effective milk removal, would prevent the huge numbers of women experiencing 'not enough milk' and would increase the numbers of women continuing to breastfeed, even without knowing about the rarer causes of breastfeeding problems.

Conclusions

In conclusion, these are the key elements which are fundamental to the future of maternity care:

- woman and baby-centred care
- local, accessible care offering continuity of care
- multidisciplinary teams working closely together
- the midwife as lead carer for most women
- GP involvement for all, with more for some women if needed
- hospitals as providers of specialized care only
- multidisciplinary, community-based education
- ongoing evaluations of care and implementation of the findings – increasing evidence-based care

- greater attention to women with special needs
- strategies to increase breastfeeding
- involvement of the family and lay services in planning and providing care
- carers, consumers, and researchers working together to address questions which are important to women.

INDEX